Principles and Practice of

INHALATION
THERAPY

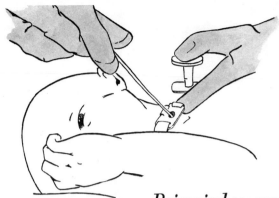

Principles and Practice of

INHALATION THERAPY

JIMMY ALBERT YOUNG, B.A., A.R.I.T.

*Director, Harvard Teaching Hospitals School
of Inhalation Therapy—Northeastern University Affiliate*

DEAN CROCKER, M.D., C.M.

*Director of Inhalation Therapy, Department of Anesthesia,
Children's Hospital Medical Center, Boston; Associate in Anesthesia,
Harvard Medical School*

Illustrated by DEBORAH RICE HAGGERTY

YEAR BOOK MEDICAL PUBLISHERS, INC.

35 EAST WACKER DRIVE · CHICAGO

Library of Congress Catalog Card Number: 78-106189

International Standard Book Number: 0-8151-2001-X

Preface

As ONE OBSERVES the historical evolution of health care, certain patterns occur again and again. One of these, which is a direct result of forces such as the "medical and technological knowledge explosion" and the greatly increased demand for services, is the emergence of groups of specialty practitioners to bridge the gap between knowledge and delivery of care.

No area of specialty illustrates this evolutionary pattern better than "Inhalation Therapy." From the early days of administration of oxygen to the development of complex mechanical devices, the duration of years has been very short indeed. This development has been so rapid that the term "Inhalation Therapy" at present is probably a misnomer. Perhaps a more appropriate term to encompass what is done would be "Life Support Systems Specialist," with particular emphasis on internal and external environmental control.

The need to train large numbers of physicians and therapists to provide this care to infants, children, and adults has been painfully apparent. The authors have been engaged in formal training programs for "Inhalation Therapy" during the past 5 years. This book is an outgrowth of the course structure of these training programs. Accordingly, appreciation is expressed to the Harvard Teaching Hospitals and Northeastern University School of Inhalation Therapy for use of course materials.

We would like to thank Rex O. Matthews, Head, Special Publications Section of the National Aeronautics and Space Administration, and also to thank the Manned Spacecraft Center, Houston, Texas, for their help and advice in the preparation of this manuscript. Much assistance was obtained from William E. Kroll of the Puritan-Bennett Corporation for graphic presentation of data. Particular thanks go to J. H. Emerson of the Emerson Company for historical notes and equipment information. Also many thanks are extended to Dr. Robert M. Smith, Dean Edmund McTerrnan, Mrs. Gretchen Riley, and others of our associates who have contributed many valuable suggestions. Miss Joan Whitney has performed yeoman services as our secretarial assistant.

We also wish to express our appreciation to the following for contributing technical information and equipment:

American Association for Inhalation Therapy
American Registry of Inhalation Therapists, Inc.
Air-Shields, Inc.
American Sterilizer Company
Beckman Instruments, Inc.
Bird Corporation
Blackwell Scientific Publications
Boeing Company
R. M. Cherniack, M.D.
L. Cherniack, M.D.
Warren E. Collins, Inc.
F. A. Davis Company
David Dimes, M.D.
Dräger/GmbH
Electric Boat Company—Division of General Dynamics Corporation
J. H. Emerson Company
Engström/Mivab Corporation
Fenwal, Inc.
Hewlett-Packard
Instrumentation Laboratory, Inc.
Journal of the American Medical Association

Mead Johnson and Company
Mine Safety Appliance Company
Minnesota Mining and Manufacturing Company
Mist O_2 Gen Equipment Company
Trier Mörch, M.D.
National Cylinder Gas—Division of Chemetron Corp.
National Fire Protection Association
North American Aviation—Division of Rockwell Corp.
Ohio Medical Products
George P. Pilling & Son Co.
Puritan-Bennett Corporation
Radiometer, Inc.
Rüsch—West Germany
Peter Safar, M.D.
W. B. Saunders Company
Shampaine Industries
The De Vilbiss Company
The Mira Corporation
Webb Associates

J.A.Y.
D.C.

Table of Contents

CHAPTER 1

Organization and Administration of Clinical Departments of Inhalation Therapy

WITH THE ADVANCES in engineering design that have evolved since 1950, major changes have taken place in the mechanical devices used in the treatment of respiratory diseases. Changes in medical, surgical, hospital administration and nursing care have occurred concurrently with the mechanical advances.

It has been clearly pointed out that the number of patients requiring respiratory care is increasing (Table 1). Patients who require respiratory care have one or more of the following defects: alveolar hypoventilation, abnormal ventilation-perfusion relationship, reduced gas transfer and hypoxia or acidosis from nonpulmonary causes. Since 1958, there has been

TABLE 1.—UNITED STATES NATIONAL HEALTH SURVEY—1962

NUMBER OF BEDRIDDEN DAYS*		REASONS FOR CONFINEMENT % OF PATIENTS	
Average male	6.9	Respiratory	49.0
Average female	8.7	Circulatory	13.2
Patients under		Digestive	8.6
5 years	5.8	Infectious and parasitic	8.1
5–14	7.8	Chronic impairments	7.5
15–24	6.3	Injuries	6.7
25–44	5.8	Genitourinary	5.3
45–64	8.8	Arthritis and rheumatism	5.1
over 65	16.7	All others	21.3

* Average person is sick in bed 7.8 days a year, and 50% of this confinement period is due to respiratory conditions.

a marked increase in the use of intermittent positive pressure breathing therapy.

Many hospitals in the past decade had so-called "oxygen" services whose main function was to control the supply of medical gases. The role of the Inhalation Therapy Department of today has changed. For a department to be clinically effective, the following categories must be well thought out and planned for:

1. Organizational functions
2. Personnel
3. Design
4. Equipment
5. Inventory
6. Records

Organizational Functions

In organizing an Inhalation Therapy Department, there should be general agreement as to its place within the hospital organization and particularly to its relationship to other departments. An Inhalation Therapy Department should have multiple functions related to respiratory care and should not be so organized as to inhibit future growth. Some of the functions should be:

1. Treatment of cardiopulmonary diseases
2. Cardiopulmonary diagnostic evaluation
3. Monitoring of ventilatory equipment
4. Chest physiotherapy
5. Maintenance of inhalation equipment
6. Controlling of medical gas supply and its usage
7. Teaching and education of medical, surgical and nursing staff in the field of inhalation therapy

The Department of Anesthesiology usually assumes the medical direction of the department. The medical problems arising in inhalation therapy are similar to those in anesthesiology and require a basic understanding of respiratory physiology. In addition, there is similarity in the equipment used in both fields. Another important factor is that the medical director of the department should be able to deal directly with the hospital administrator in matters pertaining to budget, purchasing, personnel and charges. Since the anesthesiologist's practice is located in the hospital, his availability for such day-to-day tasks is ideal. However, it is felt that any physician having proper qualifications and interest may fill the role of medical director of the department.

Departmental Personnel

The number of personnel required varies with the size of the hospital and the scope of the services offered. The department should offer 24-hour coverage, 7 days a week. The general categories of personnel should be as follows: A medical director, chief therapist, staff therapists, equipment technicians and administrative personnel. In small institutions, one person may fill more than one of these roles.

MEDICAL DIRECTOR.—The medical director must have adequate time to devote to consultation, education and administration. The qualifications for a medical director usually are:

1. Knowledge of respiratory physiology and pathology
2. Familiarity with advances in the field of respiratory therapy
3. Mechanical knowledge of equipment
4. Teaching ability
5. Familiarity with cost and accounting procedures
6. Administrative ability
7. Knowledge of intensive care procedures and techniques
8. Adequate background in research
9. A background in inventory and computer methods

CHIEF THERAPIST.—The chief therapist is considered the technical director of the department and, as such, is directly responsible to the department head. The chief therapist supervises all departmental personnel and procedures, including all records systems, and supervises disinfection, sterilization and maintenance of equipment, in accordance with accepted technical standards and nursing procedures. The chief therapist is also responsible for keeping an accurate inventory and ordering major supplies and replacement parts. The chief therapist should be familiar with all types of inhalation therapy equipment. A procedure manual is usually prepared by the chief therapist.

With the cooperation of the medical director, the organization and administration of an in-service education program is essential for both therapists and hospital personnel. The program should adequately cover the following areas:

1. Frequent reviews of respiratory anatomy and physiology
2. Pathology of the respiratory tract (i.e., ventilation-perfusion problems, clinical conditions, obstruction)
3. Current trends and advances in respiratory care (i.e., oxygen toxicity treatment, humidification and nebulization)

4. Blood gas analysis and conditions producing alterations in their values
5. Cardiopulmonary resuscitation (i.e., intubation, closed-chest cardiac massage)
6. Discussion on methods and use of monitoring devices and basic interpretation of results
7. Lung physiotherapy as an adjunct to respiratory care
8. Review of principles of ventilation and associated mechanical devices

STAFF THERAPISTS.—The personnel in this capacity are required to perform the necessary therapeutic procedures as ordered by the attending physicians or the medical director of the department. They should be completely familiar with the apparatus used in inhalation therapy. They should make rounds on all patients receiving respiratory care and should answer all pages. Whenever possible, staff therapist employment should be limited to candidates registered by the American Registry of Inhalation Therapists. When applicants with this qualification are not available, the medical director and the chief therapist have an even stronger responsibility for assuring themselves that each staff member be "fully trained and competent in the procedures to which he is assigned."

Design

Once an institution has decided to establish an Inhalation Therapy Department, the hospital administration must be prepared to provide the necessary space and facilities for immediate and future department needs. The area should not be less than 3,000 square feet for a general hospital of 500-bed capacity and about 1,000 square feet or more for smaller hospitals. The design should allow for a smooth flow of incoming and outgoing equipment. It is important that the department be located in close proximity to patient-care areas, with easy access to these areas. Figure 1 is an example of design.

Equipment

Equipment lists are available in the literature. Before the establishment of an Inhalation Therapy Department, the medical director, hospital administrator and the chief inhalation therapist should make an inventory of apparatus on hand and the needs of the future based on an evaluation of the projected usage, related to current trends and recent developments in respiratory care.

Consideration of the above factors will usually give a reasonably accurate

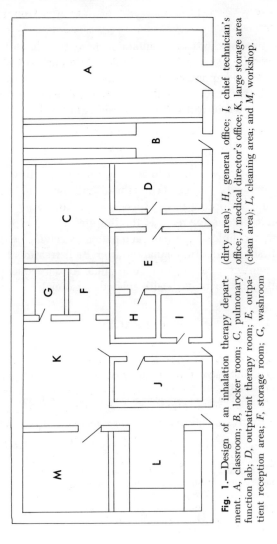

Fig. 1.—Design of an inhalation therapy department. A, classroom; B, locker room; C, pulmonary function lab; D, outpatient therapy room; E, outpatient reception area; F, storage room; G, washroom (dirty area); H, general office; I, chief technician's office; J, medical director's office; K, large storage area (clean area); L, cleaning area; and M, workshop.

estimate of capital equipment needed. Disposable items are available and offer the advantages of lower initial cost and decreased infection problems. Small alterations will occur as the service becomes established and clinical requirements change. Valuable information can be gained from observations at hospitals with established Inhalation Therapy Departments.

Inventory

Some effective methods of maintaining inventory have been used in Inhalation Therapy Departments, including assigning each item an index card on which should appear the name of the apparatus, inventory number, date of release, the ward to which it was released and the date of return. The cards can be grouped by nature of the equipment.

Records

The record system should include date, time and nature of request as minimal requirements. These data and the disposition should be maintained and kept on file, according to the specific state laws.

In addition to accounting records, the Respiratory Therapy Department should maintain a clinical record of each patient receiving care. These data are usually best recorded immediately after each treatment is rendered. This information serves as an invaluable guide for subsequent therapy by the physician, nurse or other health related personnel.

REFERENCES

Kracum, V. D., and Collins, V. J.: Inhalation therapy performs six functions, Med. Hosp., Vol. 101, No. 6, p. 104, December, 1963.

Starkweather, D. B.: Inhalation therapy department: Administrative organization, J. Am. Hosp. A., Sept. 1, 1968.

Egan, D. F.: Inhalation therapy department: Staffing and services, J. Am. Hosp. A., Sept. 1, 1968.

Lunden, S. E.: Inhalation therapy department: Physical facilities, J. Am. Hosp. A., Sept. 1, 1968.

Kracum, V. D.: Common errors in inhalation therapy: Report of a survey, J. Am. Hosp. A., June 16, 1960.

Justice, H. B.: The organization and operation of an inhalation therapy department: Items and topics, Ohio Medical Products, Madison, Wisconsin, vol. XIV, no. 1, February, 1968.

Safar, P., et al.: Respiratory Therapy (Philadelphia: F. A. Davis Company, 1965).

Symposium on Inhalation Therapy: Anesth. J., vol. 23, no. 4, 1962.

Yorzyk, W. A.; Crocker, D., and Smith, R. M.: Organization of hospital departments of inhalation therapy, J.A.M.A. 203:552, 1968.

CHAPTER 2

Respiratory System

THE RESPIRATORY SYSTEM is composed of those structures concerned with the conduction and exchange of gases between the human body and its environment. The respiratory system is composed of the *nasal cavity,* the *pharynx,* the *larynx,* the *trachea, bronchi* and *lungs.* This system supplies oxygen to the blood and removes carbon dioxide from the blood. It is through the membrane between the alveoli and the blood capillaries that oxygen diffuses into the blood and carbon dioxide elimination takes place. The act of breathing, therefore, is the act of moving air into and out of the alveoli, thereby maintaining a fresh supply of alveolar oxygen and removing carbon dioxide from the alveoli as it accumulates.

Functions of the Respiratory Structures

Air enters the nasal cavity through the *nostrils* or *nares.* The nasal cavity is divided into two chambers by a central partition, the *nasal septum.* Each of these chambers is subdivided into smaller chambers by projections called *turbinates.* Lining the nasal passages are hairs, *cilia,* which normally beat about 10–12 cycles per second and together with the mucus secretions coat the nasal epithelium and entrap and filter out dust or other finite particles. The function of the turbinates is twofold: first they increase the surface area of the nasal cavity, thereby allowing more air to come in contact with the mucous membranes; secondly, this increased surface area allows the inspired air to become thoroughly warmed before entering the trachea.

THE PHARYNX

The *pharynx,* or throat, is a tubular conducting passageway which lies behind the nasal passages and the mouth, between the base of the skull and the larynx and beginning of the esophagus. It is divided into three parts:

the *nasopharynx,* the *oropharynx* and the *laryngopharynx.* The upper portion (nasopharynx) is an air passage only. The lower portions serve the respiration and digestive tracts as a common passageway; that is, the area between the mouth and esophagus and between the nasal passages and the larynx and trachea.

The *eustachian tubes,* located on the lateral walls of the nasopharynx, communicate with the middle ear, which is a common site of infection in children. On the posterior wall of the nasopharynx is a mass of lymphatic tissue, the *pharyngeal tonsils.* During childhood, this area may become enlarged and is known as *adenoids.* The upper surface of the soft palate forms the floor of the nasopharynx.

The *palatine tonsils,* located in the lateral walls of the oropharynx, are oval, flat bodies of lymphatic tissue. The mucosa over the root of the tongue contain masses of lymphatic tissue which make up the *lingual tonsil.*

The *glottis* is the structure where the pharynx (throat) divides into the esophagus and *trachea.* Food from the mouth passes into the esophagus, and air passes into the trachea. The most important structure in the glottal area is the *epiglottis.* This is a leaflike structure of cartilage which covers the entrance to the larynx and acts as a protecting shelf to deflect food from the entrance into the air passageway (trachea). Whenever a solid material engages the pharynx, the epiglottis moves into position to cover the trachea and allows food to enter the esophagus. When air passes into the pharynx, the trachea remains open and air enters the lungs. All air going to and from the lungs must pass through the larynx. In passage, there are resultant vibrations of the *vocal cords,* which produce sounds of speech.

THE TRACHEA

The *trachea* is a tubular structure about 11.2 cm ($4\frac{1}{2}$ inches) in length, 2–2.5 cm (1 inch) in width and composed of fibrous membranes in which cartilagenous *C-shaped rings* (16–20) are embedded, which prevent collapse of the trachea. The trachea begins at the lower end of the larynx and terminates by dividing into right and left bronchi.

The walls of the right and left main stem bronchi are similar in most normal instances to the trachea. But as the bronchi become smaller and as we progress from top to bottom, we find that the cartilage in the wall of the smaller bronchi is in the form of thin irregular and isolated plates which become smaller and fewer in number with each successive branching of the tracheobronchial tree.

The trachea is lined with waving microscopic hairs, *cilia,* and *mucous glands.* The action of the cilia is a wavelike motion upward, propelling secretions and exudates of health and disease from the lungs and bronchi to the pharynx and mouth where they can be coughed up and expectorated.

THE BRONCHI

The *bronchi* are terminal branches of the trachea which transport air to the smaller structures of the lungs, the *bronchioles,* and, finally, to the *alveoli* or air sacs (Fig. 2).

THE LUNGS

The lungs are cone-shaped organs which lie in the *thoracic cavity* between a partition called the *mediastinum,* enclosed in the *pleurae.* The area at which the right and left bronchi enter the lungs is known as the *carina.* This structure is a depression on the medial surface of each lung. Upon entering the lungs, each *primary bronchus* divides into bronchi, two in the left lung and three in the right, which enter the primary lobes of the lung. Each of these secondary bronchi subdivide into smaller and smaller bronchi. Finally, after subdivision a number of times, they are called or known as *bronchioles* (1 mm in diameter or less). At this point, the C-shaped cartilage rings disappear. The bronchioles are lined like the trachea and bronchi

Fig. 2.—Anatomy of the respiratory system. *A,* right bronchus; *B,* left bronchus; *C,* terminal bronchiole; *D,* respiratory bronchioles; and *E,* alveolar air sacs.

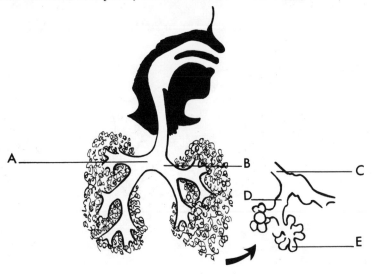

but lack the goblet cells. In the normal adult, the mucous membrane of the tracheobronchial tree secretes about one-half liter of fluid in a 24-hour period.

The bronchioles branch into terminal bronchioles: the *respiratory bronchiole*, the *alveolar duct*, the *atrium* and the *alveolar sacs*. Each terminal branch of the trachiobronchial tree ends in a pulmonary unit. The pulmonary alveoli are irregular outpouchings from a central atrium. The respiratory membrane is the only area within the lung where gas exchange occurs (Fig. 3).

The lungs are slightly asymmetrical, the left being narrower and longer due to its anatomic relationship to the heart. The right is slightly shorter and broader due to its position above the liver. The texture of the lungs is soft and spongy. They are elastic and are constantly changing their shape with each respiratory movement.

The lung divisions consist of lobes and segments. The left lung is separated by a fissure into an upper and lower lobe; two fissures divide the right lung into three lobes—the upper, middle and lower. The left main stem bronchus is not only longer than the right one, but it angles more acutely to the left of the trachea. The two lobes of the left lung have a volume about 20% less than the three lobes of the right lung, the difference being the space occupied by the heart on the left hemithorax.

The segments of the lungs are described by a universal nomenclature and numbering system (Fig. 4). The upper lobe consists of the apical poste-

Fig. 3.—Gaseous exchange at an alveolar capillary interface in the lung.

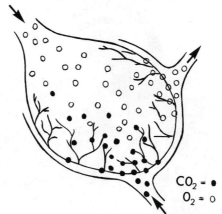

$CO_2 = \bullet$
$O_2 = \circ$

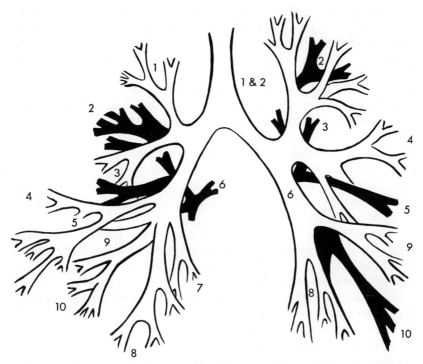

Fig. 4.—Illustration of the segments of the lungs, using the universal nomenclature and numbering system. *1 and 2*, apical posterior segment; *3*, anterior segment; *4*, superior lingular segment; *5*, inferior lingular segment. The left lower lobe consists of *6*, superior segment; *7 and 8*, anteromedial basal segment; *9*, lateral basal segment; *10*, posterior basal segment. The right upper lobe consists of *1*, apical segment; *2*, posterior segment; *3*, anterior segment. The right middle lobe consists of *4*, lateral segment; *5*, medial segment. The right lower lobe consists of *6*, superior segment; *7*, medial basal segment; *8*, anterior basal segment and lateral basal segment; and *10*, posterior basal segment.

rior segments 1 and 2, anterior segment 3, superior lingular segment 4 and the inferior lingular segment 5. The left lower lobe consists of the superior segment 6, anteromedial basal segment 7 and 8, lateral basal segment 9 and the posterior basal segment 10. The right upper lobe consists of the apical segment 1, posterior segment 2 and anterior segment 3. The right middle lobe consists of the lateral segment 4 and the medial segment 5. The right lower lobe consists of the superior segment 6, medial basal segment 7, anterior basal segment 8, lateral basal segment 9 and the posterior basal segment 10.

The Thoracic Cavity

The *thoracic cavity* is the space within the walls of the thorax or chest. Its walls are formed by the ribs and muscles. The floor of the thoracic cavity is formed by another dome-shaped muscle, the *diaphragm*. The roof is formed by the muscles at the root of the neck.

As mentioned previously, the thoracic cavity is divided into two pleural cavities by the *mediastinum* (Fig. 5). In each of the pleural cavities is found a lung. The lung itself is covered by a serous membrane called *pleura*. The pleura actually consists of two layers, visceral and parietal. The *visceral pleura* covers the lungs. The *parietal pleura* forms the lining of the thoracic cage. Thus, lungs never directly touch the ribs or muscles, rather the two pleurae touch each other, providing an almost frictionless surface on which to rub.

As we have seen, the body requires a method to obtain fresh oxygen and rid itself of carbon dioxide. Also, at this point, it should be mentioned that excess moisture and heat are also partially eliminated through the lungs. These will be discussed in Chapter 15.

The *physiology of breathing* has two aspects: inspiration, the taking in of air, and expiration, the expulsion of air. This is brought about by changing the size of the thoracic cavity by utilizing the respiratory muscles to increase or decrease the pleural space. Remember, the thoracic cavity is a closed system—there is no communication with the outside. The lungs hang inside pleural space, and they do communicate with the outside environment with the help of the respiratory structures previously described. When the pleural space enlarges, a reduction in pressure within it allows the

Fig. 5.—Thoracic cavity is divided into two pleural cavities by the mediastinum. A, parietal pleural; B, visceral pleural; C, mediastinum; and D, diaphragm.

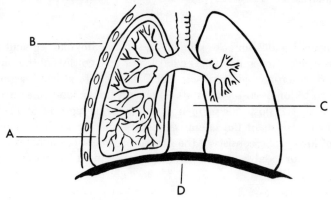

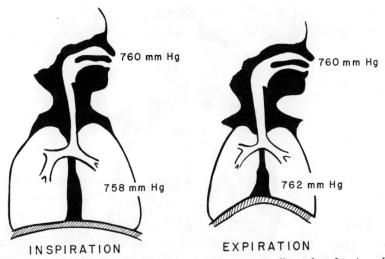

760 mm Hg

760 mm Hg

758 mm Hg

762 mm Hg

INSPIRATION

EXPIRATION

Fig. 6.—During quiet breathing, the intrapulmonic pressure will vary from 2 to 4 mm Hg below atmosphere during inspiration and 2 to 4 mm Hg above during expiration.

elastic lungs to expand with air. Conversely, when the pleural space is decreased, it puts pressure on the lungs and air is expelled.

The pressure that is found between the two pleurae in the thoracic cavity is known as *intrapleural* or *intrathoracic* pressure. This pressure is a little less than that in the pulmonary passageways. This difference is known as *subatmospheric pressure*. This keeps the lungs in a state of moderate expansion at all times (Fig. 6). If this pressure difference is not kept intact, then the lungs will collapse. This occurs when an opening is made in the thoracic wall. The pressure between the pleura is then equalized and the lung collapses. This condition is known as a *pneumothorax*. Shift of the mediastinum also may occur when abdominal contents are present in the chest (Fig. 7).

MUSCULAR ACTIVITY

As we have seen, changes in the size of the pleural space allow the lungs to expand. The change in the size of the thorax is brought about by the action of the respiratory muscles (Fig. 8).

INSPIRATION.—The diaphragm is a dome-shaped muscle forming the floor of the thoracic cavity. When the muscle contracts, it flattens its dome and increases the vertical diameter of the thorax. This increases the negative pressure already present, and the air on the outside, having a higher pres-

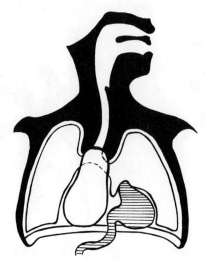

Fig. 7.—Mediastinal shift in herniation of abdominal viscera.

sure, rushes in. This is known as *diaphragmatic breathing* or *abdominal breathing*.

The pleural space can also be enlarged by raising the sternum and the ribs. This is known as *thoracic* or *costal breathing*. The contraction of the intercostal muscles raises the ribs and sternum and thus increases the *anteroposterolateral* diameter of the chest.

Fig. 8.—The lung moves in accordance to the thoracic cavity's movements during breathing. It maintains its position adjacent to the thoracic wall due to its own elastic properties.

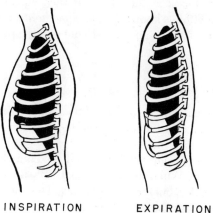

INSPIRATION   EXPIRATION

The result of these two actions constitutes normal breathing. Contraction of the diaphragm and of the intercostal muscles increases the pleural space. By increasing this space, the negative pressure in the lung is increased by about −3mm Hg.

EXPIRATION.—Normal expiration is a passive process. When inspiration has ceased, the muscles simply relax. The result is a decrease of pleural cavity size; and ribs, sternum and diaphragm press the lungs, raising intrapulmonary pressure by +3 mm Hg. This forces air out of the lungs. The above refers only to normal respiration. There may be forced inhalation exchange and transport of gases.

The principal process in the exchange of gases is *diffusion*. Briefly, this is the tendency which the molecules of gas have to become uniformly distributed. When there is a difference in the number of gaseous molecules per unit of space, these molecules tend to move from an area of higher number to one of the lower number. Each gas acts independently of the other; that is, oxygen acts independently, regardless of the amount of carbon dioxide.

When fresh air is drawn into the lungs, there is a higher percentage of oxygen in the inspired air than there is in the blood. Therefore, diffusion of oxygen into the blood occurs (Fig. 9). Just the opposite is true of carbon dioxide. There is, because of the body chemistry, a higher percentage of carbon dioxide in the blood than in the air. Therefore, diffusion occurs from

Fig. 9.—Alveolar gas exchange. *A*, pulmonary artery; *B*, capillary Po_2, 40 mm Hg; *C*, pulmonary vein; *D*, capillary Pco_2, 45 mm Hg; and *E*, pulmonary artery.

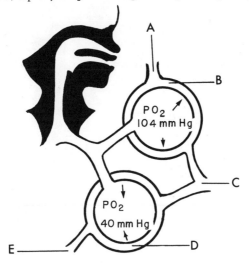

the blood stream into the lungs. These events take place each time air is inspired and expired. Let us examine the mechanics of these actions more closely.

Mechanics of Breathing

It is necessary to understand clearly the distinction between respiration, the exchange of gases between a cell and its environment (which in man consists of the three phases of external respiration, transportation by the circulation of blood, and internal respiration), and breathing, which is defined as the mechanical process of air uptake into the lungs (inspiration) and air expulsion (expiration). Since the lung capillaries are constantly removing oxygen from and putting carbon dioxide into the alveoli, the need for replacing the air in the lungs is obvious.

In man, the ribs, chest muscles and diaphragm are so constructed and arranged as to be easily movable, allowing the volume of the chest cavity to be increased or decreased. When it is necessary to increase the lung volume during inspiration, the rib muscles contract, drawing the anterior end upward and outward, an action made possible by the hingelike connection of the ribs with the backbone (Fig. 10). At the same time, the floor of the chest cavity, the diaphragm, forcefully contracts, decreasing its convexity and consequently increasing the size of the cavity. Since the space is closed, the increase in volume results in a lowering of the pressure

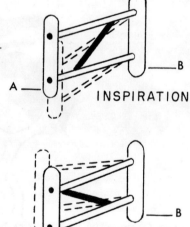

Fig. 10.—Illustration of the mechanics involved during inspiration. *A*, spinal column; *B*, sternum.

in the lungs, and when it falls below atmospheric pressure (760 mm Hg), gases from the atmosphere enter the upper airway into the trachea, air sacs and finally into the alveoli. That volume of air expelled from the lungs during expiration is due primarily to the elastic recoil of the lungs but, to some extent, to the weight of the chest wall. During inspiration, the lungs are distended as they are filled with a mixture of gases. When the rib muscles relax, the ribs are allowed to return to their original position, and the simultaneous relaxation of the diaphragm permits the abdominal structures to push it upward to its previous convex shape. These factors decrease the chest volume and allow the distended, elastic lung to contract and expel the air which has been inhaled.

During physical exercise, this passive expiration of the relaxing rib diaphragm muscles is not rapid enough to expel the normal volume of air before the next inspiration must start, so that the size of the chest cavity is reduced by muscular contraction. Besides the muscles which raise the ribs for inspiration, there is another set of muscles with fibers going at right angles to the first, which lowers the front ends of the ribs and thus decreases the thoracic volume.

The muscles of the abdominal wall also contract, forcing the abdominal organs up against the diaphragm and further increasing the elastic contraction of the lungs. The chest walls play an inactive part in forcing the air out of the lungs: the decrease in the size of the thoracic cavity simply allows the lungs to contract by means of their own elasticity. Coughing and sneezing are types of forced expiration in which a forceful contraction of the muscles of the abdominal wall push the abdominal viscera against the diaphragm, decreasing the thoracic volume suddenly and causing a rapid expulsion of air and/or sputum from the lungs.

The trachea, pharynx and other air passages play no active, muscular part in the process of air uptake: they function simply as conduction channels.

At rest, the normal male adult breathes in and out about 500 ml of air each breath (tidal volume). When this volume has been expelled, however, another 1.5 L can be expelled forcibly by contraction of the abdominal muscles. After this, there still remains about 1 L of air which cannot be expelled (residual volume). During normal breathing, therefore, a reserve of some 2.5 L of air remains in the lungs, with which 500 ml of fresh air is mixed on each inspiration (functional residual volume).

Although about 500 ml of air is breathed in with each inspiration, only about 350 ml actually reaches the alveoli because the last 150 ml inhaled remains in the conduction passages where no exchange of gases between lungs and circulating blood can occur. This volume of air is the first to be expelled on the next expiration. The last 150 ml expelled from the alveoli on each expiration also remains in these tubes, and this air, although high in carbon dioxide content, is the first to be drawn into the alveoli on the next inspiration. With each breath, then, only about 350 ml of fresh air reaches the pulmonary units to mix with the approximately 2.5 L already there. The 150 ml of space in the air passages is known as *anatomic dead space*. If this dead space is increased by rebreathing through a long tube, the air going into the lungs will soon be depleted of its oxygen, with fatal consequences.

The Physical, Chemical and Neurogenic Control of Respiration

Respiration normally occurs quietly and unconsciously and the only muscles involved in a quiet inspiration are the diaphragm and the external intercostal muscles (Fig. 11). During inspiration, the chest is enlarged and air enters the lungs: the glottis widens and the bronchioles dilate. The contraction of these inspiratory muscles provides the force necessary to overcome the elastic recoil of the lungs and thorax and also the force to overcome the frictional resistance during the flow of air through the tracheobronchial tree.

Alveolar pressure is lower than atmospheric. The contraction of the inspiratory muscles as they enlarge the thorax, lowers the intrathoracic pressure. A lowering of this pressure enlarges the alveoli, expands alveolar gas and lowers the alveolar gas pressure to below atmospheric pressure, allowing the air to flow into the alveoli.

At the end of inspiration, the muscles relax and no longer exert a force

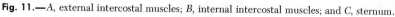

Fig. 11.—*A*, external intercostal muscles; *B*, internal intercostal muscles; and *C*, sternum.

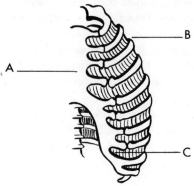

which distends the thorax and lungs; the tissue of the thorax and the lungs recoils, the internal intercostals contract, the glottis narrows and the bronchioles diminish their caliber. Thus expiration takes place.

During a deep breath or a forced respiration, the accessory muscles come into action. The accessory muscles for inspiration are:

Serratus magnus	Rhomboideus
Pectoralis	Trapezius
Scalenus	

During the expiration, the anterior abdominal wall contracts and drives the diaphragm into the chest.

RESPIRATORY CENTERS

Respiration is controlled by centers located throughout the reticular formations of the pons and medulla. Their role is not exactly known in humans, but they can control respiration directly. Control of rhythmic respiratory movements is performed by these centers:

Inspiratory center   Expiratory center   Pneumotaxic center

INSPIRATORY CENTER.—In the presence of adequate carbon dioxide and oxygen tension, the inspiratory center discharges steadily without intermission along a descending path to the spinal cord, stimulating the motor neurons and producing inspiration.

This inspiratory effort comes to an end when anoxia becomes sufficient to paralyze the activity of the cells of the center. If a state of deep inspiration develops, apneusis, the lungs will be kept inflated and fatal asphyxia may develop.

EXPIRATORY CENTER.—Descending fibers from the expiratory center stimulate the spinal cord motor neurons which innervate the muscles of expiration. The medullary respiratory center passes an automatic rhythm of alternate discharges and impulses from both inspiratory and expiratory components.

Stimulation of inspiration and expiration probably involves a reciprocal innervation. For example, when inspiration motor neurons are stimulated, the antagonistic expiratory spinal motor neurons are reciprocally inhibited, and vice versa.

PNEUMOTAXIC CENTER.—Located in the upper pons, this center converts respiration into a rhythmic pattern of inhibiting the continuous discharge of the inspiratory center into discharges and rest. It has been suggested that when the inspiratory center discharges impulses, these impulses also pass to the pneumotaxic center.

THE VAGUS NERVE

In the wall of the alveoli of the lungs, there are extensive ramifications of vagal afferent filaments. These receptors are stimulated when lungs are stretched during inspiration. The frequency of these impulses will increase as the lung-stretch becomes greater and their impulses disappear when expiration begins.

It has been proved that vagal afferent nerves in conjunction with the pneumotaxic center convert the steady discharge of the inspiration center into the rhythmic alternation of inspiration and expiration.

During inspiration, as lungs are stretched, impulses pass by the vagus. As more impulses arrive along the vagus, inhibition occurs as more of the cells of the inspiratory center come into an inhibition state, until all activity ceases.

Afferent vagal impulses continue to reach the inspiratory center and maintain inhibition for some time, producing a pause at the end of inspiration. As reverberation subsides, the inspiratory center frees from inhibition and resumes its discharges.

FACTORS INFLUENCING RESPIRATION

Respiration is determined by the amount of physical, chemical, and nervous influences which are integrated and coordinated in the respiratory centers.

There are some factors which cause changes in ventilation either by acting directly on medullary respiration centers or indirectly via the nervous activity. The respiratory centers are capable of responding to changes in neurologic stimuli or chemical stimuli (pH and carbon dioxide) which vary the output of their impulses and control the ventilation volume. Impulses are conducted to the motor portion of the upper spinal cord via the motor nerves to the respiratory muscles. Any abnormality in this chain will produce abnormal volumes of ventilation.

Regulation of ventilation due to chemical changes is originated from the activity of two chemoreceptors which sense changes in the composition of two body fluids:

1. Carotid and aortic bodies sense changes in arterial oxygen tension, hydrogen ion and carbon dioxide tension, probably its acid-forming properties. Arterial receptors function to maintain carbon dioxide tension and hydrogen ion constant.

2. Medullary hydrogen ion receptors on the ventrolateral medulla sense changes in the cerebrospinal fluid hydrogen ion. These medullary hydrogen

ion receptors act to maintain the cerebrospinal fluid hydrogen ion, the extracellular fluids and the hydrogen ion of the brain constant.

Medullary hydrogen ion receptors are of primary importance only in acute changes of arterial carbon dioxide; carbon dioxide diffuses rapidly into the cerebrospinal fluid, increasing the hydrogen ion content.

With chronic changes in levels of breathing and in arterial and cerebrospinal fluid carbon dioxide tension, active transport across the blood barrier restores the pH of cerebrospinal fluid to normal, resetting the chemoreceptors to normal activity, despite an elevated or diminished carbon dioxide tension. Arterial carbon dioxide tension and pH are the principal stimuli in regulating the respiration.

Alteration of carbon dioxide tension and the pH of capillary blood thought to contain chemoreceptors are not depressed by a fall in oxygen tension of the blood but will be depressed if there is a lack of oxygen.

Air contains amounts of carbon dioxide (0–.3%); if there is a gradual increase of carbon dioxide from its normal volume (around 40 mm Hg tension), ventilation is also increased, at first the depth and then the frequency. If inspired air contains higher carbon dioxide than normal, alveoli cannot eliminate carbon dioxide; therefore, its content rises. When arterial blood leaves the lung, its carbon dioxide tension rises and breathing is stimulated.

Pulmonary ventilation is soon changed if there is an increase in the inspired air of carbon dioxide, although alveolar and arterial carbon dioxide tension will stay almost normal.

If the inhaled carbon dioxide exceeds the alveolar air, carbon dioxide hyperventilation occurs; but it cannot compensate fully for this rise. Alveolar carbon dioxide rises, and at this state (6–12%) some symptoms appear— mental confusion, headache, rise in blood pressure and tachycardia. An increase of more than 12% inspired carbon dioxide will bring ventilation to its maximum (around 90 L per minute).

If higher concentrations of carbon dioxide are inhaled, it leads to depression. If 40% carbon dioxide is inhaled over a period, depression of ventilation occurs, followed by bradycardia, unconsciousness and death.

Alveolar hypoventilation, caused by severe lung impairment or paralysis of respiratory muscles, as in hypercapnia, reduces responsiveness to the respiratory center. The tissue solubility of carbon dioxide is greater than oxygen; therefore, diffusion is much greater and will produce extreme depression.

If the respiratory center is also depressed due to hypoxia or drugs, such as morphine or barbiturates, depressant effects of carbon dioxide may occur at a lower concentration. If in such cases carbon dioxide is used to stimulate, ventilation may lead to further depression.

HYDROGEN ION CONTENT.—Changes in hydrogen ion concentration of the blood change the pulmonary ventilation, which tends to restore the blood reaction to normal. Its alteration of pH increases ventilation more when it results from alteration of other acids.

Gary suggested that a steady-state ventilation is directly proportional to the algebraic sum of the partial effects of the arterial hydrogen ion and carbon dioxide tension. For effective control, the hydrogen ion and bicarbonate ion must be coordinated. The carbon dioxide tension is regulated primarily by ventilatory responses to the peripheral and central input to the respiratory centers. These responses are determined by the hydrogen ion content in the arterial blood and cerebrospinal fluid. The changes in carbon dioxide and pH in metabolic acidosis and alkalosis are reflected by chemoreceptors inducing hyper- or hypoventilation.

METABOLIC ACIDOSIS AND ALKALOSIS.—In acute acidosis, the activity of the arterial hydrogen ion receptors is increased; breathing increases and the arterial cerebrospinal fluid carbon dioxide tension decreases, cerebrospinal fluid pH rises and depresses the activity of the medullary hydrogen ion receptors.

An active transport mechanism restores cerebrospinal fluid pH and the medullary hydrogen ion receptors activity to normal; the increased ventilation originates from an increase in activity of the peripheral hydrogen ion chemoreceptors.

In correction of acute acidosis, a decrease of peripheral chemoreceptor activity will decrease ventilation and also decrease cerebrospinal fluid pH. Therefore, ventilation will not return to normal, as has been frequently observed after correction of diabetic or renal acidosis, because of the increased activity of medullary hydrogen ion chemoreceptors. To restore ventilation to normal depends on the restoration of the bicarbonate ion and hydrogen ion of the cerebrospinal fluid to normal.

In metabolic alkalosis, the mechanisms are the same, but the acid-base pathways are in the reverse direction. Compensation following a shift in the arterial pH is dependent on active regulation of the cerebrospinal fluid bicarbonate ion or hydrogen ion, the main need being the restoration of cerebrospinal fluid hydrogen ion concentration to normal.

Respiratory alkalosis and hypoxia increase the arterial CO_2 tension and cerebrospinal fluid tension. When the cerebrospinal fluid bicarbonate ion falls, it restores cerebrospinal fluid pH to normal.

RESPIRATORY ACIDOSIS.—If one is exposed to high altitudes for a few days, alveolar ventilation increases and alveolar carbon dioxide tends to fall. This is in proportion to oxygen tension adaptation to respiration by newcomers to altitude, and it has been shown that the arterial blood remains alkaline in the first stages of acclimatization.

Renal excretion does eventually restore blood pH to normal. Mild respiratory alkalosis might lower bicarbonate concentration of the environment of medullary hydrogen ion receptors. Respiratory acidosis occurs in patients with chronic or acute respiratory insufficiency who can no longer maintain adequate pulmonary ventilation. Major structural and functional derangements in the organs of the cardiorespiratory system allow excessive amounts of carbon dioxide to accumulate in the lungs, body and body tissues. The patient becomes hypercarbic and hypoxic.

Chronic acidosis develops most often in patients who have chronic emphysema, asthma or bronchiectasis. Gradual deterioration of the lung tissues impairs pulmonary function, diminishes gas exchange and leads to carbon dioxide retention. Compensation is accomplished by first increasing the minute ventilation so that the acidosis develops slowly. Often body buffers also bind up acid ions.

A compensatory metabolic change is thus created in the direction of alkalosis. The ultimate result is the restoration of hydrogen ion concentration toward normal with very high plasma bicarbonate and low chloride concentration and a high total carbon dioxide. This compensated state can exist for years. Although pH is near normal, the total body buffers are completely taken up by hydrogen ions.

ACIDEMIA.—Pulmonary ventilation is increased, eliminating carbon dioxide faster and making it fall below normal. The alveolar carbon dioxide tension regulates the amount of bicarbonate in the arterial blood. As the alveolar carbon dioxide is decreased, the arterial carbon dioxide and carbonic acid content falls. Hydrogen ion concentration in the blood increases and normal blood reaction is restored.

ALKALEMIA.—When the hydrogen ion concentration of the blood falls, the pulmonary ventilation is decreased, carbon dioxide is retained, increasing alveolar carbon dioxide, arterial carbon dioxide and carbonic acid. Hydrogen ion concentration in the blood increases and normal blood reactions are restored. High-buffer base (respiratory acidosis, metabolic alkalosis) may make the respiratory centers less sensitive to changes in carbon dioxide tension. Low-buffer base (metabolic acidosis, respiratory alkalosis) may increase the sensitivity of the centers. Drug stimulants such as amphetamines, if given in large quantities, induce hyperventilation, leading to severe respiratory alkalosis. Drug depressants, such as narcotics and tranquilizing agents, and anesthesia depress the respiratory center, diminishing respiration, leading to respiratory acidosis.

OTHER FACTORS AFFECTING THE CONTROL OF VENTILATION.—Blood flow/ventilation ratio is regulated by the pH and carbon dioxide tension. The rate by which carbon dioxide is eliminated from the cells is determined by the activity of the centers, which depends on its blood supply.

An example of the factors involved may be seen by examining the so-called Cheyne-Stokes respiration. This type of respiration consists of periods of breaths and apnea (caused by hypoxia and depression of the respiratory centers). It is commonly seen in patients with brain damage or congestive heart failure.

Hypoxia decreases the oxygen tension and increases the carbon dioxide tension which stimulates the chemoreceptors to initiate respiration.

Hypoxia is relieved by the oxygenation of the blood; the arterial oxygen tension rises and carbon dioxide tension falls. This increase of arterial oxygen tension removes the stimulus to the respiratory centers and respiration is stopped again. Meakins and Davies defined Cheyne-Stokes respiration as a want for oxygen, diminished carbon dioxide and time required for pulmonary blood to reach the respiratory center, resulting in the periodic Cheyne-Stokes respiration.

1. Hyperventilation with increased tidal volume followed by
2. Diminuation followed by
3. Periods of apnea

Cheyne-Stokes respiration differs from Biot's respiration in that there is no waxing or waning of tidal volume when breathing occurs. Carbon dioxide tension in Cheyne-Stokes respiration is usually low and ventilation results in higher levels of alveolar ventilation than that required for carbon dioxide elimination.

REFERENCES

Brock, R. C.: *The Anatomy of the Bronchial Tree* (London: Oxford University Press, 1954).
Dunnill, M. S.: Postnatal growth of the lung, Thorax 17:329, 1962.
Engel, S.: *Lung Structure* (Springfield, Ill.: Charles C Thomas, Publisher, 1962).
Hayward, J., and Reid, L. McA.: Observations on the anatomy of the intrasegmental bronchial tree, Thorax 7:89, 1952.
Thoracic Society of Great Britain: The nomenclature of bronchopulmonary anatomy, Thorax 5:222, 1950.
Comroe, J.: *Physiology of Respiration* (Chicago: Year Book Medical Publishers, Inc., 1965).
Ciba Foundation Symposium: *Pulmonary Structure and Function* (Boston: Little, Brown & Company, 1962).

CHAPTER 3

Respiration and the Atmosphere

Composition of Air

TEMPERATURE by definition is a measure of the intensity of heat and is no indication of the quantity involved. These are several temperature scales:

1. Fahrenheit
   a) Freezing point—32° F
   b) Boiling point—212° F

2. Centigrade
   a) Freezing point of water is 0° C
   b) Boiling point of water is 100° C

As you may have noted, the difference between the freezing point and the boiling point is 180° on the Fahrenheit scale but only 100° on the Centigrade scale. So if we had a temperature reading of 20° Centigrade and we wanted to convert it into degree Fahrenheit, we would use the formula:

$$\text{Degrees F} = (\tfrac{9}{5} \text{ Tc}) + 32 = (\tfrac{9}{5} \times 20) + 32 = 68° \text{ F}$$

or conversely:

$$\text{Degrees C} = \tfrac{5}{9} (T_F - 32)$$

As we mentioned, the term "temperature" is an indication of the intensity of heat in an object and indirectly reflects the amount of movement of the molecules which make up the body. As the molecular movement slows down, a point is reached at which there is no molecular movement and this is said to be *absolute zero*, and on the Fahrenheit scale is 459.6° below 0° F.

This is an important relationship and one which physicians, medical students, nurses and respiratory therapists should remember, because any calculation involving the ratio of temperatures must be done on an absolute temperature basis. This means that 460° must be algebraically added to the temperature in degrees Fahrenheit in order to determine the number of degrees above absolute zero.

On the Centigrade scale, the point of absolute zero is −273.1 below 0° C.

Heat.—Whereas temperature in degrees is an indication of the intensity of heat, the *British Thermal Unit* or *BTU* is the accepted unit of heat quantity.

A. BTU is frequently defined as the amount of heat required to raise 1 pound of water through 1° F.

B. A more accurate definition is that 1 BTU equals $\frac{1}{180}$ of the amount of heat required to raise the temperature of a pound of water from 32° F to 212° F.

E X A M P L E : Given 50 pounds of water and 50 pounds of cast iron, each to be heated through a temperature rise of 100° F, determine the heat added to each substance: average amount of heat required to raise the temperature of 1 pound of water through 1° F = 1 BTU. Heat added to water = 1 × 50 × 100 = 5,000 BTU. Average amount of heat required to raise the temperature of 1 pound of cast iron through 1° F = 0.12 BTU. Heat added to cast iron = 0.12 × 50 × 100 = 600 BTU.

In this example, the weight of material and the temperature rise were the same in each case, but the quantity of heat added differed considerably due to the nature of the substances. Had the same amount of heat been added to the cast iron as was added to the water, the temperature rise of the iron would have been 5,000 ÷ (50 × 0.12) = 833° F.

Specific heat.—The specific heat of any substance is the ratio of the heat required to raise a unit weight of the substance 1° F to the quantity of heat required to raise the temperature of the same weight of water through 1° F.

E X A M P L E : Find the quantity of heat required to raise the temperature of 100 pounds of ice from 0° F to 32° F. Specific heat of ice = 0.5.

$$100 \times (32-0) \times 0.5 = 1,600 \text{ BTU}$$

Pressure.—Air is such a commonplace thing that we are seldom conscious of its existence. We must, however, realize that air has *weight, exerts a pressure* and everything that we do takes place in an ocean of air. The pressure exerted by the atmosphere is termed *atmospheric pressure.*

The pressure of the atmosphere varies with the elevation above sea level, weather conditions, etc., and since it is such a variable quality, it has been necessary to define *standard atmospheric pressure* so that it can serve as a basis for comparison in engineering and other formulas. This standard atmospheric pressure is supposed to be measured at sea level and by definition is equivalent to 29.92 *inches Hg per square inch*. This means that a column of air 1 square inch in cross section and extending up into the sky to the limit of our atmosphere would exert just enough weight to counterbalance the weight of a column of mercury 1 square inch in cross section and 29.92 inches in height.

The height of mercury standing in the tube will be exactly equal to the pressure of the atmosphere pushing down on the surface of the mercury in the beaker.

As a matter of fact, atmospheric pressure is frequently measured by an instrument using mercury, precisely as shown in the above illustration, and this device is referred to as a *mercurial barometer*. There is another type of barometer in general use which uses no fluid. Instead, the pressure of the air is measured by a linkage which is attached to the elastic side of a box or chamber which has been exhausted of air. This type of instrument is called an *aneroid barometer,* which means "no fluid."

In the above illustration, we talked about the pressure of air as measured in terms of inches of mercury, but we should also be familiar with the other units in which air pressure is frequently measured. Standard atmospheric pressure (which is theoretically the air pressure at sea level) is also equal to 14.7 pounds per square inch and this gives us a relationship of $14.7/29.92 = 0.491$ pounds per square inch for each inch of mercury column.

In many pressure determinations, the unit "inches of mercury" is too large for the value of the pressure being measured, and so we need a smaller unit of measurement "inches of water." Since mercury is 13.6 times as heavy as water, then 1 inch of mercury = 13.6 inches of water (Fig. 12). Standard atmospheric pressure of 29.92 inches of mercury is, therefore, equivalent to approximately 407 inches of water per square inch. When pressure is measured in a steam boiler, for example, the pressure is measured above or below the atmosphere and such pressure is always expressed as gauge pressure and is frequently abbreviated *PSIG,* meaning *pounds per square inch gauge.*

In order to determine the absolute pressure or the pressure above zero, it is necessary to add algebraically the gauge pressure to the atmospheric or barometric pressure. Absolute pressure is frequently abbreviated *PSIA, pounds per square inch absolute.* One must always be sure that each pressure is expressed in the same units.

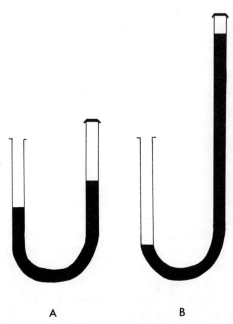

A

B

Fig. 12.—Measuring pressures with two types of fluids; the construction of the two tubes is the same. The difference is in the type of liquid used. The recorded movement is either in mm Hg. or cm of water. In example **A,** mercury is used and in example **B,** water is used. The difference in absolute height shows **B** to be approximately 13 times the height of **A** due to the increased density of the mercury.

A manometer is used to measure the amount of mercury or water that is being supported (Fig. 13). The manometer consists of a U-shaped glass tube half filled with mercury. One tube is left open to the atmosphere, while pressure is applied to the other. The total distance the mercury moves in relation to the millimeter marks on the meter stick indicates the applied pressure. Since one tube of the manometer is exposed to the atmosphere, this device also reads pressures above or below the atmospheric pressure.

Air is drawn into the tracheobronchial tree and forced out strictly in relationship with the pressure gradient between the atmosphere and the volume of air in the lungs and not by active dilation and contraction of the lungs.

During exhalation, the diaphragm and the intercostal muscles relax and the thoracic cavity decreases; the elastic lung recoils, and the intrapulmonic (lung) pressure increases to above atmospheric pressure. (According to Boyle's law (Fig. 14), if one decreases the volume of a gas container, the temperature remaining constant, there will be an increase in the pressure

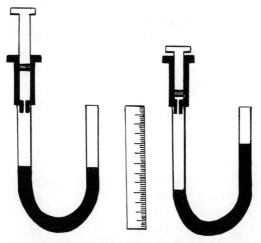

Fig. 13.—Mercury manometer used to measure applied pressure. The total distance the mercury moves in relation to the millimeter marks on the meter stick is the applied pressure in mm Hg.

of the gas within that container.) During a normal respiratory cycle, the lungs play a passive role. The volume changes they undergo and the intake and elimination of gases are brought about through pressure changes in the thoracic cage. Intrapulmonic pressure or the pressure applied to the lungs from inside is, therefore, practically atmospheric pressure and is

Fig. 14.—Application of Boyle's law. These two syringes connected to pressure gauges indicate that by moving the plunger in, the same number of molecules are compressed into a smaller space, causing more frequent collisions and a greater force applied to each surface; thus, an increase in pressure occurs.

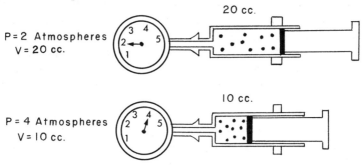

P = 2 Atmospheres
V = 20 cc.

20 cc.

P = 4 Atmospheres
V = 10 cc.

10 cc.

TEMPERATURE CONSTANT

usually given as 760 mm Hg. The outside of the lungs is protected from atmospheric pressure by the chest wall.

Although intrathoracic (intrapleural) pressure varies with thoracic conditions, this pressure is usually about 752 mm Hg, or less than that of the atmosphere, and is, therefore, subatmospheric pressure at the end of inspiration and 754 mm Hg at the end of expiration, as recorded by a mercurial manometer connected with the intrapleural cavity.

As mentioned earlier, the large oxygen pressure gradient between the alveoli and the blood capillaries allows oxygen diffusion to occur very rapidly under normal conditions.

Blood combines with oxygen in two ways: (1) in physical solution in the watery parts of the blood as dissolved oxygen and (2) in chemical combination with hemoglobin as oxyhemoglobin. In each instance, the amount of oxygen taken up depends directly on the partial pressure to which the plasma or blood is exposed. The oxygen from the alveoli diffuses into the blood. On entering the circulating blood, oxygen immediately goes into simple solution in the plasma. If blood consisted merely of plasma without red blood cells, the amount of oxygen it could take up in ordinary breathing would be small. For example, 100 cc of arterial blood normally contains 0.3 cc of oxygen in simple solution. However, a special chemical compound, hemoglobin, is present in red blood cells. One gram of this chemical compound is capable of combining or associating with 1.34 ml of oxygen; thus, if 100 ml of blood contains 15.6 Gm of hemoglobin, it can combine chemically with $15.6 \times 1.34 = 20.9$ ml of oxygen. However, the actual amount of oxygen combined depends on the partial pressure of oxygen in the circulating blood.

The amount of oxygen in combination with hemoglobin is not linearly related to the partial pressure of oxygen. If whole blood is exposed to ten different containers of ten different oxygen tensions ranging from 10 to 100 mm Hg and the amount of oxygen combined with hemoglobin (total oxygen minus dissolved oxygen) is measured in each when equilibrium is achieved, the values (see Fig. 148, p. 263) will be observed. A graph of oxygen content (or % saturation) against Po_2 is not a straight line but an S-shaped curve which has a steep slope (between 10 and 50 mm Hg Po_2) and a very flat portion (between 70 and 100 mm Hg Po_2) (see Fig. 148, p. 263).

Although hemoglobin is capable of combining with 1.34 ml of oxygen per Gm, it does not always hold this maximal amount. For example, the hemoglobin of a normal healthy adult male breathing room air holds only about 97.5% of the maximum (97.5% saturated). However, whenever, this person breathes oxygen at very high pressures (3 or 4 atmospheres), as much oxygen can sometimes be transported in the dissolved state as in combination with hemoglobin. In other words, the more oxygen available (increased Po_2) in the atmosphere, the more oxygen that can be carried by the blood, hence a higher percentage saturation.

The next phase is the absorption of oxygen from the blood into the tissue cells. A small portion of oxygen is lost from the arterial blood before the capillaries are reached, and the blood reaches the periphery with a fairly high oxygen content. The oxygen tension (Po_2) of the tissue cells is relatively low; a flow of oxygen from the plasma across the capillary membrane results. In other words, when the partial pressure of a gas is different in two areas of a system, a diffusion "gradient" exists between the two parts. Hence, the gas diffuses from the area in which its partial pressure is high to that in which its partial pressure is low. This activity continues until the pressure is the same in both parts of the system.

Thus far, we have introduced only one part of the inhalation phase of respiration. Let us now look into the second part as well as other phases of respiration.

In adults at sea level, each inspiration carries toward the lungs about 500 ml (called tidal volume) of a mixture of 20.93% oxygen, 79.03% nitrogen and .04% carbon dioxide. As this inspired air is carried toward the alveolar spaces in the lungs for ultimate mixing with the blood in the pulmonary capillaries, two changes occur in its composition. It becomes mixed with gas (anatomic dead space gas) which has a lower oxygen and high carbon dioxide content, and it also becomes saturated with water vapor in the lungs. The molecules of the different gases will in time distribute themselves evenly throughout the space in which they are found.

Each gas in a mixture of gases will behave as though it were present alone. Its molecules will become distributed evenly throughout the mixture, and its pressure will depend on its concentration without regard to the concentration of the other gases. Thus, the total pressure of a mixture of gases is equal to the sum of the pressures of the individual gases. For example, the atmosphere exerts a pressure of 760 mm Hg. The gases of which it is composed, oxygen, nitrogen and carbon dioxide, exert their own partial pressure (in the same proportions as their concentrations) 159 mm Hg (20.93% of the total pressure), 600 mm Hg (79%) and 30 mm Hg (0.4%), respectively. The word "tension" is used interchangeably with "partial pressure," and it refers to the stress exerted by the gas molecules on the wall of a closed space or vessel.

Since the oxygen tension of the tissue cells is low and the oxygen tension in the arterial blood is high, there is obviously a pressure gradient or slope in the partial pressure of oxygen. Thus, oxygen diffuses out of the arterial blood and into the tissue cells until equalization of tension occurs.

The arterial blood reaches the capillaries with an oxygen tension of about 100 mm Hg. Each 100 ml of blood normally contains about 20 ml of oxygen; however, only 0.3 ml is in physical solution in the plasma. Since the tension of oxygen in the tissue cells is lower than that in the plasma, oxygen is always diffusing from the blood plasma into the cells.

When the blood reaches the capillaries, the oxygen molecules, held in the plasma under a tension of 95 mm Hg, are forced through the capillary wall because the tension outside the wall is lower; oxygen then moves into the tissue cells. The tension of oxygen in the plasma rapidly falls, leading to a dissociation of oxygen from combination with hemoglobin.

The utilization of oxygen by the tissue cells is the fourth phase of respiration. The rate of utilization of oxygen by the cell is determined by the activity of the cells, the rate of blood flow and amount of oxygen in combination with hemoglobin and plasma.

The circulation is so adjusted in resting tissues that the cells get all the oxygen they need, but, as a rule, there is a large margin for further increase both in the rate (or volume) of total blood flow through the tissue and in the total capillary surface over which it is exposed for the diffusion of gases.

The average amount of oxygen given up to the tissue cells of the body from each 100 ml of blood is usually about 5 ml. A normal adult utilizes about 250 ml of oxygen per minute. Even after the tissues have received all their requirements, the venous blood is still 70–75% saturated with oxygen under normal conditions.

Carbon dioxide is produced in living cells at varying rates, depending on activity and metabolism of the body. It is much more soluble in water than is oxygen (2.7 volumes per cent). It also forms carbonic acid in the presence of water. This reaction is reversible but is known to proceed slowly at body pH of 7.4.

Carbon dioxide diffuses into the plasma and then from the plasma into the erythrocytes, where an enzyme, carbonic anhydrase, catalyzes the formation of carbonic acid ($H_2O + CO_2 \rightarrow H_2CO_3$), which then reacts in many ways with substances in the erythrocytes. One of the ways considered important in the theory is as follows: $H_2CO_3 + KHb \rightleftarrows KHb + KHCO_3$. As oxyhemoglobin gives off oxygen to the tissues, the hemoglobin offers a greater number of basic ions to form compounds with the H_2CO_3, and, hence, more $KHCO_3$ are formed in the cells. This results in a relatively high concentration of HCO_3^- ions in the erythrocytes. Most of these HCO_3^- ions diffuse back into the plasma and form carbonates there, chiefly $NaHCO_3$ (necessitating the "chloride shift" to erythrocytes where bases combine with the chloride ions leaving bases in plasma to neutralize the

HCO_3 ions). Carbon dioxide also forms carbamino compounds, carbohemo-globin, with hemoglobin. Varying quantities of carbon dioxide reaching the blood cause its pH to vary and, in consequence, limit the amount of carbo-hemoglobin that can be carried; hence, the main factor in the ability of the blood to take up carbon dioxide in the tissues and give it off in the lungs is that the hemoglobin gives off oxygen in the tissues and, becoming less acid in consequence, takes in another available acid, carbonic acid, to replace it. Also, when in the lungs, oxygen is available and the carbon dioxide can escape, so there is again an exchange. This time oxygen takes the place of the carbon dioxide in the erythrocytes.

Hyperbaric Oxygenation

The mechanism of oxygen transport from the pulmonary unit to its ultimate destination in the cells is basic to life in the mammalian organism. Since the discovery of oxygen and its critical importance has become more evident, a variety of modalities have been improvised and used to provide additional oxygen or to decrease the metabolic needs of tissues struggling against an overwhelming burden of relative anoxia.

Within the past decade, the use of hyperbaric oxygenation has proved to be an important and imaginative step forward in increasing the volume of oxygen transported in blood. Exposure of man to high atmospheric pressure is not new. For many years, caisson and underground workers and deep-sea divers have been subjected to pressurized air above ambient pressures at sea level, but the over-all basic understanding of the effects in man has been limited. The most significant studies have been concerned with the primary causes and ultimate management of decompression sick-ness, oxygen toxicity and inert gas narcosis. The convulsive effect of hy-perbaric oxygen was first described by Bert, in 1878, and the adverse pulmonary effect by Smith, in 1899. Historically, man has been subjected to increased air pressures for varying periods, often days, for a variety of diseases, but this practice was abandoned by its proponents, whose obser-vations and claims were empirical and from which no basic scientific data emerged.

The degree of oxygenation that can be achieved by breathing 100% oxygen under hyperbaric conditions is impressive, according to our present thinking. The increase in partial pressure of alveolar gas (oxygen) from approximately 104 mm Hg, breathing 100% oxygen at three atmospheres, has important physiologic implications. One can think of situations in which this technique might be useful: to sustain life without red blood cells; to supply oxygen by diffusion to areas rendered ischemic by vascular occlusion; or to combine hyperbaric oxygenation with hypothermia for performance of surgery under conditions of total circulatory arrest.

Physiologic Basis

Under normal conditions, the partial pressure of oxygen is about 159 mm Hg in inspired air, reduced by uptake of oxygen, the addition of water vapor and carbon dioxide to about 104 mm Hg in alveolar gas. Administration of 100% oxygen at one atmosphere can increase the alveolar gas tension nearly sevenfold to about 670 mm Hg.

When oxygen is administered to a healthy individual at normal pressure, the oxygen tension, Pa_{O_2}, of arterial blood increases to the new alveolar level. The hemoglobin, normally at 97.5% saturated with oxygen, becomes fully saturated. Moreover, additional oxygen becomes physically dissolved in the blood. The over-all oxygen content of arterial blood is elevated from 20 volumes per cent (ml of oxygen per 100 ml of blood) to about 22 volumes per cent.

If a normal healthy adult or infant is placed in a hyperbaric chamber and exposed to increased ambient pressure while breathing oxygen, the alveolar oxygen tension will be increased correspondingly, and the oxygen tension and content of arterial blood will also rise. If the rise in alveolar oxygen tension is maximum, the Pa_{O_2} will increase 760 mm Hg with each atmosphere (14.7 pounds per square inch) of increase in ambient pressure. The increase in arterial oxygen content will be equal to about 2 volumes per cent per atmosphere. Since the hemoglobin is already fully saturated, this increase will be in the form of physically dissolved oxygen. Thus an ambient pressure of 3 atm (atmospheres, absolute) will yield an arterial Po_2 of over 2,000 mm Hg and an increase of about 6 volumes per cent in arterial oxygen content above the normal level.

Pulmonary Ventilation

One of the most common causes of hypoxia is insufficiency of the volumes of air breathed in and out the alveoli. This condition can be corrected by controlled or assisted ventilation with or without oxygen. One important aspect of hyperbaric oxygenation which can be injected at this point is that the use of pure oxygen greatly reduces the volume of ventilation required for adequate oxygenation. The fact that the level of CO_2 remains unchanged limits the effectiveness of this technique. It still may be practical, however, if CO_2 can be reduced by the use of injected buffers such as sodium bicarbonate or THAM.

DISTRIBUTION OF INSPIRED GAS

It is a well-known fact that hypoxia can result from gross nonuniform ventilation and perfusion in the lungs. A well-perfused, but poorly ventilated, area will rapidly reduce the alveolar Po_2 and result in poorly oxygenated arterial blood. The administering of high-oxygen concentration in this instance is valuable, as has been indicated. However, if only a small fraction of blood flow goes to the lung areas with essentially no ventilation, oxygen at normal pressure may be of little help. This procedure cannot add sufficiently to the oxygen content of blood from ventilated areas to provide enough compensation. Hyperbaric oxygenation, on the other hand, may be of great benefit.

ALVEOLAR DIFFUSION

Pulmonary edema and fibrosis of alveolar membrane will cause hypoxia due to the inability of gases to diffuse across the capillary membrane. In many instances, oxygen given at normal pressure may correct this situation; in severe diffusion defects with shunting, hyperbaric oxygenation may be indicated.

RIGHT-TO-LEFT SHUNTS

A right-to-left shunt is a condition whereby venous blood in returning to the lung fails to pass through adequately ventilated areas. It is encountered in many congenital cardiac abnormalities and in pulmonary diseases. In conditions in which there might be a 50% shunt with a mixed venous blood oxygen content of 14 volumes per cent and only half of this blood was being oxygenated to the normal 20 volumes per cent in the lungs, the mixed arterial oxygen would be only 17 volumes per cent. Oxygen under high pressure would be indicated to increase the oxygen content by 6 volumes per cent.

Despite its many advantages, hyperbaric oxygen has some disadvantages, such as possible lung damage due to oxygen toxicity and central nervous system disturbance leading to convulsions.

Continuous exposure to high concentrations of oxygen at normal pressure generally produces reduction in vital capacity and substernal distress within less than 24 hours (Comroe, Dripps, Dumke and Deming, 1945). Further exposure results in dyspnea and increasing evidence of pulmonary hyperemia and edema.

Convulsions develop after varying periods of exposure to oxygen at pressures higher than 2 atm. This phenomenon will vary greatly between individuals. The greatest source of experience is the oxygen tolerance test administered to all candidates for United States Navy diving training. This test consists of breathing pure oxygen at 2.8 atm for 30 minutes at rest. The incidence of convulsions is approximately 2%. Onset has been known to occur in as little as 15 minutes. It appears that a critical level exists near 3 atm, but available data give little suggestion of the probable limits of tolerance at that pressure.

Broader realization and potential benefits of hyperbaric oxygen will surely depend on the extent to which oxygen toxicity can be circumvented. The need for more basic research in the area is great.

CIRCULATION

The over-all function of the heart, which is a double pump, is to adjust the circulation throughout the body in accordance to the metabolic need of the cells. This fine adjustment is accomplished by chemical and nervous control, which enables these needs to be met by adjustments of the pulse rate and the pulse amplitude, which increases and decreases the velocity and volume of blood in the tissue capillaries. Thus, the cellular requirements are met by the numerous changes in the number, size and area of the open capillaries and in the temperature and minute volume of the blood in these capillaries.

The heart, as was mentioned previously, is a double pump, hollow organ, weighing well under a pound, and it is slightly larger than the average adult male fist. Its tough muscular wall (myocardium) is surrounded by a fiber-like bag (pericardium) and is lined by a thin, strong membrane (endocardium). A wall (septum) divides the heart cavity up the middle into a "right heart" and a "left heart." Each side of the heart is divided again into an upper chamber (atrium) and a lower chamber (ventricle). Valves in each chamber regulate the flow of blood through the heart and to the pulmonary artery and the aorta. The right side of the heart supplies the pulmonary system with blood, whereas the left side supplies the systemic system.

One pump, the right heart, receives blood which has just come from the tissues of the body after delivering nutrients and oxygen. It pumps this dark bluish red blood, desaturated, to the lungs where the blood rids itself of carbon dioxide and picks up a fresh supply of oxygen. The second pump, the left heart, receives this "reconditioned blood" from the lungs and pumps it out through the great trunk-artery, the aorta, to be distributed by smaller arteries to all parts of the body.

To make this somewhat clearer, a detailed summary of the movement of blood through the right heart and lungs as well as through the left heart and to the somatic capillaries is shown in Figure 15.

During diastole of the atria, the relaxation phase of the heart with accompanying dilation, blood enters via the superior and inferior vena cava, coronary sinus and other small vessels and fills the right atrium and ven-

Fig. 15.—The heart is a hollow organ. Its tough, muscular wall (myocardium) is surrounded by the pericardium and is lined by a thin, strong membrane (endocardium). A wall (septum) divides the heart down the middle into a "right heart" and a "left heart." Each side of the heart is divided again into an upper chamber (atrium) and a lower chamber (ventricle). Valves regulate the flow of blood through the heart and to the pulmonary artery and the aorta.

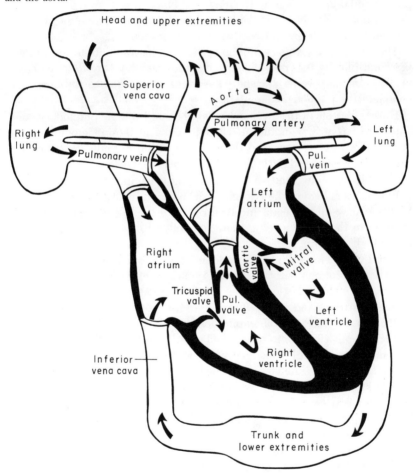

tricle, which for the sake of simplicity may be thought of as a single chamber with the tricuspid valve open.

The right atrium contracts, atrial systole, and forces the blood over the open valve into the ventricle, which has been passively filled with blood and now becomes distended.

After a 0.1-second pause, the right ventricle contracts and the pressure exerted by the blood behind the cusps of the tricuspid valve closes it.

There is a rise of pressure within the right ventricle to a point slightly higher than that in the pulmonary artery, thus allowing the pulmonary valve to open.

The pulmonary artery divides into the right and left branches and transports blood into the lungs. In the lungs, the blood passes through capillaries that surround the alveoli of the lungs. Blood gives up carbon dioxide, and the red blood cells are enriched with fresh oxygen.

The venules, tiny veins continuous with capillaries, unite to form larger veins until finally two pulmonary veins from each lung are formed. These veins, pulmonary veins, transport the oxygenated blood to the heart and complete the pulmonary circulation.

During diastole of the atria, oxygenated blood from the pulmonary veins enters the left atrium and fills it. The left ventricle, most efficient muscular part of the heart, relaxes, and the pressure within its walls decreases, the mitral valve opens and the blood enters the left ventricle and fills it. Systole of the atrium begins, and ventricular filling is completed.

Blood enters behind the two cusps of the mitral valve and closes them. Ventricular systole is begun, intraventricular pressure rises and exceeds the pressure in the aorta, causing the aortic valve to open, and blood enters under high pressure.

Blood then is forced into the conducting or elastic arteries, innominate, subclavian, common carotids, internal femoral, etc.

These stretched elastic arteries recoil, pushing blood onward into the muscular arteries and finally into the arterioles, smallest arteries leading to their distal ends into the capillaries.

These capillaries fuse to form venules which in turn unite to form veins, then larger veins, until blood finally reaches the right atrium and the circuit begins again. This is known as systemic circulation as opposed to pulmonary circulation, which is sometimes called the lesser circulation. The pulmonary circulation carries the blood which has been used by the tissues of the body.

We have talked about circulation to various parts of the body except to the heart. How does the heart receive its blood supply? Blood supply to the heart muscle is a function of the coronary arteries. These arteries branch off the aorta close to the heart. They fill during diastole and empty during systole of the heart. Usually during normal conditions in healthy adults, the rate of blood flow through these vessels is from 50 to 75 ml of blood per 100 Gm of heart muscle, 300 Gm per minute, depending on the heart rate and heart volume. Since the cardiac output in healthy adults has been estimated to be 4000 ml per minute, therefore, about 10–12% of the cardiac output flows through the coronary arteries. Blood leaving the coronary arteries is returned to the heart via the coronary sinus which branches into the right atrium.

THE HEART BEAT.—The first visible sign of heart contraction is noted where the superior vena cava empties into the right atrium. The sinoatrial node (S–A) is located in the wall of the right atrium near the entrance of the superior vena cava. From this node, fibers extend throughout the wall of the atria.

The S–A node is often called the pacemaker of the heart because waves of contraction pass over the muscle of both atria from this spot. The two atria, left and right, contract simultaneously, driving the blood into the ventricles. The wave of contraction further spreads over the ventricles, causing them to contract simultaneously, also driving blood into the arteries. How is it possible to produce a wave of contraction in a muscular tissue such as the atria and have it continue over to the ventricles, which are not continuous with that of the atria? The connecting pathway is furnished by the atrioventricular node (A–V node), which is located in the lower part of the interatrial septum. From the S–A node, an excitation wave spreads throughout the musculature to the atria and to the A–V node to the ventricles.

THE ELECTROCARDIOGRAM.—During contraction of the heart, electrical changes continuously take place in heart muscle fibers. Viable cardiac muscle fibers are electrically negative to resting fibers. The electrical differences in parts of the heart which occur constantly can be led off from the surface of the body by electrodes placed on specific areas of the extremities and connected to a galvanometer.

Each lead will show the potential differences in the heart activity as recorded at the body surface. This procedure is called the electrocardiogram. Normal recording (Fig. 16) will show an electrical heart cycle with a peaked elevation called the P wave, which is caused by the spread of excitation from the S–A node out over the atria and to the A–V node. The QRS deflections are recorded as the electrical impulse spreads down the A–V bundle and out over the ventricles (ventricular systole). The T wave is recorded as ventricular excitation ends.

The cardiac cycle in healthy state consists of three distinct phases: (1) a period of active contraction called the systole; (2) a period of dilation

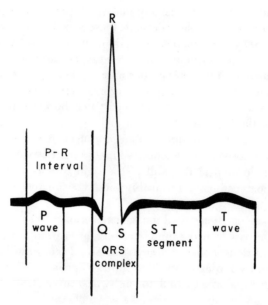

Fig. 16.—A normal tracing of an electrocardiographic lead, showing its components.

called the diastole; and (3) a period of rest. In healthy man, the average heart rate at rest is 70–72 beats per minute. When the heart rate is faster than the normal, the rest period is the phase that is shortened, thus allowing the heart to receive decreasing periods of rest, which could have its effect after a period of time.

The ultimate cause of the heart beat is unknown. Many cardiologists favor the regulatory theory, that the contractions are due to the built-in power of contraction possessed by the muscle cells of the heart and that the stimulus which excites the contraction is a chemical one dependent on the presence of definite proportions of inorganic salts in the blood.

Although the heart contracts automatically and with built-in rhythm, the continuously changing frequency and volume of the heart is regulated by the following factors:

1. Nerve impulses
2. Chemical substances in the blood
3. Physical factors, temperature and pressures within the heart and the great vessels

Sensory regulation of the heart beat is controlled by the cardiac center located in the medulla oblongata. Afferent nerves carry sensory impulses from the heart to the central nervous system via the spinal cord. Depressor fibers are also present. These fibers carry impulses from receptor cells lying in the base of the aorta. These depressor fibers are also sensitive to pressure changes. Pressor fibers increase the heart rate. The heart also receives nerve impulses through two sets of efferent fibers, the right and left vagus nerves, of the parasympathetic division and the accelerator nerves sympathetic division.

Efferent fibers of the vagus (10th cranial nerve) are preganglionic fibers ending in a small ganglion in the wall of the heart. Here they synapse with postganglionic neurons, the fibers of which are distributed to the S–A and A–V node. Impulses carried by these fibers are inhibitory; they slow down or stop the beat of the heart. Stimulation of the afferent nerves results in a quickened heart beat.

Chemical factors in regulation of the heart beat include (1) increase in P_{CO_2} causing vasoconstriction, (2) decrease in P_{O_2}, increasing heart rate, (3) increased rate and depth of contractions and (4) digitalis slows heart beat by depressing conduction in the A–V bundle, causing a slowing of ventricular activity, excessive dosage and may cause heart block.

REFERENCES

Comroe, J., *et al.: The Lung* (Chicago: Year Book Medical Publishers, Inc., 1962).

Cherniack, R. M., and Cherniack, L.: *Respiration in Health and Disease* (Philadelphia: W. B. Saunders Company, 1961).

Comroe, J.: *Physiology of Respiration* (Chicago: Year Book Medical Publishers, Inc., 1965).

Lilienthal, J. L., Jr., and Riley, R. L.: Circulation through the lung and diffusion of gases, Ann. Rev. Med. 5:237, 1954.

National Research Council, Division of Medical Sciences Committee on Hyperbaric Oxygenation: *Fundamentals of Hyperbaric Medicine*, 178 pp. (Washington, D. C.: The Council 1966, Publication No. 1298).

Adams, W., and Veith, I.: *Pulmonary Circulation* (New York: Grune & Stratton, 1959).

Rankin, J.: *Evaluation of Alveolar Capillary Diffusion in Clinical Cardiopulmonary Physiology* (New York: Grune & Stratton, 1960), pp. 624–634.

Severinghaus, J. W., and Stupfel, M.: Alveolar dead space as an index of distribution of blood flow in pulmonary capillaries, J. Appl. Physiol. 10:335, 1957.

CHAPTER 4

Manufacture, Transport and Storage of Gases

ALTHOUGH THAT which is presented here is recognized as standard material, the authors feel that its presentation at this point is necessary for a complete understanding of the chapters that follow. Prior to 1868, there was little need for compressed gases, especially in anesthesia, since the gases used at that time consisted of ether and chloroform and these agents were given as vapors in atmospheric air. Of the many compressed gases, oxygen was most often used, although its vital importance was unknown at that time. The compression of gases after 1868, however, created many hazards due to the high pressures needed to compress the gas. Standards of purity and regulations for safe practice had to be devised.

In the United States, the Interstate Commerce Commission drew up standards regulating the manufacture of medical gases. The Compressed Gas Association and the National Fire Protection Association further defined safe practice in the manufacture, packaging and handling of these gases. All gas cylinders must be made of chrome-molybdenum steel to insure a high total expansion limit and relative light weight. The cylinder contents must be identified by permanently attached labels or stencils naming the contents and giving their proportions.

All post-type cylinder valves shall be pin indexed in accordance with Compressed Gas Association recommendations (Fig. 17). All large cylinder valves shall conform with Compressed Gas Association valve outlet standards. Large cylinder valves must conform with CGA thread specifications. For low-pressure medical gas connections (Figs. 18 and 19), a thread system called DISS is used. Cylinder valve seats must be fabricated of special plastic material to insure excellent sealing characteristics with a high resistance to ignition. A Teflon plastic seal should be used as a packing on cylinder valves to provide "self-sealing" protection against leakage of gas past the

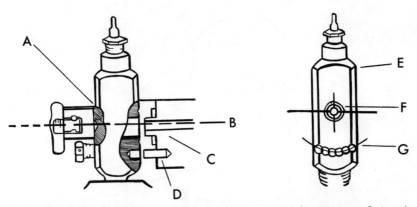

Fig. 17.—Yoke outlet with cylinder valve yoke connections showing pin indexing. *A*, valve indent for yoke-adjusting screw; *B*, yoke gas inlet; *C*, yoke block; *D*, pin placement for pin index system; *E*, cylinder valve head; *F*, valve gas outlet; *G*, variation in holes in valve stem dependent on specific gas for pin indexing.

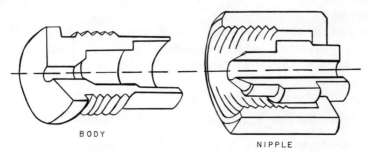

BODY

NIPPLE

Fig. 18.—Diameter-index safety system for low-pressure medical gas connections. The small bore in the body matches the grooves in the nipple, making a specific connection.

Fig. 19.—Diameter-index safety system standard low-pressure connections for air and vacuum. **A,** connection # 1160 air; **B,** connection # 1220 suction.

A   B

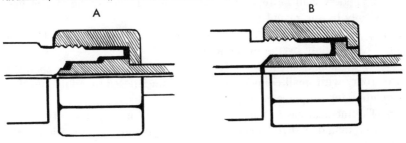

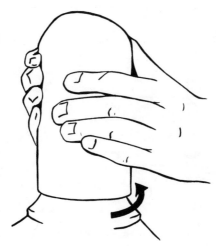

Fig. 20.—Protective metal caps should be replaced on the cylinders when they are not in use.

valve stem. A valve outlet washer (Gasloc seal) is used, which has a high-ignition temperature, and shall be supplied with each cylinder having a post-type valve. The valve is capped to protect it from grease or dirt (Fig. 20).

Recommended Safe Practices

1. Cylinder valves shall be inspected for safe and easy operation and proper pin indexing.

2. Cylinders shall be checked for damage, moisture and foreign odors, and the hydrostatic-test date on the shoulder cylinders shall be hydrostatically tested at least once every 5 years to check for leaks or structural weakness.

3. Cylinders shall be repainted with accepted color coding when necessary only by the manufacturer.

4. Cylinders shall be weighed empty, tagged and then labeled. This also is to be done only by the manufacturer.

5. All cylinders shall be purged by drawing a vacuum of at least 25 inches of mercury with small cylinders filled on a pin-indexed manifold and then reweighed for proper contents.

6. The medical gas in the cylinders is tested for proper purity.

7. Full cylinders shall be checked for leakage and easy operation of the valves.

8. Cylinder valve outlet shall be sealed against dirt and other foreign material.

9. Cylinders shall be properly wrapped and packaged during shipment both for protection and to retain good appearance.

In order to prevent explosion, the following procedures should be followed in the storage and handling of compressed gases. These requirements refer to the storage of flammable medical gases and piping systems for nonflammable medical gases.

1. Storage of gases should be systematic and shall be segregated from areas of storage of other medical equipment (Fig. 21).

2. Separate cylinder or manifold enclosures shall be provided for flammable gases and for oxidizing gases. All storage rooms or manifold enclosures for medical gases in excess of 1,500 cubic feet shall be vented to the outside.

3. Provisions shall be made for racks to protect cylinders from damage and to prevent injury.

4. The storage area should have a conductive flooring and a fireproof light.

5. The Compressed Gas Association has the following standards:

   a) Never permit oil, grease or highly flammable material to come in contact with oxygen cylinders, valves, regulators or fittings.
   b) Never lubricate flowmeters, regulators or gauges with oil or any other flammable substances.
   c) Never handle medical gases with oily hands, greasy gloves or rags.
   d) Always clear the particles of dust and dirt from cylinder valves by slightly opening and closing the cylinder valve before applying and fitting.
   e) Open the high pressure valve on the gas cylinder before bringing to patient area.
   f) Open the the valve slowly with the face of the gauge on the regulator pointed away from any person (Fig. 22).
   g) Never drape anything over the gas cylinder.
   h) Never interchange fittings used for another gas.
   i) Never mix gases.
   j) Always use a reducing valve to deliver gases from a cylinder.
   k) Never use equipment that is in need of repair or cylinder with valves which do not operate properly.
   l) Return all defective gas cylinders to the manufacturer or authorized agent for replacement.

The physical properties of the most commonly used gases in inhalation therapy may be seen in Table 2.

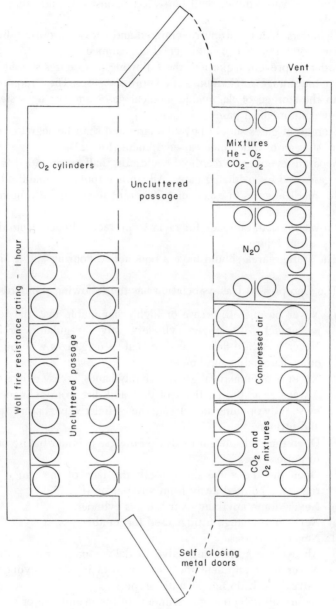

Fig. 21.—Suggested storage room arrangement for medical gases.

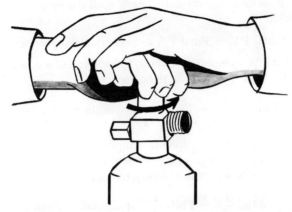

Fig. 22.—Open the cylinder valve slowly for the first time and be certain that the outlet is pointing away from you or others.

A thorough knowledge of the general gas laws is fundamental to an understanding of many of the problems involved in their use. At sufficiently low pressures and high temperatures, all gases have been found to obey three simple laws. These three laws relate the volume of a gas to the pressure and temperature. The laws which are called the "ideal" gas laws are described below:

Boyle's law: When the temperature is kept constant, the volume of a

		OXYGEN	CARBON DIOXIDE	HELIUM
Symbol		O_2	CO_2	H_2
Molecular weight		32	44.01	4.00
Cylinder color		Green	Gray	Brown
Physical state in cylinder at 70° F		Gas	Liquid	Gas
Specific gravity of gas (air = 1 at 25° C)		1.11	1.53	0.14
Critical temperature		118.8° C	88.41	− 450.33
Boiling point		− 182.96° C	− 78.43	− 268.9
Cylinder fillings	E	165	420	131
(Gal)	G	1,400	3,200	1,100
Gas	E	1.83	6.56	0.1875
Weight (lb)	G	15.50	50.0	2.0

TABLE 2.—PROPERTIES OF MEDICAL GASES

given mass of an ideal gas varies inversely with the pressure to which the gas is subjected.

$$\text{Initial P.V.} = \text{Final } P_2V_2 \text{ at constant temperature}$$

Charles' law: At a constant pressure, the volume of a given mass of gas varies directly with the absolute temperature.

$$\text{Initial } \frac{V_1}{T_1} = \text{Final } \frac{V_2}{T_2} \text{ at constant pressure}$$

when T_1 and T_2 denote the absolute temperatures of the gas.

Gay-Lussac's law: At a constant volume, the pressure of a given mass of gas varies directly with the absolute temperature.

$$\text{Initial } \frac{P_1}{T_1} = \text{Final } \frac{P_2}{T_2} \text{ at constant volumes}$$

General gas law: Any of the above three gas laws can be used to derive the general gas law which applies to all possible combinations of changes.

$$\text{Initial } \frac{P_1V_1}{T_1} = \text{Final } \frac{P_2V_2}{T_2} \text{ a constant for a given mass gas used}$$

Density of a gas: As the volume of a given mass of gas increases, the mass per unit volume (i.e., the density) decreases proportionally. Therefore, the density of a gas varies inversely with its volume.

Dalton's law: The total pressure of a gaseous mixture is equal to the sum of the partial pressure of the components. The partial pressure of a component of a gas mixture is the pressure which that component would exert if it alone occupied the entire volume.

The compression of a gas to a liquid state is the most economic form of supply and smallest volume; but the physical characteristics limit the conditions under which this may be achieved (Fig. 23). Compressed oxygen is always supplied as a gas since condensation to a liquid requires a pressure of 51 atmospheres (735 PSI) at a temperature usually below 118.8° C, the critical temperature above which condensation cannot occur. Carbon dioxide is compressible to a liquid at 50 atmospheres and at 50° C. In the use of oxygen, there is a gradual decrease in pressure as the oxygen is consumed, and the cylinder contents can be determined from the pressure on the regulator; at a given temperature when the pressure is reduced to half the original pressure, the cylinder will be approximately half full. With nitrous oxide gas, as long as any liquid remains and until the cylinder is about 75% exhausted, the cylinder pressure is equal to the vapor pressure and, therefore, does not indicate the amount of gas remaining.

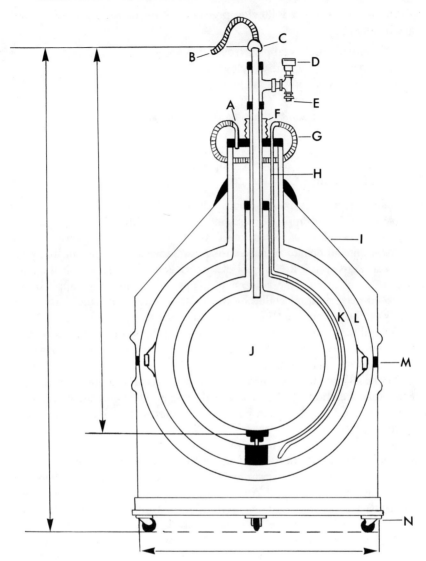

Fig. 23.—Cross-section illustration of an oval, small-volume storage flask for liquid helium, which is insulated by liquid nitrogen at −320° F, using a double-vacuum layer. A, nitrogen vent; B, pressure relief valve; C, liquid helium fill and discharge; D, helium pressure gauge; E, helium pressure relief valve (set at 7 PSIG); F, bellows seal; G, rubber tubing; H, liquid nitrogen line; I, outer casing; J, liquid helium reservoir; K, liquid nitrogen reservoir; L, vacuum; M, support; N, caster-mounted dolly.

PRECAUTIONS.—The following precautions are to be taken when gases are in use:

1. Remove paper wrappers from cylinder
2. Secure in place with a cylinder carrier
3. Open valves completely
4. Open valve slowly
5. Position cylinder so that identifying labels are clearly visible

Regulatory Authorities for Compressed Gases in the United States and Canada

Manufacturing companies who produce and transport compressed gases or persons using compressed gases must comply with a number of governmental safety rules and regulations in the United States and Canada. Gases used for inhalation are usually strong oxidizing agents and, in many instances, increase the fire hazard of materials, including medicinal agents present in or around the equipment. These regulations are supplied and enforced by regulatory bodies on the federal, state or provincial and local levels of the government in the two countries previously mentioned.

Federal regulation is concerned chiefly with the shipment of compressed gases by land, water or air between states or provinces. This regulatory body also sets specifications for shipping containers and various shipping practices. Regulations so far as storage and use of compressed gases are concerned functions of the state and province, although they may extend in some cases to certain transportation policies within the area, province or state.

Let us now look at the major regulatory bodies on each level of government in Canada and the United States.

FEDERAL REGULATORY AUTHORITIES.—The two most important agencies governing the shipment of compressed gases in North America are the Interstate Commerce Commission (ICC) of the United States and the Board of Transport Commissioners of Canada (BTC). These two agencies issue requirements for transporting compressed gas by rail in the case of gases which classify as "dangerous" commodities in interstate or interprovince commerce. All gases must be shipped in containers which comply with certain codes and specifications. The containers must be equipped with safety devices as stipulated, tested by methods identified, filled within listed maximal amounts and, in some instances, be boxed and transferred in a prescribed manner.

At the turn of the century, the United States Congress charged the Interstate Commerce Commission with the promulgation of regulations, including container specifications for the safe transportation of dangerous commodities by rail and authorized the ICC to utilize the services of the Bureau of Explosives of the Association of American Railroads. This bureau began working in close cooperation with the ICC and has continued to do so through to the present time.

Presently, this bureau acts as a central point of coordination and communication for the railroads on the one hand and the ICC and the BTC on the other. This bureau also serves all three bodies as a central office for registration, licensing and inspection.

Since the Bureau of Explosives represents both Canadian and United States railroads, substantially identical requirements have been adopted by the BTC for Canada and by the ICC for the United States concerning compressed gas shipment by rail across state or province border lines. Canadian needs and interests are thus taken into account in the setting of ICC regulations, as are the United States' needs and interests in the setting of BTC regulations. Thus, compressed gas cylinders, tank cars and portable tanks can be shipped freely between the two countries, and the shipping, charging, labeling and other practices authorized for the one country largely meet the requirements of the other.

One major difference between the ICC and the BTC is that the ICC regulates interstate motor vehicle transport of designated gases as well as rail transport in the United States, whereas the BTC regulates only rail shipment of gases in Canada. The Canadian Provincial Governments set the regulations in gas shipment by motor vehicles rather than the Canadian Federal Government.

The complete regulations of the ICC, including those applying to compressed gases, are published under the following title:

Agent T. C. George's Tariff No. 15 Publishing Interstate Commerce Commission Regulations for Transportation of Explosives and other Dangerous Articles by Land and Water, in Rail Freight Service, and by Motor Vehicle (Highway) and Water, including Specifications for Shipping Containers.

OTHER AREAS OF FEDERAL REGULATION.—A few special areas of the compressed gas field are subject to further regulation by other federal government agencies in the United States and Canada, such as in the labeling and purity requirements prescribed for gases used in medicine under national laws concerning drugs. In the United States, an area of importance arose with the enactment of the Hazardous Substances Labeling Act; the specific provisions of this act apply to those gases under pressure which will be used in the home, for instance, aerosol propellants. The act does not apply generally to compressed gases. Further information may be secured from the Federal Food and Drug Administration in the United States.

STATE OR PROVINCIAL REGULATION.—Regulations for storage, use and, in some instances, transportation, vary widely in the states of the United States and the Canadian Provinces. These governments generally have developed regulations applying to compressed gas through their chief fire safety office, pressure vessel authorities or industry and labor commission. However, it may prove to be the Railway Commission or the Industrial Accident Commission which has developed the main body of applicable regulation. Certain states have adopted the ICC regulations in full or in part.

Also, many of the states have based their fire codes for precautions with liquefied petroleum gas on the recommendations of the National Fire Prevention Association given in NFPA pamphlet No. 58, entitled: "Storage and Handling of Liquefied Petroleum Gases."

Also, widely reflected in state as well as local regulation is NFPA pamphlet No. 51, "Standard for the Installation and Operation of Oxygen-Fuel Gas Systems for Welding and Cutting."

LOCAL REGULATIONS.—Municipalities, towns and other local governments in the United States and Canada have also adopted a variety of regulations pertaining to compressed gas storage, use and shipment. These regulations are usually issued and enforced by such officials as the fire commissioner, the chief of the buildings and grounds department or zoning commissioner.

The Commercial Manufacture of Oxygen

Unlimited volumes of oxygen are separated from the air by inexpensive methods. Air is thus considered to be the best commercial source of oxygen; although water is extremely abundant too, it cannot compete with air as a commercial source of oxygen, simply because the electrical energy required to decompose water into hydrogen and oxygen is expensive. ·

The air we breathe is a mixture of gases, but its chief components are oxygen, nitrogen, carbon dioxide and relatively small amounts of inert gases. These gases are always present in any sample of air in the proportion of about 20.93% by volume of oxygen, 79.04% by volume of nitrogen and 0.03% by volume of carbon dioxide.

If the air is completely free of moisture, these gases constitute about 99.9% of the sample. Water vapor, argon and traces of other inert gases are present in samples of air in proportions that will vary with the barometric pressure and the geographic location.

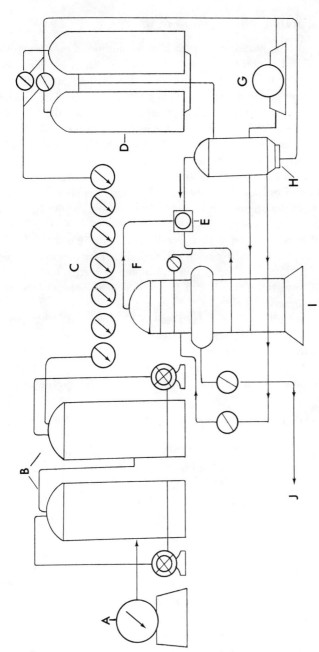

Fig. 24.—Schematic illustration of oxygen-manufacturing process. The process for the production of oxygen from liquid air in commercial quantities was developed about 1895. In the above schema, air is drawn in and treated to remove oil, water, carbon dioxide and all other impurities present. The purified air then is liquefied by means of compression and expansion, interspersed with cooling. The liquefied air is fractionated under controlled conditions at −300° F to produce oxygen which is more than 99.5% pure. The purified oxygen is compressed into cylinders at 1,800–2,400 PSI. A, air inlet; B, scrubbers; C, seven-stage compression; D, exchangers; E, liquid nitrogen cooler; F, low-pressure column; G, air liquifier; H, expander; I, high-pressure column; J, pure liquid oxygen.

Method of Separation of Oxygen from the Air

The most important and most frequently used method of obtaining oxygen is fractional distillation (Fig. 24). The volume of air is liquefied, and the air is converted from the gaseous state to the liquid state by means of low temperatures and high pressures. Then the nitrogen and oxygen are separated by fractional distillation. This method is based on the fact that nitrogen is more volatile than oxygen. Since nitrogen is more volatile and thus has a lower boiling point, $-195°$ C, than that of liquid oxygen, $-182.9°$ C, when liquid air is partially evaporated, the more volatile nitrogen escapes more rapidly than the less volatile oxygen. The vapor that is the by-product of evaporation contains a larger percentage of nitrogen than was present in the original liquid air, and the remaining liquid contains a larger percentage of oxygen.

The vapor that is given off is then condensed and re-evaporated. The new vapor that is given off will contain still higher percentages of nitrogen, and the remaining liquid will contain a still higher percentage of oxygen. This method is repeated a number of times, and finally the oxygen and nitrogen are separated.

The oxygen and nitrogen manufactured by the fractional distillation method are then stored and shipped in steel cylinders under pressures of about 2,000 pounds per square inch.

Oxygen in the liquid state is stored and shipped in large quantities at atmospheric pressure and at a temperature below the boiling point.

Air

Air is a natural product of the earth's atmosphere. It is nonflammable, colorless and odorless and consists of a mixture of gaseous elements, such as oxygen, water vapor, a small percentage of carbon dioxide and minute traces of other inert gases. Liquefied air containing carbon dioxide exhibits a milky color, and, when carbon dioxide is removed, it appears transparent with a bluish-tinted cast.

Air is used for many practical applications, such as medical, scientific, industrial, fire protection, undersea and aerospace maneuvers. To meet the desired needs, air is purified or compounded synthetically and shipped in specified cylinders as a nonliquefied gas at high pressures. Listed on the facing page is the composition of dry air at sea level.

Air, when used in human respiration, must meet specified purity requirements. Thus, it was necessary for the Compressed Gas Association,

Element Component	% by Volume	% by Weight
Nitrogen	78.3	75.5
Oxygen	20.99	23.2
Argon	0.94	1.33
Carbon dioxide	0.03	0.045
Hydrogen	0.01	—
Helium	0.0004	—
Krypton	0.00005	—
Xenon	0.0000006	—

CGA, to specify and define nine grades of gaseous air and two grades of liquid air, according to differing maximal limits for particular trace constituents.

Dry air is noncorrosive and can usually be contained in equipment constructed with common commercial metals. Air of known purity and composition is either compressed from the atmosphere and purified by chemical and mechanical means. It can also be made synthetically from its already purified components, namely, nitrogen and oxygen.

In commercial use, liquid air is the chief source of all the atmospheric gases. The method for its removal is termed fractional distillation.

Air Containers

Compressed air is always shipped under ICC regulations in specified cryogenic cylinders. These cylinders are specially vented and insulated and are similar to those used in the shipment of liquid nitrogen and hydrogen. Compressed air can be shipped at pressures below 25 PSIG. The maximal filling limits at 70° F authorized for compressed air under the present regulations are the authorized service pressures marked on the cylinders. They must also meet special requirements up to 10% in excess of their marked service pressures.

Compressed air may be shipped in any cylinders authorized by the ICC for nonliquefied compressed gas. These include cylinders meeting ICC specifications 3A, 3AA, 3B, 3C, 3D, 3E, 4, 4A, 4B, 4BA and 4C; in addition, continued use of cylinders meeting ICC specifications 3, 7, 25, 26, 33 and 38 is authorized, but new construction is not authorized.

Lastly, all cylinders authorized for compressed air service must be requalified by hydrostatic retest every 5 years, with the following exceptions: ICC–4 cylinders every 10 years; no periodic retest is required for cylinders of types 3C, 3E, 4C and 7.

Oxygen

Oxygen is colorless, odorless and tasteless. Oxygen in its physical state in compressed gas cylinders such as ICC–3A or 3AA exists as a nonliquefied gas; in ICC–4L cylinders, it exists as a pressurized liquid gas. Other physical characteristics show that the number of gallons in 1 ounce at 1 atmosphere and at 70° F is 5.65 and the number of liters in 1 ounce at 1 atmosphere at 70° F is 21.39. The specific gravity at the above figures shows that oxygen compared with air is 1.1053 and is nonflammable.

The normal cylinder-filling limit of a nonliquefied gas is 1,800–2,400 PSIG at 70° F, depending on the type of cylinder. Pressures in nonliquefied charged cylinders of oxygen will vary. At any given temperature, the pressure will decrease proportionately as the cylinder content is withdrawn. The pressure minimum and maximum is 75–235 PSIG in ICC–42 cylinders. The pressure within the cylinder during normal operation is 75 PSIG, but, during nonusage, pressure will increase very slowly over a period of 3–5 days to 235 PSIG, after which the gas will be vented out at a rate of 2–5 cubic feet per hour.

Carbon Dioxide-Oxygen Mixtures

Mixtures of carbon dioxide and oxygen, carbogen, are available in a number of different compositions ranging from 5% carbon dioxide equaling 95% to 30% carbon dioxide equaling 70% oxygen. These mixtures exist in the cylinder as nonliquefied gas of homogenous composition. The cylinder for these gases is usually charged to a pressure of 1,500–2,200 PSIG at 70° F, depending on the type of cylinder. The pressure in the cylinder will increase or decrease according to the temperature and/or the contents withdrawn.

One ounce of the mixture within the range of compositions given above is equivalent to about 5.4 gallons at normal atmospheric pressure and temperature.

Helium-Oxygen Mixtures

Various mixtures of helium and oxygen are available commercially, the most common mixture containing 80% helium and 20% oxygen. These gases exist in the cylinder in the nonliquefied state. They are normally charged in cylinders to a pressure of 1,650–2,000 PSIG at 70° F, depending on the type of cylinder.

One ounce of this mixture is equivalent to about 19 gallons at normal atmospheric pressure and temperature.

Carbon Dioxide

The chemical formula for carbon dioxide is CO_2. This gas is colorless, odorless, slightly acid and appears in the physical state (in a full cylinder) in a liquefied form below 88° F and in a nonliquefied form at 88° F and higher.

The number of gallons in 1 ounce at 1 atmosphere at 70° F is 4.08. The number of liters in 1 ounce at 1 atmosphere and at 70° F is 15.44, with a specific gravity of 1.529.

Pressures in cylinders of carbon dioxide charged to a "filling density" (the per cent ratio of the weight of gas in a container to the weight of water that container will hold at 60° F) of 68% will vary with temperature. In any cylinder of carbon dioxide gas at temperatures below 88° F, the pressure will remain constant, varying only with temperature as long as liquid and vapor are both present. At temperatures of 88° F or higher, the pressure at a given temperature will decrease proportionately as the cylinder contents are withdrawn.

Marking and Labeling Cylinders

All cylinders built to ICC or BTC specifications must be marked permanently with symbols stamped into the shoulder (part sloping up to the neck or into the top head or the neck of the cylinder) (Fig. 25).

EXAMPLE: ICC–3A   2015
462   Spun
XY   Manufacturer's Name
CGA   5–68

These above marks first give the ICC or BTC specification to which the cylinder has been made (in the example above, ICC–3A specification). Immediately following is the service pressure for which the cylinder was built (2,015 PSIG in this instance). Next in order appears the serial number of the individual cylinder ("462"). CGA is the owner's stamp. Other markings required include the date of final inspection, indicating the month and year of the initial qualifying test (5–68). The date stamp is placed so that the dates of subsequent retestings for required requalification can be added later to the shoulder top head or neck of the cylinder. Moreover, the ICC and BTC codes specify that the word "spun" or "plug" be stamped near the specification mark when an end closure has been made by one or the other of these means. The name of the manufacturer must be a part of the permanent stamp. Lastly, if a plus sign is given immediately after the

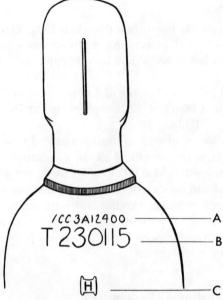

Fig. 25.—Marking and labeling of cylinders. *A*, ICC specifications–ICC 3A1; immediately following that is the service pressure 2,400 PSIG; *B*, serial number of individual cylinder; *C*, owner's stamp.

test date marking of a 3A or 3AA cylinder, it means that the cylinder can be charged up to 10% in excess of the marked service pressure (up to 2,200 PSIG at 70° F).

Federal Food, Drug, and Cosmetic Act

The shipment of medical gases in interstate commerce is also regulated by the Federal Food, Drug, and Cosmetic Act. Under this Act, the medical gases must conform to the standards of the Pharmacopeia of the United States or National Formulary and must be labeled appropriately.

The Pharmacopeia defines the standards and methods of testing the quality, purity and potency of the following gases: carbon dioxide, cyclopropane, ethylene, helium, nitrogen, nitrous oxide and oxygen.

The Act further states that the gases mentioned must be packaged and labeled as stated in the Pharmacopeia and that each cylinder must bear a label containing the name and address of the manufacturer, packer or distributor as well as an accurate statement of the quantity of the contents and a statement of the explosiveness of the item.

Color Coding

A color code to aid in the identification of small as well as large cylinders is used by the Medical Gas Industry, the American Society of Anesthesiologists and the American Hospital Association. The following color codes are in use today:

Kind of Gas	Color
Oxygen	Green and white
Carbon dioxide	Gray
Nitrous oxide	Light blue
Cyclopropane	Orange
Helium	Brown
Ethylene	Red
Carbon dioxide and oxygen	Gray and green
Helium and oxygen	Brown and green

It should be emphasized that color coding should be used only as a guide in identifying gases and that the primary identification for gas cylinder content is the label.

REFERENCES

National Fire Protection Association: NFPA Pamphlet 56, Code for the Use of Flammable Anesthetics, 60 Batterymarch St., Boston, Mass. 02110, 1968.
———: NFPA Pamphlet 565, Non-flammable Medical Gas Systems, 60 Batterymarch St., Boston, Mass. 02110, 1967.
———: NFPA Pamphlet 76, Essential Hospitals Electrical Services, 60 Batterymarch St., Boston, Mass. 02110, 1967.
Compressed Gas Association: Handbook of Compressed Gases (New York: Reinhold Publishing Corporation, 1966), p. 398.

CHAPTER 5

Oxygen Administration

History of Oxygen

IN THE EARLY 1600s, experiments with animals in leakproof chambers started investigational work to find out in detail what happened if living things were deprived of a vital atmospheric element which supported life. What the element was to be called was still a mystery. In 1666, Robert Boyle, an investigative analyist, postulated that there were in the atmosphere "numberless exhalations of the terraqueous globe. The difficulty we find in keeping flame and fire alive . . . without air renders it suspicious that there may be dispersed through the rest of the atmosphere some odd substance either of a solar, astral, or other foreign nature; on account of whereof the air is so necessary to flame!" In his message in the Philosophical Transactions for September 12, 1670, he suggested that whenever there was a lack of whatever the substance was, it possessed a destructive factor, and he reported occurrences of aeroembolisms in experimental animals subjected to low pressure.

In 1774, oxygen was discovered by an Englishman, Joseph Priestley, even though he failed to realize the significance of "dephlogisticated air," erroneously believing that the spark necessary for combustion had been removed. His famous remarks bear repetition: "My readers will not wonder that having ascertained the superior goodness of dephlogisticated air by mice living in it . . . I should have the curiosity by breathing it, drawing it through a glass siphon, and by this means I reduced a large jar full of it to the standard of common air . . . but I fancied that my breath felt peculiarly light and easy for some time afterwards. Who can tell but that in time, this pure air may become a fashionable article in luxury. Hitherto, only two mice and myself have had the privilege of breathing it."

Preceding the discovery of oxygen, another Englishman, Joseph Black, had investigated carbon dioxide, but it wasn't until 1775 and 1794 that the French scientist Lavoisier presented the fundamental principles of breathing. Lavoisier proved that oxygen was absorbed through the lungs and that carbon dioxide and water were eliminated through expiration and that nitrogen remained in the lungs. The first person to use oxygen therapeutically was Thomas Beddoes, in 1880, at his first Pneumatic Institute at Bristol. At that time, he treated patients with heart disease and asthma by using face pieces of oiled silk to contain oxygen.

During World War I, the effective therapeutic use of oxygen was achieved by Haldane in the treatment of pulmonary congestion and edema due to gas poisoning.

Many studies in the early 1900s by Paul Bert, Haldane, Bancroft, Krogh, Bahr, Van Slyke, Henderson, Campbell and Poulton contributed to the knowledge of the mechanism of breathing.

Regulation of Gas Flow

The ultimate process of removing or administering any gas from a cylinder or piped system requires two distinct actions:

1. Reduction of the pressure to atmospheric conditions
2. Precise control of the flow of the gas in liters per minute

The term "regulator" will be used to indicate the instrument which accomplishes the two actions described above. Most of the commercial regulators today are built with two gauges. A gauge by definition is an instrument of measure. The gauge nearest the cylinder measures pressure of the gas in pounds per square inch and thus indicates the volume of gas in the cylinder. The second gauge measures gas flow from the regulator in liters per minute and is designated as the "flow control" or flow gauge.

Pressure as defined here is the force applied to, or distributed over, a surface, measured as force per unit area. We might also say that pressure is a result of molecular energy.

The molecule is the smallest form of matter in which a substance may occur in the natural state. Molecules may be further subdivided into atoms and subatomic particles. There are about thirty billion billion molecules in 1 ml of air.

Robert Brown, a Scottish scientist, described the phenomenon of molecular energy expressed as motion. He observed pollen grains suspended in water vibrating constantly although the water was motionless.

He postulated that the molecules of water, moving due to their own energy, were constantly bombarding the pollen grains causing their erratic motion. The concept is known as the *Brownian movement* and is the basis for the kinetic theory of matter, which states that all molecules are in a state of constant motion.

We may most easily demonstrate pressures exerted by gases using the kinetic theory (Fig. 26). Imagine that we have captured a quantity of gas within a rigid container of a fixed size. Since we know that molecules have mass and are constantly in motion, we can state that the frequency with which these molecules of mass strike the walls, exerting a force, determines the pressure on any given surface area. If there are very few molecules of gas present in our container, the pressure would be low due to fewer collisions with the walls and other molecules.

If we add more molecules and keep the temperature constant, the frequency of the collisions would increase and the pressure would be raised. The pressure scale used for recording high pressure is the pounds per square inch scale.

The term "pounds per square inch" (PSI) simply means a weight (pounds) exerting a force over an area (square inch). The weight of air in the atmosphere around us exerts a nearly constant pressure of 14.7 PSI at sea level. This scale is widely used in many areas. For example, the gas station fills your car tires until a pressure of 25 PSI is reached. In the hospital, oxygen is purchased stored in a cylinder at 2,200 PSI.

The most common method of recording this pressure is with a hollow metal tube called a Bourdon tube. As gas molecules are forced into the Bourdon tube, the increased pressure causes the tube to straighten. This straightening action rotates a needle pointer reflecting the applied pressure.

It is obvious that the high pressure of the gas source must be reduced

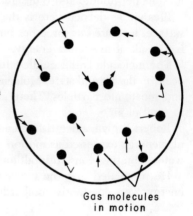

Fig. 26.—Kinetic theory. Gases in a container are in constant motion. The frequency with which the molecules strike the walls of the container, exerting a force, determines the pressure on any given surface.

Gas molecules
in motion

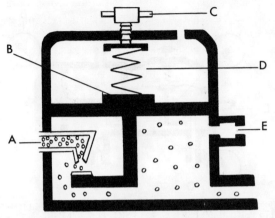

Fig. 27.—Cross-section of a single-stage pressure regulator. A, high-pressure source; B, diaphragm; C, adjusting screw; D, spring compression; E, 100 PSIG.

before it may be administered. Opening the cylinder valve would produce a flow of gas with such a force that it would be harmful and useless for therapeutic purposes. A device is needed to reduce and regulate the pressure to a steady, workable pressure similar to that in a piping system. A high-pressure regulator will give the precise control that is necessary.

Figure 27 is a cross-section of a simplified high-pressure regulator. The area "high-pressure" source (A) is connected to a high-pressure cylinder.

When the cylinder valve is opened, gas molecules enter the regulator body through a nozzle, forcing a padded seat away from it. This seat is attached to a central diaphragm which has a spring of adjustable compression about it. The combined force of the spring and the high-pressure gas pushing the seat away from the nozzle allow gas to flow into the regulator body so long as the outlet is open. When the outlet is closed or resistance is encountered, the number of gas molecules within the regulator body increases. These molecules exert a force on the large diaphragm, which is great enough to overcome the spring tension and the gas flowing against the seat. When this occurs, the pressure has been increased in the lower chamber to a value high enough to force the diaphragm upward and close the regulator's high-pressure source inlet.

The diaphragm is able to move upward readily because the chamber above the diaphragm is open to the atmosphere. The amount of compression placed on the spring by the adjusting screw determines the amount of pressure required to move the diaphragm upward. In Figure 27, the spring is set so that 50 PSI must be present in the lower chamber. Tight-

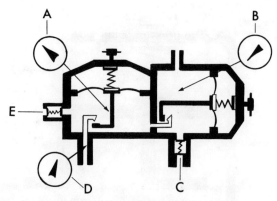

Fig. 28.—Cross-section of a two-stage pressure regulator showing pressure reduction in two stages. A, 175 PSIG; B, 50 PSIG; C, 100 PSIG; D, 2,200 PSIG; E, 225 PSIG. The first stage, A, is preset at 175 PSIG. The second stage, B, 50 PSIG, which is adjustable, works with a constant pressure of 175 PSIG rather than one which is changing in the cylinder.

ening or loosening the adjusting screw will increase or decrease the operating or regulated pressure.

The assembly on the right side of the regulator is an excess pressure escape. This is a simple spring-loaded device which opens when pressure inside the regulator exceeds established limits, allowing excess pressure to slowly escape instead of building up and possibly damaging the regulator.

There are several means of controlling the flow of a gas from the regulator; the most commonly used features the flow-adjusting screw on the bonnet of the regulator. Another is a needle valve built into the regulator. A valve by definition is a movable part which opens or closes a passage. The term usually refers to the object on the top of the cylinder.

There are three types of reducing regulators:

1. The single stage
2. The two stage
3. The three stage

In the one-stage regulator, pressure reduction and control of gases are accomplished by a single variable mechanism. The two-stage regulator (Fig. 28) has two mechanisms for reducing the pressure, one preset and the other variable for control of the gas flow. The two- and three-stage regulators are preferred to the one-stage because they are easier to maintain and their reliability is greater.

There are three types of flowmeters (Fig. 29):

1. The Bourdon
2. The Thorpe tube
3. The pressure compensated

The Bourdon flowmeter consists of a chamber open at one end to atmosphere through a known size orifice, which is usually .018 inches in diameter. The opposite end of the chamber opens into a hollow, curved metal tube. This flowmeter is a pressure gauge, adjustable between 0 and 115 pounds per square inch, which has been recalibrated in liters per minute and which operates against a fixed orifice size. Pressure of the gas entering the chamber is controlled by an adjustable needle valve positioned between the flow scale and the gas source. The more the needle valve is opened, the greater the flow inside the flow scale chamber. As the pressure of the gas source enters the chamber, it moves up the hollow tube, causing the distal end of the tube to move outward. The tip of this tube is attached by a small gear system to an indicator needle on the face of the flowmeter. The more the needle valve is opened, the more the tip of the hollow tube moves outward and, consequently, the higher the indicated flow in liters per minute on the meter flow scale.

The fixed size of the outlet orifice (Fig. 30) allows a known flow of gas to pass through it for each increment of pressure difference between the chamber and the opposite end of the orifice. The increments of pressure are marked on the face of the meter in liters per minute rather than in pounds per square inch gauge.

Fig. 29.—*Thorpe flowmeter:* A, inlet pressure (from piping system); B, calibrated flow scale; C, needle valve (at inlet of flow tube); D, outlet. *Bourdon flow gauge:* A, inlet pressure; B, dial-type flow scale; C, needle valve (at inlet of flow gauge); D, restricted orifice (fixed size). *Pressure compensated flowmeter:* A, inlet pressure; B, needle valve (at outlet of flow tube); C, calibrated flow scale; D, outlet.

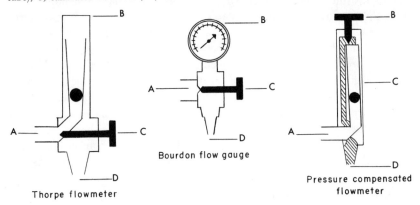

Bourdon flow gauge

Thorpe flowmeter

Pressure compensated
flowmeter

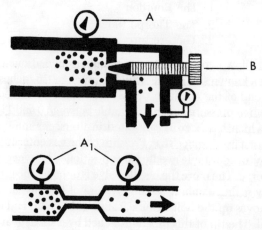

Fig. 30.—Flow of gases through an orifice. *A*, pressure gauge; *B*, needle valve. As the flow of gases decreases, the number of molecules will also decrease and will exert less force; therefore, the pressure below the constriction will be less than the pressure above, as shown in the lower figure (A_1). In the upper figure, the needle valve can be adjusted to any number of constrictions or orifice sizes, but there is always a pressure drop across the needle valve.

All Bourdon flowmeters (Fig. 31) will record the flow of gas accurately, as long as there are no restrictions applied to the outlet orifice. Because there is a direct relationship between the orifice size and the calibration of the flow scale, a unit of this type would indicate maximal flow delivered, even when the outlet orifice is closed off completely, since pressure of the inlet gas source would still be against the flow scale. The patient will receive a flow of gas less than that indicated on the flow scale.

All Thorpe tube types of flowmeters in use today can be classified as either pressure compensated or uncompensated. The uncompensated Thorpe tube flowmeter has the needle valve placed between the gas source and the calibrated flow scale. The tube is calibrated for a free flow of gas to the atmosphere. In the use of uncompensated Thorpe tube flowmeters, the pressure change occurs at the needle valve between the inlet gas source and the flow tube. If a humidifier, nebulizer or any device that offers restriction is attached to the outlet orifice, the flow of gas delivered to the patient will be somewhat less than that indicated on the calibrated flow scale. This reduction in gas flow delivered is brought about due to an increase in pressure of the gas at the outlet, causing compression of gas within the tube which forces the flow indicator ball downward. As this gas passes the restriction offered by the devices added to the outlet orifice, it expands. The indicated flow under these conditions is incorrect.

The pressure-compensated flowmeter is calibrated for operation at 50 pounds per square inch gauge and 70° F. Inlet pressure is applied through the calibrated flow scale to a needle control valve which is always positioned so that the pressure change occurs between the top of the calibrated flow scale and the flowmeter outlet, which is downstream from the flow scale. Back pressure will cause the ball to drop because the amount of gas passing the restricting orifice is less. The amount of back pressure can never be greater than the pressure within the tube. The flowmeter will accurately indicate the flow delivered.

Accurate pressure and flow gauges are absolutely necessary. An inaccurate pressure gauge either permits oxygen to run out before the gauge registers zero or leads to a change of the cylinder before all oxygen is used. Accuracy of pressure gauges may be checked by the following procedures:

1. Compare with control pressure gauge.

2. On a full industrial cylinder, the gauge should read 2,000 or 2,200 pounds, depending on the cylinder at a temperature of 70° F (21° C).

3. Oxygen should remain in the cylinder after the gauge has been turned off and the pointer reaches zero, as determined by trial and error. Attach the regulator to a cylinder of gas and turn on the cylinder valve. Adjust flow to 6 L per minute and turn the cylinder valve off. The flow should continue until after the pointer of the pressure gauge reaches zero.

A flow gauge may be tested by the following procedures:

1. Flow the oxygen through a tested separate flow gauge.

Fig. 31.—Bourdon flowmeter (uncompensated). A, 10 L/min with no restriction; B, 8 L/min when attached to humidifier; C, flowmeter indicates maximal flow when outlet is completely occluded.

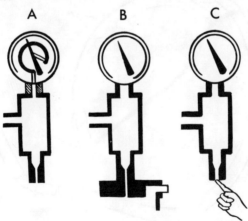

2. Turn the oxygen into a basal metabolism apparatus calibrated by volume with the recording device running and calculate the flow.

3. Allow the oxygen to flow at a given rate for a period of time and note the fall in cylinder pressure. Flow in liter per minute times the number of minutes should equal the drop in pressure in pounds times three. In the large cylinders, 1 pound of pressure is equal to 3 L.

Testing the flow-regulating mechanism:

1. Attach regulator to a full cylinder.

2. Adjust the flow to 4–8 L per minute.

3. Close the cylinder valve. The flow on a two-stage regulator should remain constant, but it may vary slightly. The single-stage regulators often show a wide variation in the rate of flow.

Oxygen Nasal Cannula

To deliver moderate oxygen concentrations. Oxygen concentrations: 35–50% in inspired air. Usual flow rate: 6–8 L per minute.

The oxygen nasal cannula is a safe, simple and comparatively economic method of delivering moderate-to-low concentrations of oxygen (Fig. 32). It may be used at liter flows as low as 1 L per minute in patients with severe chronic lung disease when high concentrations of oxygen may further depress respiration by relieving the hypoxic drive of the respiratory center

Fig. 32.—Disposable nasal oxygen administration set. *A*, nasal cannulae; *B*, humidified oxygen inlet.

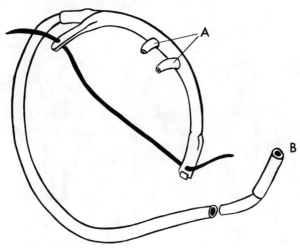

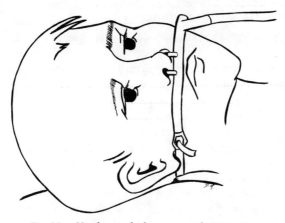

Fig. 33.—Nasal cannula for oxygen administration.

of the brain. There is little danger of carbon dioxide retention with this device, even at very low flows.

It has been demonstrated that the patient who tends to breathe through his mouth does not significantly decrease the concentration of oxygen in the inspired gas, providing he does not have bilateral nasal obstruction.

The oxygen nasal cannula is well tolerated by the patient and usually does not produce nasal irritation. It cannot be used for any type of aerosol therapy because the lumen of the cannula is too small and the aerosol particles tend to conglomerate and "fall out" in the tubing.

EQUIPMENT

Plastic nasal cannula with connecting tubing attached, humidifier and flowmeter as regulator if to be used with oxygen cylinders (Fig. 33).

TECHNIQUE

1. Tell the patient what you are going to do and why. Reassure the patient.
2. Fill the humidifier with sterile distilled water.
3. Attach cannula tubing to outlet on the humidifier. Set the flow rate at 6–8 L per minute.
4. Place tips of the cannula in water to make sure they are not obstructed.
5. Place the cannula with the tips in the patient's nose and adjust flow to the rate prescribed by the physician.
6. The tubing should be fastened conveniently to the pillow or bed clothes.
7. Place "No Smoking" signs in the patient's room.

Oxygen Face Mask (Rebreathing)

To deliver high oxygen concentrations of 60–90% at a usual flow rate of 6–8 L per minute.

The lightweight plastic oxygen face mask effectively delivers high concentrations of oxygen (Fig. 34). The liter flow may be adjusted to meet the patient's individual demands by watching the reservoir bag. The oxygen flow is regulated so that the reservoir bag does not completely collapse when the patient inspires.

High concentrations of oxygen with the face mask are indicated in the acute phase of the following diseases:

1. Mycocardial infarction
2. Pulmonary edema
3. Massive pneumonia
4. Pulmonary embolism
5. Carbon monoxide poisoning
6. Shock

EQUIPMENT

1. Plastic face mask with reservoir bag and tubing.
2. Humidifier and flowmeter or regulator, if to be used with oxygen cylinder
3. Distilled water.

Fig. 34.—Illustration of a patient receiving oxygen via a rebreathing-type mask.

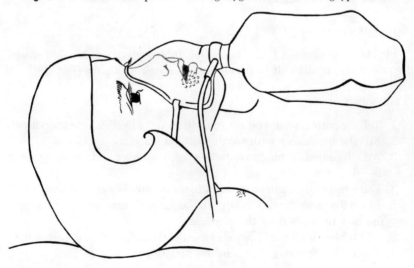

Technique

1. Fill humidifier with sterile distilled water.
2. Attach tubing to outlet on the humidifier.
3. Check out the system by turning the liter flow rate to 6–8 L per minute.
4. Place the face mask on the patient's face and adjust the straps.

Fig. 35.—OEM meter mask. *A*, oronasal face piece with one-way expiratory flutter valve. *B*, oxygen inlet tube. *C*, unidirectional mica valve, which prevents rebreathing. It may be "seated" or removed if rebreathing is desired, as with helium-oxygen therapy. *D*, accessory mica inlet valve, which permits room air to enter when there is inadequate oxygen flow. *E*, rubber collecting 1- or 2-L-size bag. *F*, disk, metered for positive pressure (1–4 cm water) in expiration only. Expiratory one-way flutter valve seated. *G*, oxygen concentration meter (40–95%), which also serves as a humidifier. *H*, special-gauge rubber connecting tubing.

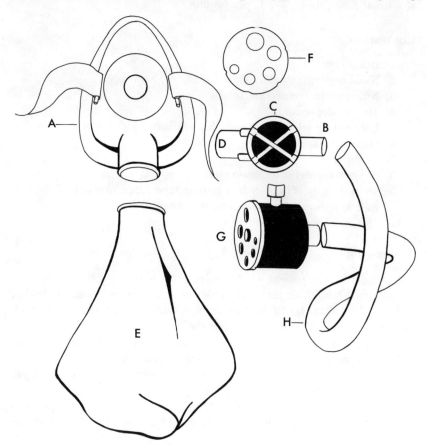

5. Observe the reservoir bag, being certain that it does not collapse during any inspiratory cycle.
6. Secure the tubing to the pillow or bed clothes.
7. Place "No Smoking" sign in patient area.
8. Reassure the patient and make him as comfortable as possible.

A nonrebreathing face mask (i.e., OEM) has been available for many years (Fig. 35). The authors feel, however, this technique has limited usefulness today.

Oxygen Catheter

To deliver moderate oxygen concentrations of 35–50% (in the inspired air) at a usual flow rate of 4–7 L per minute.

EQUIPMENT

1. Humidifier
2. Nasal oxygen catheter (sizes 10, 12, 14, French)
3. Nine feet of connecting tubing
4. Tongue depressor
5. Lubricating jelly (water soluble, nonflammable)
6. Distilled water (500 cc)
7. Flashlight
8. Oxygen regulator or flowmeter
9. Short length of 3/4-inch adhesive tape (approximately 3 inches) split lengthwise from one end to center
10. "No Smoking" sign

TECHNIQUE

1. Explain to the patient what you are going to do. Plug flowmeter with the attached humidifier into wall outlet or attach to the oxygen cylinder.
2. Fill humidifier jar to the 500-cc mark with distilled water and check unit to be certain it is working properly.
3. Attach tubing to humidifier and the catheter to the connecting tubing.
4. With the catheter, measure the distance from the tip of the patient's nose to the lobe of his ear and mark this point with a small piece of tape. Adjust flow rate to 2–3 L per minute.
5. Place a small amount of lubrication on a sterile 4 × 4 gauze pad and pass the catheter lightly through the lubricant. Put the tip of the catheter

into a glass of water and allow the oxygen to bubble through to be certain that the openings are patent.

6. Keeping your fingers at the point you have marked off insert the catheter into the nose and advance the tube gently. If you meet any resistance try the opposite nostril.

7. If the patient is responsive, instruct him to swallow. If he can swallow without gagging, the catheter is not inserted too deeply. If the patient gags on swallowing, pull the catheter out a short distance until he can swallow without gagging (Fig. 36). Be certain that the catheter is not in esophagus.

8. If the patient is unresponsive, depress tongue and observe the location of tip of catheter. The tip should be visible but must not be lower than the tip of the uvula (Fig. 37). Adjust accordingly.

9. To keep the catheter in position place unsplit end of adhesive tape on nose with split ends hanging from tip of nose. Place the catheter between split ends, encircle catheter one time with each end, bringing both ends back to nose (Fig. 38).

10. Adjust flow rate to the desired or ordered rate.

11. Loop an elastic band around the connecting tubing and pin it to the bedding, leaving enough tubing to allow patient to move about in bed.

Fig. 36.—Insert the nasal catheter slowly to the measured depth. Observe the position of the catheter through the patient's mouth, then withdraw it about $\frac{1}{4}$ inch. A, catheter tip.

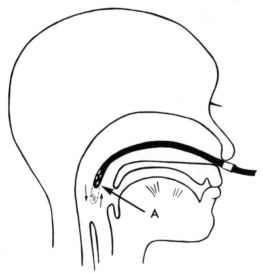

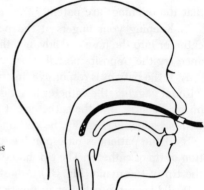

Fig. 37.—Illustration of correct position of nasal oxygen catheter as related to the uvula.

12. Reassure the patient and instruct him about exerting too much effort. Make patient comfortable.

13. Place "No Smoking" sign at entrance to patient's room.

Care of the Patient with a Nasal Catheter

1. Apply a nonflammable bland ointment about the nostrils every 4 hours or as necessary.
2. Give mouth care every 4 hours.
3. Give fluids frequently.
4. Watch the patient's vital signs and check the oxygen flow and position of catheter.

Fig. 38.—Tape the catheter at the end of the nose, using ½-inch adhesive tape split at the end and individually wrapped around the catheter.

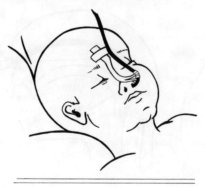

5. Check the water level in the humidifier every 4 hours.
6. Always have a clean catheter at the bedside.
7. Change the catheter every 8–12 hours, or more often if nasal secretions make it advisable. Use alternate nostrils at each change.
8. If the patient is producing large amounts of nasal secretions and has upper airway obstruction, he should be changed to heated aerosol oxygen administration.

Oxygen Analyzers

Shampaine/OEM

Description

1. Analyzing chamber
2. Drying chamber
3. Sample inlet tube
4. Aspirator bulb
5. Battery to supply electrical power
6. Switch button
7. Oxygen concentration scale

As the aspirator bulb is squeezed, it draws a small amount of atmosphere from within administering apparatus through sample inlet tube, drying chamber and into the analyzing chamber.

Principle of operation.—It is based on the fact that changes in oxygen concentration of an atmosphere surrounding a platinum wire will affect its electrical resistance because thermal conductivity of this atmosphere varies directly with the amount of oxygen present. Electrical resistance of two coils of platinum wire surrounded by normal air is compared with that of a set of coils surrounded by the atmosphere to be tested.

Beckman Analyzer

Description

1. Analyzing chamber
2. Drying chamber
3. Sample inlet tube
4. Aspirator tube
5. Batteries to supply electrical power
6. Switch button
7. Oxygen concentration scale

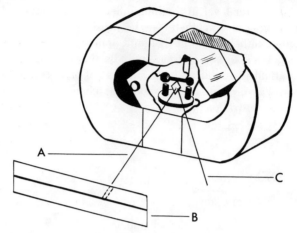

Fig. 39.—*A*, schema of a Pauling-type paramagnetic oxygen analyzer; *B*, beam of light reflected onto a translucent scale; *C*, mirror suspended between poles of a magnet.

Principle of operation.—This is based on the fact that oxygen is strongly attracted to a magnetic field; measurement of magnetic susceptibility of a gas sample indicates amount of oxygen present. Inside the analyzer, a test body is suspended between poles of a magnet. As characteristics of magnetic field change, the test body moves. A mirror mounted on the test body reflects a beam of light on to a translucent scale (Fig. 39). Position of light indicates oxygen concentration.

The drying chamber consists of a glass tube filled with indicator-type silica gel crystals.

Mira Oxygen Analyzer

Description

1. Analyzing chamber
2. Humidity-control chamber
3. Sample inlet tube
4. Aspirator bulb
5. Battery to supply electrical power
6. Switch button
7. Oxygen scale

As aspirator bulb is squeezed, it draws a small quantity of gas from within apparatus through sample inlet tube, humidity-control chamber and into the analyzing chamber.

Principle of operation.—This is based on the fact that changes in oxygen concentration of an atmosphere surrounding a platinum wire will affect its electrical resistance, because thermal conductivity of the atmosphere varies with the amount of oxygen present. Electrical resistance of two coils of platinum wire surrounded by normal air is compared with that of a set of coils surrounded by atmosphere to be tested.

The humidity-control chamber consists of a glass tube filled with indicator-type silica gel crystals in the moist state. Crystals remove water from samples that are too wet and impart moisture to those that are too dry.

REFERENCES

Seedor, M. M.: *Therapy with Oxygen and Other Gases* (New York: Teachers College Press, 1967).

Bendixen, H. H., *et al.: Respiratory Care* (St. Louis: C. V. Mosby Company, 1965).

Safar, P., *et. al.: Respiratory Therapy* (Philadelphia: F. A. Davis Company, 1965).

Wells, R. E., Jr.; Perera, R. D., and Kinney, J. M.: Humidification of oxygen during inhalation therapy, New England J. Med. 268:644, 1963.

Nash, G.; Blennerhasset, J. B., and Pontoppidan, H.: Pulmonary lesions with oxygen therapy and artificial ventilation, New England J. Med. 276:368, 1967.

Campbell, E. J. M.: Oxygen administration, Anesthesia 18:503, 1963.

Smith, L.: Pathologic effects due to increase of oxygen in air breathed, J. Physiol. 24:19, 1899.

Comroe, J. H., Jr., and Betelho, S.: The unreliability of cyanosis in the recognition of arterial anoxemia, Am. J. M. Sc. 214:1, 1947.

Eldridge, F., and Gherman C.: Studies of oxygen administration in respiratory failure, Ann. Int. Med. 68:569, 1968.

Meyer, J., *et al.:* Inhalation of oxygen and carbon dioxide gas, Arch. Int. Med. 119:4, 1967.

Beck, G. J.; Nanda, K., and Bickerman, H. A.: Effect of oxygen on patients with pulmonary emphysema, J.A.M.A. 179:403, 1962.

CHAPTER 6

Humidity Therapy

CELSUS RECOMMENDED the use of heated mist for laryngeal inflammation during the late Hippocratic and Galenic eras. During that time, as well as the present time, inhalation of mist was used unwisely. The first aerosolizer was developed in 1857 by Sales-Gerons, a Frenchman who is referred to as the "Father of Atomization." In 1858, the modern version of the nebulizer was developed by Beigson.

Before we can discuss pulmonary water balance in patients with respiratory diseases, it is necessary to review briefly the terminology used today, which can be quite confusing.

Relative humidity is the amount of water vapor actually present in a volume of air, compared with the amount of water vapor necessary to saturate fully that volume of air at the same temperature. Absolute humidity is expressed as the number of grains by weight of water per pound of dry air and is thus a figure which can remain constant, despite variations in temperature or pressure of the atmosphere.

Nebulization, or the production of mist as opposed to relative humidification, is the production of particles of water, with or without medication, suspended in air. The suspension of particulate matter in a volume of gas is referred to as an "aerosol." One of the most important factors about an aerosol is the droplet size. The number of droplets that can be generated, the per cent that will deposit in various locations and the amount of medication carried are all a function of droplet size.

Atomization and nebulization have been and, in many instances, still are used interchangeably but differ in meanings. Atomization is a method of breaking liquids or solids into small particles for the ultimate purpose of suspension into a stream of gas. An extremely wide assortment of particle sizes are produced, many of which are too large to be of therapeutic value. Nebulization is the production of mist which is brought about by adding baffles. The baffle knocks down the larger droplets, and only those light enough to float around will eventually emerge.

During the poliomyelitis epidemic of 1958, an amazingly high incidence of tracheal crusting and atelectasis became quite apparent. The crusting and obstruction were occurring despite cold mist therapy with wetting agents and occasionally steam inhalation. Measures were sought to correct these conditions.

Among the devices that were used to provide possible solutions to humidity deficits were steam generators and bubbling devices. The steam generators had many advantages, the most important being the decrease in water loss from the tracheobronchial tree; however, they had many obvious disadvantages. These steam generators not only produced water vapor, but a detrimental amount of heat, which caused discomfort to the patient by increasing the room temperature as well as the patient's temperature. Because of the increased metabolic demands on the human body caused by increased temperatures, therapists and physicians gradually used steam generators less as treatment for humidity deficits in patients with respiratory diseases.

Many types of bubble devices were used in conjunction with gases (Fig. 40). The limiting factors with these devices were that they produced vapor only, and their potential water output was limited to the amount of water vapor that could be absorbed by the gas flowing through it. Vapor was produced from bubble devices by means of evaporation. Water molecules passed into the bubbles of air from around their entire surface area. The volume of gas, degree of agitation and the total time of exposure to water determined the resultant humidity. These devices were effective to a great degree, but due to evaporation (cooling effect) as the gas passed through the water, the temperature of the water fell well below ambient or room temperature. Thus, as the patient's ventilatory demands increased, high flow rates of gas were necessary, thereby further decreasing the water temperature and the relative humidity.

To limit aerosol evaporation, the addition of hydroscopic agents such as propylene glycol was recommended, but evidence has shown that such solutions increase the size of the droplet particles and make them too large. Certain antibiotics have also been given to patients in aerosol form. Although some portion of these do reach the alveoli and are absorbed into the blood stream, those alveoli which are involved in the disease process probably are not penetrated. The improvement following administration by aerosolized antibiotics is due to the blood stream carrying of the drug to the infected areas of the lung, and more effective blood stream levels can certainly be obtained by giving the drug parenterally.

There have been many methods developed over the years in hope of loosening retained secretions within the tracheobronchial tree. The use of

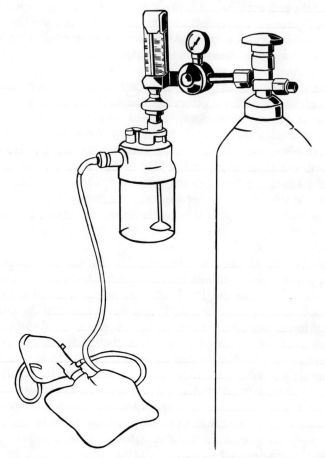

Fig. 40.—Bubble-jet humidifier, regulator-universal flowmeter combination with large "H" cylinder of oxygen, disposable rebreathing mask and small-bore disposable tubing.

wetting agents or detergents, beginning with ethyl-alcohol aerosol, has been tried. Despite an early burst of enthusiasm, controlled studies have shown that the effects of inhaling detergent aerosols are indistinguishable from those of inhaling water droplets alone. Trypsin, pancreatic dornase, sulfur-containing compounds and others have been used, all with questionable success. In the case of isoproterenol, there is at present little doubt that it is effectively administered by means of aerosol, although its effect is far above the alveolar level.

The development of the nebulizer (Fig. 41) has made it possible to control temperature and particle size to a great degree. The liquid is broken up into small particles. The nebulizer consists of a container which holds the liquid, a housing which incorporates a gas jet, a capillary tube which picks up the liquid and a baffle which regulates the particle size. The nebulizer uses a high-pressure gas source which forms a jet stream as it passes through the nozzle. As the jet air stream passes across the top of a tube with a small diameter extending up from a liquid reservoir, the resultant suction action of the jet draws up liquid which is baffled off a ball, producing droplets of various micron sizes. The number of small droplets in the gas stream generally depends on the pressure driving the jet. The over-all performance depends in a complex way on the velocity of the jet and the ratio of gas to liquid flow.

A quantitative knowledge of the relationship between the dose of an inhaled aerosol and the effective dosage rate at the critical site within the lungs is needed. With the treatment of respiratory diseases, it is not only necessary to know the atmospheric concentration and the volumetric rate but also the rate of delivery of the aerosol into the respiratory system. Neither is it sufficient to understand in a qualitative way that the respiratory system has selective properties for the trapping of inhaled particulates of various sizes and densities. In order to establish a quantitative dose-response situation at the site of the problem, the physician, nurse or respiratory therapist must first estimate how much of the inhaled aerosol is initially deposited and at what sites within the ventilation system, how rapidly and to what degree the deposited particles are cleared from the respiratory tract and lungs and, finally, what fraction of the retained material reaches the critical sites within the lungs to initiate a beneficial response. It is beyond the scope of this presentation to go into the logistics of nebulization, but it can and does point out the need for a more quantitative and qualitative procedure in aerosol therapy.

Fig. 41.—Sidearm and mainstream nebulization. A, gases from the generator enter nebulizing chambers; B, gas inlet to nebulizer jets; C, fine aerosol or dense mist is delivered from the sidearm and mainstream nebulizers, respectively.

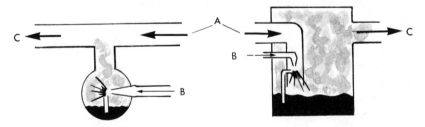

Aerosol Therapy

Indications for humidifying inspired gases range from absolute to marginal. The air must be humidified at all times for patients with a tracheostomy, debilitated patients who breathe through their mouths, patients with chronic respiratory diseases and for patients who have undergone extensive surgery with dry anesthetic gases. Some of the purposes of aerosol therapy are:

1. To thin secretions
2. To obtain both a bronchodilator and a decongestant effect
3. To soothe inflamed mucous membranes
4. To combat systemic dehydration
5. To deliver droplets to areas of the lungs which are effected

The performances of some modern humidifiers and nebulizers are ineffective since they operate at below room temperature, due to evaporative cooling, and produce about 45–50% relative humidity. In treating patients with respiratory diseases, it is important to remember that in most instances breathing is rapid and shallow. Large droplets of mist will not move well beyond the upper airways, and, therefore, humidification or aerosol therapy must be carefully adjusted to give optimum delivery to all segments of the tracheobronchial tree that are affected. In general, a maximal density of small-to-medium droplets, generally by an efficient nebulizer operated at high pressure, is needed to give adequate treatment in short period of time.

It has been shown by Tovell, Segal and others that the size of the particles (Fig. 42) determines their usefulness in inspired atmospheres. Particles smaller than 3 μ in diameter reach the alveolar ducts; and particles smaller than 0.5 μ enter the air sacs, but almost half, because of their extreme lightness, are borne out again in the expired air. A particle size between 0.5 and 3 μ is, therefore, the most usable for providing particulate water throughout the lung.

Breathing with rapid inspiratory flow, breathing through the nostrils or causing inhaled mist to be deposited in the mouth will increase upper airway deposition of larger droplets, hence deposition of larger droplets will be decreased in the remaining portion of the tracheobronchial tree. Shallow breathing, on the other hand, will decrease retention of smaller droplets in the more peripheral portions of the respiratory tract. Usually 100% of large droplets, 40 μ or above, are retained in the respiratory tract, and about one-half of the droplets below 1 μ are exhaled. Ultimate deposition

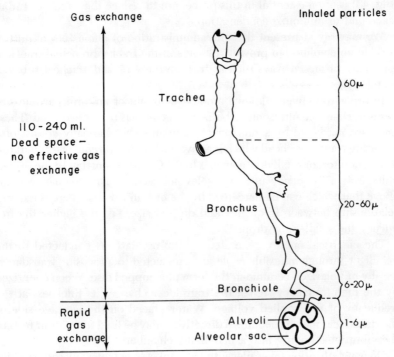

Gas exchange

Inhaled particles

Trachea

110-240 ml.
Dead space –
no effective gas
exchange

60μ

Bronchus

20-60μ

Bronchiole

6-20μ

Rapid
gas
exchange

Alveoli
Alveolar sac

1-6μ

Fig. 42.—Diagram of the tracheobronchial tree, illustrating the deposition of particle sizes.

of fine droplets is dependent on the time they spend in the lungs: Essentially all the small droplets of 1–3 μ will be deposited if the breath is held long enough after a maximal inhalation.

In controlling the droplet diameter of aerosol, the degree of baffling, settling, turbulence and the driving pressure of the nebulizer play important roles. High-pressure gas forms a jet stream as it passes through a nozzle. This jet stream of gas passes across the tip of a tube extending up from a liquid reservoir, the suction of the jet stream produces a negative pressure, and liquid is drawn up through a tube and thrown against a baffle plate, resulting in a fine spray.

This fine spray usually contains an extreme range of particle sizes. The over-all performance depends on the velocity of the jet and the ratio of gas to liquid flow. The highest mist density with minimal waste is achieved by making the delivery to the patient as direct as possible, with most baffling taking place in the nebulizer. The use of smooth, large-bore tubing

(Fig. 43) is often essential in this procedure to reduce the effects of turbulence and to minimize condensation.

We may say at present that the administration of a fine aerosol mist of considerable volume to provide a lavage of the tracheobronchial tree, and especially of any airways such as tracheostomy or endotracheal tubes, is useful.

In order to deliver a known amount of liquid of uniform particle size per unit time, the ultrasonic nebulizer (Fig. 44) has been developed. These units are marketed by a number of companies but basically consist of a vibrating transducer head which is activated by a high-frequency generator. The generator, or oscillator, converts line AC electric current to the proper voltage at a frequency in megacycles per second. This frequency is far above that which can be perceived by the human ear, and there is a direct relationship between frequency and droplet size, i.e., the higher the frequency the smaller the droplet.

The electrical energy generated by the oscillator is conducted to the nebulizer through a flexible cable and connected to a focusing transducer, usually of polarized ceramic in the form of a cupped disc. When energized by the high-frequency signal, the transducer changes its thickness at the frequency of the applied voltage. Water placed on the concave side of the transducer may be nebulized directly or may be used to transmit further the vibrational energy into a nebulizing chamber.

Once nebulization takes place, the aerosol is swept away by some carrier gas, usually a compressed air blower, or oxygen. This may be utilized in environmental control systems, respirators or directly to the patient's mask. At present, it is fair to say that much more investigational work is required

Fig. 43.—Plastic disposable aerosol mask to be used with large-bore corrugated tubing.

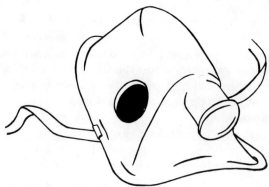

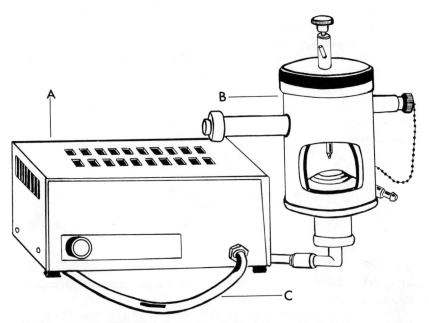

Fig. 44.—MIVAB HNE ultrasonic nebulizer U-700, designed specifically for use with the Engstrom Respirator, model 150 or model 200. It consists of three basic parts: *A*, ultrasonic generator; *B*, the nebulizing chamber; *C*, the line cord. The unit is designed to supply ultrasonic energy at a frequency rate of 3 mc to the transducer with constant power output. The nebulizing chamber is mounted together with the transducer and supplies vibrating energy with a maximal output of 18 watts at the surface of the transducer head.

before the final development and utilization of these techniques are determined.

Correcting Humidity Deficits

In order to correctly understand the humidity deficit, it is important to know the amount of moisture that is needed and the amount of moisture that is being delivered to the airways.

It has been estimated that a healthy afebrile adult looses about 40 ml of water per day from the respiratory tract (Fig. 45). Patients with elevated temperatures and with poor fluid balance will have a "humidity deficit." During hyperpnea, the water lost from the lungs may be as great as 200 ml daily. Oxygen is supplied as a dry gas which must be humidified. In order to correct humidity deficits of the lungs, it is important to super-

WATER BALANCE

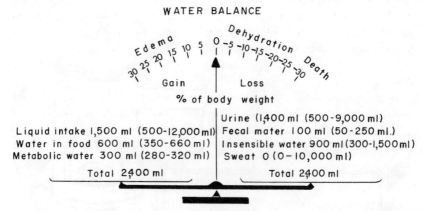

Liquid intake 1,500 ml (500-12,000 ml)	Urine (1,400 ml (500-9,000 ml)
Water in food 600 ml (350-660 ml)	Fecal mater 100 ml (50-250 ml.)
Metabolic water 300 ml (280-320 ml)	Insensible water 900 ml (300-1,500 ml)
	Sweat 0 (0-10,000 ml)
Total 2,400 ml	Total 2,400 ml

Fig. 45.—The general character of water balance, showing standard values for gain and loss. Extremes are shown in parentheses.

saturate the inspired air. A convenient technique to use is the modern heated nebulizer with an adjustable temperature control.

Therapy gas is generally administered for one of two reasons: The patient needs the beneficial effects of the gas itself (oxygen), or compressed air is used simply to carry medication into the tracheobronchial tree. In either case, one primary factor should be remembered—gas from a high pressure cylinder or a liquid oxygen cylinder is completely dry. Administering dry gas to a patient is not only irritating to his tissues, but it may be life threatening in time if not corrected.

Air in the alveoli is always 100% saturated with water vapor at body temperature. Where does this water come from when we are breathing dry gases? Most of it comes from the mucosa of the nasal passages and the remainder from the tracheobronchial tree. In the process of breathing, the mucosa continually gives up moisture. For a normal, healthy person there is no cause for concern because the mucosa is replenished with water taken into the body orally.

For the patient who is febrile, dehydration of the mucosa is an acute situation. If moisture lost in humidifying the inspired air is not replenished as rapidly as needed, many problems within the respiratory system result.

Thick, viscid secretions form which cannot be eliminated by either expectoration or reabsorption into the body tissue. Moisture is required to prevent this drying condition. Whether gases are being given for their benefits alone or for medication they are carrying into the respiratory tract, they should contain moisture at all times.

The maximal amount of water that air can hold in the vapor state depends on the temperature of the air. The chart (see Glossary) shows the maximal amount of water that one cubic meter of air is capable of holding at a given temperature. We can see from the figures on the chart that the warmer the air or gas the greater the amount of water it is capable of holding.

By using the formula for obtaining relative humidity which is expressed as a percentage of the amount of water in the air compared with what the air is capable of holding, we can compute the percentage relative humidity of a given volume of air at a given temperature.

$$(\% \text{ Relative Humidity } = \frac{\text{actual } H_2O}{\text{potential } H_2O} \times 100)$$

Assume for the moment that we have just turned on the radio and the weather forecaster closes with the following report: "The forecast for tomorrow is fair and warmer; the present temperature is 41° and the relative humidity is 50%." What he has actually stated is that the air at 41° is holding about 50% or one-half of its potential. Referring to the chart (see Glossary), the potential for 41° air is 6.80 Gm. Therefore, the actual water vapor content present is 3.40 Gm.

Assume that we take this same air into your house and warm it to a comfortable 68° F. What will be the relative humidity?

$$\%RH = \frac{3.4}{17.30} \times 100 = 19.6\%$$

Therefore, by using the formula, we find that warming the 41° F air to 68° F drops the relative humidity from 50 to 19.6%. Pursuing this further, we find that if the same volume of air was warmed to 98.6° F, it would have a 7.7% relative humidity.

You can clearly see that for any gas to be 100% humidified at 98.6° F it must contain 43.90 Gm per cubic meter, or per 1,000 L since they are the same. Yet, 7% relative humidity air at 98.6° F contains only 3.4 Gm per cubic meter. To be fully saturated, 40.4 Gm would have to be supplied by the patient's airways per every 1,000 L of air breathed.

A minute volume of 6,000 ml × 60 minutes = 360 L per hour. In about 3 hours (3 × 360 = 1080), the patient would breathe 1,000 L. Since grams and milliliters of water are practically equal, we can say that this patient would have to supply from his airway about 40 ml of water every 3 hours. From the above, it is obvious that some method must be provided to offset the humidity deficit when gas is being administered. The following techniques have proved to be effective in eliminating these humidity deficits.

HEATED AEROSOL

The purpose of heated aerosol is to supply to the patient's airway an atmosphere of gas or gases which are completely saturated with water vapor at body temperature, to aid in thinning sputum and to increase the moisture content of the total airway.

The length of the treatment is usually 30 minutes every 4 hours, when by oral-pharyngeal route, but it is used continuously when large amounts of thick sputum are present. When used with a patient with a tracheostomy, the treatment is continuous, usually at a 40% concentration of oxygen, except during conditions when the patient is acutely hypoxic, when 100% oxygen concentration is indicated. In patients with severe chronic lung disease, respiratory depression should be watched for while using 100% oxygen concentration.

TECHNIQUE

1. Inform the patient what you are about to do and why.
2. Place "No Smoking" signs in patient areas.
3. Fill the nebulizer bottle with 500 ml of distilled water.
4. Clamp the nebulizer to the bed or table by means of a universal clamp and bracket. Because water will condense in the corrugated tubing, this method is used to reduce the amount of water collecting in them. The nebulizer is best placed below the level of the patient, and there should be no loops in the tubing (Fig. 46).

5. The back pressure compensated flowmeter is connected to a high pressure line and the nebulizer.
6. The flowmeter is plugged into the oxygen outlet.
7. The oxygen dilutor is set at 40%, unless 70% or 100% is indicated.
8. The immersion heater is then plugged in and checked for temperature control.
9. The corrugated tubing is placed on the outer part of the nebulizer with the aerosol mask attached to the distal end.
10. The oxygen is set to flow at 6 L per minute.
11. A vapor will be seen coming from the delivery tube and adjusted to comfortably fit the patient.
12. The patient is instructed to lift the mask, expectorate and then replace the mask.
13. A sputum box is left near the bedside.

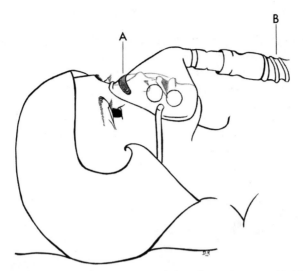

Fig. 46.—Translucent polyethylene mask with large-bore inlet. *A*, malleable clamp; *B*, large-bore corrugated tube.

14. Slow, deep breathing is the most effective breathing pattern that can be used when the patient is receiving this form of therapy.

PRECAUTIONS

1. There must be no smoking in the area where this unit is being used. "No Smoking" signs are posted.

2. The nebulizer should not be used without water in the nebulizer reservoir jar or the gas delivered will be extemely dry, contributing to patient dehydration and drying of respiratory tissues (Fig. 47).

3. The immersion heater (Figs. 48 and 49) is equipped with a three-prong grounding plug for use with 110–120 volts, 25, 50 and 60 cycle alternating current only. If three-hole grounding outlets are not available, the grounding adaptor should be connected to a suitable ground, such as a cold water pipe. Always unplug the heater from electrical outlet when not in use. Do not place the heater on scorchable surface until cool. Do not touch the barrel of the heater with bare hands until the electrical cord has been disconnected for 5 minutes.

4. The immersion heater has been factory sealed to preclude moisture. It should not be disassembled under any circumstances.

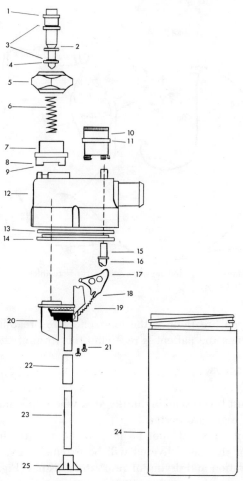

Fig. 47.—Puritan aerosol nebulizer assembly. *1,* tailpiece assembly; *2,* "O" ring; *3,* washers; *4,* retaining ring; *5,* wing nut; *6,* spring; *7,* dilution knob; *8,* dilution insert; *9,* "O" ring; *10,* plug; *11,* "O" ring; *12,* cap; *13,* gasket; *14,* gasket-retaining ring; *15,* push button; *16,* quad-ring; *17,* pivot arm; *18,* cleaning wire; *19,* spring; *20,* jet-body assembly; *21,* two screws; *22,* siphon tube (tygon); *23,* siphon tube (metal); *24,* glass jar; *25,* filter assembly.

DILUTION CONTROL

The dilution control can be set to mix oxygen and air for concentrations of 40 or 70% oxygen, or the control can be set to deliver 100% oxygen. When the unit is set up to 40% setting, the nebulizer is mixing three parts

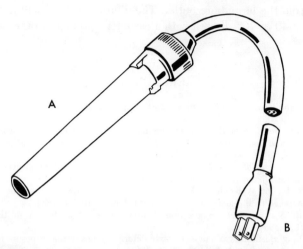

Fig. 48.—A, immersion heater equipped with, B, three-pronged grounding plug for use with 110–120 volts, 25, 50 and 60 cycle alternating current only.

room air to one part oxygen flow of 8 L per minute. We are mixing 24 L of room air. This gives us a total flow emitting from the nebulizer of 32 L per minute. The 32 L is, of course, able to carry more water vapor and water particles than the original 8 L. To set the percentage of oxygen, lift control knob from recess and set concentrations desired opposite 100% oxygen arrow. (Make certain that control knob resets in recess.) The 40 or 70% oxygen concentrations should be used only with an unrestricted 3/4 inch large-bore breathing tube no longer than 5 feet when nebulizing

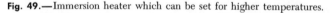

Fig. 49.—Immersion heater which can be set for higher temperatures.

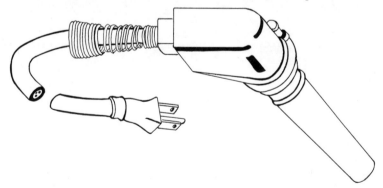

directly from the large-bore outlet. The dilution control will not function when set at 40 or 70% if used with a catheter, cannula or other restricting attachment.

REFERENCES

Hatch, T. F., and Gross, P.: *Pulmonary Deposition of Inhaled Aerosols* (New York: Academic Press, Inc., 1964).

Safar, P., *et al.: Respiratory Therapy* (Philadelphia: F. A. Davis Company, 1965).

Green, H. L., and Lane, W. R.: *Particulate Clouds, Dusts, Smokes, and Mists* (2d ed.) (Princeton, N. J.: D. Van Nostrand Co., Inc., 1964).

Comroe, J. H., Jr., *et al.: The Lung* (Chicago: Year Book Medical Publishers, Inc. 1962).

Dautrebande, L.: *Microaerosols* (New York: Academic Press, Inc., 1962).

Dautrebande, L., and Walkenhorst, W.: Deposition of microaerosols in the human lung with special reference to the alveolar spaces, Health Physics 10:981, 1964.

Levine, E. R.: A more direct liquefaction of bronchial secretions by aerosol therapy, Dis. Chest 31:155, 1957.

Modell, J. H., *et al.*: Blood gas and electrolyte determinations during exposure to ultrasonic nebulized aerosols, Brit. J. Anaesth. 40:20, 1968.

CHAPTER 7

Sterilization

Control of Microorganisms
during and after Inhalation Therapy

IT IS NECESSARY TO POINT OUT means of preventing transmission and contamination and of providing inhibition and destruction of microorganisms often encountered in the treatment of patients with respiratory disease.

The inhibition or destruction of microorganisms can be brought about by physical agents and by chemical substances. There are various methods used now in controlling the growth of microorganisms associated with inhalation therapy equipment while it is providing respiratory care to patients. There is, indeed, a host of agents available to control microbial growth, but the nature of their action against microbes varies, and each has limited practical application. (Some of them merely inhibit growth and metabolic activity, whereas others actually destroy the cells.)

The over-all results produced by various agents, chemical or physical, can best be known and described in terms of the processes and substances used in controlling microbial population. The terms defined below will help in understanding the processes and substances used against microorganisms.

1. *Sterilization:* The process of destroying all forms of life. Sterility in the microbiologic sense is making objects free from living microorganisms. This means complete absence of all microorganisms and is not used in a relative sense.

2. *Disinfectant:* Any agent, usually a chemical, that kills the growing forms of disease causing microorganisms, usually referring to destruction of infectious agents.

3. *Antiseptic:* A substance that opposes sepsis or prevents or arrests the growth or action of microorganisms either by inhibiting or destroying them.

4. *Germicide or microbicide:* An agent that destroys the growing forms but does not necessarily destroy the resistant spore forms of germs; in

practice a germicide can be said to be a disinfectant, but germicides are used for all kinds of germs and in any place.

5. *Bactericide:* Any agent that destroys bacteria. Similarly, the terms fungicide, virucide and sporicide refer to agents that kill fungi, viruses and spores.

6. *Bacteriostasis:* Any condition in which the multiplication of bacteria is prevented.

7. *Microbistatic:* Any agent that has the ability to inhibit the growth of microorganisms.

8. *Antimicrobial agent:* Any agent that inhibits the growth and activity of microbes.

THE PATTERN OF DEATH OF BACTERIA

In the process of destruction of bacteria by chemical or physical means, death usually does not occur instantaneously to the entire population. The death rate for a particular organism under uniform conditions will follow a definite, predictable pattern. Irrespective of the initial population under uniform conditions, the number of organisms will be reduced by the same percentage during each equal period of time. That is, the percentage of cells dying per unit of time is constant, regardless of the number of cells present (Fig. 50). The fact is known as the "logarithmic death rate."

Sometimes the application of a chemical agent produces a condition of bacteriostasis that can be mistaken for bactericidal action.

Some chemical substances are bactericidal at high concentrations and bacteriostatic at low concentrations.

CONDITIONS INFLUENCING MICROBACTERICIDAL ACTION

1. *Concentration and kind of chemical agent used.*—Within certain limits and depending on the chemical substance used, the more concentrated the substance, the more rapid is its action on microorganisms.

2. *Intensity and nature of physical agent.*—Microorganisms death rates vary with the intensity and nature of the physical agent to which they are exposed. Usually, the more intense the physical agent (the more heat or radiation), the faster it will kill microorganisms.

3. *Time.*—Usually, the longer the contact time between the organisms and the agent, the greater is the number of organisms destroyed.

4. *Temperature.*—An increase in the temperature, when used with another agent such as a chemical substance, increases the death rate of microorganisms.

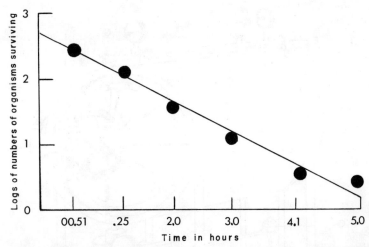

Fig. 50.—Logarithmic death curve of bacteria: Based on the exposure time to physical or chemical agents, and according to the number of organisms present, death will occur at a constant rate.

5. *Kind of organisms present.*—Microorganisms differ in their susceptibility to chemical and physical agents. Generally, the growing vegetative forms are most susceptible, whereas the spore forms are extremely resistant.

6. *Number of organisms.*—Usually the larger the microbial population, the longer the time required to kill all the microorganisms under uniform conditions.

7. *Nature of material bearing the organisms.*—The chemical and physical properties of the medium carrying the organisms have an influence on the rate of microbial destruction.

Mode of action, inhibition or death

1. Damage to cell wall
2. Alteration of cell permeability
3. Alteration of colloidal nature or protoplasm
4. Inhibition of enzyme activity
5. Interference with synthetic process

Control by physical methods

Temperature

1. Vegetative cells can be killed at temperatures from 50° to 70° C (moist heat) for a 5–10-minute exposure time.

2. A temperature of 70°–80° for 5–10 minutes is required to kill spores.

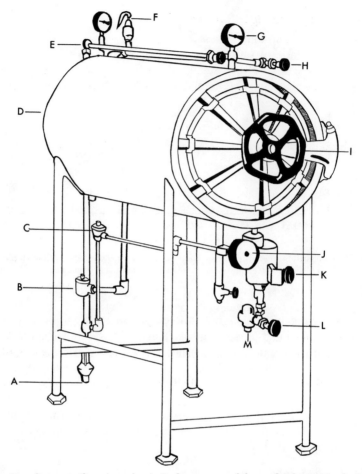

Fig. 51.—Steam sterilizer (autoclave). As the pressure of the confined steam in the jacket rises, the temperature rises. At a pressure of 15 pounds per square inch gauge, the temperature is 121° C, which will produce sterilization of materials in 30 minutes. A, vapor drain; B, jacket return trap; C, chamber trap; D, jacket; E, exhaust to atmosphere; F, safety valve; G, pressure-control indicator for jacket; H, operating valve; I, door release; J, indicating thermometer; K, high-low pressure regulator; L, steam supply valve; M, steam strainer.

3. Vegetative cells of many fungi are destroyed by moist heat, 60° C for 5–10 minutes.

4. Most bacterial spores are killed only by exceptionally high temperatures: 100° C and above for extended periods.

Methods of applying high temperatures

Moist heat: Steam under pressure

Heat in the form of saturated steam under pressure is most practical and dependable for sterilization but cannot be used for sterilization of all equipment used in inhalation therapy due to the material from which this equipment is made (Figs. 51 and 52).

Killing and inhibiting by chemical means

The ideal disinfectant does not exist for any and all purposes. In choosing any chemical agent for disinfection, the following evaluation should be made:

1. Toxicity to microorganisms: The capacity of the substance to kill microorganisms is the first requirement to be considered. The substance should have a broad spectrum of activity at a high dilution, low concentration.

2. Solubility: It should be soluble in water or in tissue fluids for effective action.

3. Stability: The substance should not lose its germicidal action due to changes resulting from standing for periods of time.

4. The disinfectant should be nontoxic to man and other animals.

5. Homogeneous: The preparation should be uniform in composition.

6. Capacity to avoid combination with extraneous organic material.

Fig. 52.—Steam sterilization utilizing the "gravity displacement" system. Steam enters under pressure at the rear of the sterilizer, forcing the heavier air down and forward until it is discharged from the chamber port at the front of the sterilizer.

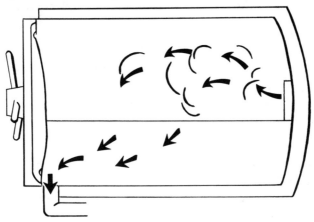

7. Toxicity to microorganisms at room or body temperatures.
8. Should have the capacity to penetrate.
9. Noncorroding and nonstaining features are desirable.
10. Deodorizing ability while destroying organisms.
11. Detergent capacities.
12. Availability.

Major Groups of Chemical Antimicrobial Agents

1. *Phenols.*—A carbolic acid or phenol is used as a standard against which other disinfectants are compared in order to arrive at an evaluation of their bacterial activity.

2. *Alcohol.*—Alcohol is used extensively as a skin disinfectant. It is effective for general usage in concentrations between 50 and 70%. Although alcohol cannot be relied on to produce a sterile condition, it is useful in reducing the microbial flora of the skin and small inanimate objects that may be used in contact with the mucous membranes or openings of the body such as the mouth.

Alcohols are protein coagulants as well as dehydrating agents, which account for their germicidal activity. They can be used for soaking the mouthpiece and small volume micronebulizers used in inhalation therapy.

3. *Iodine solutions.*—Iodine is one of the oldest effective germicides. Iodine tincture U.S.P. (2% iodine) shows high bactericidal efficiency and possesses sporicidal and fungicidal activity. Relatively new are compounds called iodophors. These are organic compounds of iodine in which the iodine is loosely combined with some surface active agent. These iodine solutions can be used for disinfection of most of the equipment used in inhalation therapy, where staining is not objectionable. The cost is relatively high if large quantities are used. The iodine solutions will lose their effectiveness if left standing for a period of time, usually clearing of the brown color of the solution indicates its loss of effectiveness as a detergent.

4. *Chlorine compounds.*—Either in the form of a gas or in certain chemical combinations, these are effective and widely used as disinfectants. Tubercle bacilli are not destroyed by concentrations safe for skin. Chlorine compounds are highly irritating to mucosal tissue, will corrode metal and will break down the properties of rubber goods.

5. *Soaps and synthetic detergents.*—Soaps are sodium or potassium salts of the higher fatty acids, and, as a general group, they are mildly germicidal and exhibit selective action against microorganisms. For example, the pneumococci and some streptococci are relatively susceptible to the action

of soaps, whereas staphylococci, gram-negative rods and acid-fast bacteria display considerable resistance. Soaps, especially those with hexachlorophene, are quite effective as a hand scrub.

6. *Quaternary ammonium compounds.*—These are used exclusively for disinfection in most hospitals. These compounds will usually lower surface tension of solutions. The bactericidal power of the quaternaries is exceptionally high against gram-positive bacteria, and they are also quite active against gram-negative organisms.

7. *Formaldehyde.*—Formaldehyde is a gas that is stable only in high concentrations at elevated temperatures and is soluble in water. The U.S. Pharmacopeia solution contains 37% (by weight) of gas in water. A 5% solution is usually germicidal and sporicidal in the presence of moderate amounts of organic matter. Formaldehyde is a powerful deodorant and has an objectionable odor. Also, it is irritating to skin and mucous membranes. All equipment disinfected with formaldehyde should be rinsed thoroughly in sterile running water before using.

8. *Ethylene gas sterilization.*—This method has made it possible for the first time to sterilize most of the equipment used in inhalation therapy. Although its use is complex and often expensive, it is considered to be the most effective method available in the sterilization of equipment, large and small.

The advantages of ethylene oxide in sterilization are its effectiveness against all types of organisms when used properly. The concentration must be in the nature of 800–1,000 mg/L. The gas has the ability to penetrate through small orifices and through wrappings of cloth and certain plastics.

Some of the disadvantages are that sterilization of equipment is quite expensive because of the high price of ethylene oxide and because of the large size of equipment (Fig. 53).

Techniques for cleaning and disinfecting

1. Collect the contaminated equipment from patient areas; place in plastic bags when possible; and take to dirty area of inhalation therapy department for cleaning.

2. The operator should wear gloves during the cleaning process.

3. The equipment should be disassembled and rinsed well immediately after bringing to dirty area.

4. The disassembled equipment is placed in a large sink or container with detergent cleaning solution and soaked for a period of time. After soaking, the equipment is scrubbed with brushes under running water and allowed to soak for 15–30 minutes more in a detergent solution.

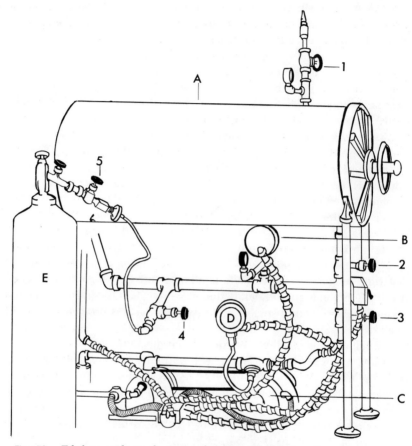

Fig. 53.—Ethylene oxide sterilizer. *A*, ethylene oxide chamber; *B*, mercury pressure switch; *C*, mercury immersion vacuum pump; *D*, mercury pressure switch; *E*, ethylene oxide gas cylinder; *1*, chamber air inlet valve; *2* and *3*, chamber shutoff balancing valve; *4*, chamber opening balancing valve; *5*, single-stage liquid-gas reducing valve.

5. After soaking, the equipment should be rinsed under running water, the operator being certain that no residue of detergent is left on the equipment.

6. After rinsing, the equipment is then hung or placed to dry in a designated portion of the cleaning area.

7. After the equipment is air dried, it is packaged in the proper plastic bags for gas sterilization or steam autoclaving. The date of sterilization is placed on the plastic or cloth container.

8. After having been sterilized, the equipment is then stored in the proper place in the clean area for use after a 24-hour aeration period.

9. All equipment must remain sealed while not in use.

Microbiology of Air

The microbial flora of the air, especially in health care institutions, is normally not free from pathogenic organisms. Although air is not considered a medium for growth of microorganisms, air is a carrier of particulate matter, dust and droplets of varying particle sizes which may be laden with microbes. The relative numbers and types of microorganisms found in the air in the wards, intensive care units, recovery room and respiratory care units are determined by the source of contamination. For example, organisms are sprayed by coughing of hospital personnel and the patients. Airborne microorganisms may be carried on particles of dust, in large suspended droplets and in droplet nuclei which result from evaporation of smaller droplets.

The ultimate fate of airborne microorganisms is governed by a complex set of circumstances, including the atmospheric conditions (e.g., humidity, sunlight and temperature), the size of the particles bearing the microorganisms and the nature of the organisms, i.e., the degree of susceptibility or resistance of an organism to the new physical environment.

We have discussed the importance of proper cleaning and sterilizing techniques in hospitals. With the ever-increasing use of ventilators, nebulizers and humidifiers during respiratory insufficiency in patients, airborne microorganisms constitute a hazard in terms of contamination of this equipment in the hospital complex. The purpose of this section is not to provide any mechanical solution to the problem but to point out some techniques and procedures of decreasing the microbacterial count in the presence of the patient requiring respiratory therapy.

During prolonged oxygen administration, it is important to provide adequate humidification to avoid drying of mucous membranes and their secretions. This is especially important during controlled or assisted ventilation of patients with tracheostomies or when the normal body-humidifying mechanisms have been bypassed. During controlled ventilation, there are three general types of humidifiers that are used in conjunction with ventilators: (1) jet-type or nebulizer humidifier that delivers air which is saturated at operating temperature in addition to a mist of fine particles of liquid; (2) cascade-type humidifiers; and (3) ultrasonic nebulizers, which are special nonjet-type aerosol generators that are capable of putting out three to five times the output of conventional nebulizer systems. These

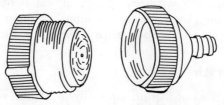

Fig. 54.—Swinnex porous millipore filter composed of pure and biologically inert cellulose esters for absolute surface retention of all particles and organisms larger than the filter pore size (usua

humidifying devices are capable of producing varying particle sizes of aerosols into the pulmonary system (0.5–25 μ).

Many ventilators that are commonly used today entrain varying volume of air through filters or some filtering device (Fig. 54).

All nebulizers and ventilator systems are subject to contamination by airborne or resident organisms of the environment, such as bacteria, algae, yeasts, spores and molds. The organisms that have been found most often in reservoir and ventilator systems are of the pseudomonas variety.

The degree of microbial contamination of indoor air is usually influenced by ventilation rates, overcrowding and the nature and degree of activity of the individuals occupying or entering the quarters. The airborne microorganisms in the hospital complex are carried on dust particles or in droplets expelled from the nose and mouth during coughing, sneezing, and talking. Bed clothes of patients may be heavily contaminated with microorganisms; hence, bedmaking adds many microorganisms to the circulating air. Tubercle bacilli have been isolated from the dust of hospitals; diphtheria bacilli and hemolytic streptococci have been found in floor dust near patients or carriers harboring these organisms.

Since many infectious organisms may be airborne, air hygiene and measures to reduce the microbial population of air during respiratory care is of great importance. One solution would be to use sterile gases; but why use sterile gases when the atmospheric air is contaminated as well as the equipment that is used to administer these gases?

METHODS OF CONTROLLING MICROORGANISMS IN AIR EQUIPMENT

1. *Ultraviolet radiation.*—Ultraviolet lighting systems have great potential in the ward, intensive care units, operating rooms and respiratory care units. Many types of germicidal lamps are available which emit a high percentage of radiations in the 2,500–2,600 region. Because of their limited

penetrating power, these rays are effective only when they make direct contact with the organisms. Skillful installation of the lamp is a must in order to permit the circulating air to make direct contact with the radiation of greatest germicidal or bactericidal intensity.

2. *Chemical agents.*—Certain chemical agents can be used in nebulizers and ventilators or sprayed in the rooms of patients. Dilute acetic acid solution (1 : 16) can be aerosolized through humidifiers or ventilators for 5–10 minutes once daily. In effect, the chemical is dispersed as an aerosol and manifests its antimicrobial action through contact with the suspended particles carrying organisms.

3. *Filtration.*—Air filters are generally made from cotton, glass or other fibrous material. Many ventilators of today use filters that are relatively effective, depending on (1) the rate of air blown through the filter; (2) the size of the particles to be filtered; and (3) the nature of the filter material. One of the difficulties in using air filters is the rapidity with which they become clogged if the air contains an appreciable amount of dust. The filters and entraining devices should be cultured and cleaned on a daily basis while in use.

MISCELLANEOUS METHODS AND PRACTICES

1. Change all humidifiers and nebulizers and replace with sterile one at least once a day.
2. Routine cultures of equipment while in use.
3. Change patient supply systems daily (i.e., tubing and exhalation valve).
4. Air samples of room air twice a week.
5. Change ventilator weekly and replace with clean one.
6. Disinfect the outside of the ventilator daily with a chemical agent.
7. Culture the pipeline gas or gases periodically for contaminants.
8. Floor and air cultures should be done once or twice a week, in respiratory care units, recovery rooms as well as open wards.
9. Culture of hands, ears, nose, throat, hair and clothing of all persons giving constant care to patient.
10. Use of sterile techniques at all times and following proper precaution procedures.
11. Isolation techniques should be used and emphasized to protect the health care worker as well as the patient, relatives and friends.

REFERENCES

Sykes, G.: *Disinfection and Sterilization* (Princeton, N. J.: D. Van Nostrand Co., Inc., 1958).
Finch, W. E.: *Disinfectants: Their Values and Uses* (London: Chapman & Hall, Ltd., 1958).

Cowan, S. T., and Rowatt, E.: *The Strategy of Chemotherapy* (London: Cambridge University Press, 1958).

Tyler, V. R.: Gas sterilization, Am. J. Nursing 60:1596, 1960.

Opfell, J. B., *et al.:* Penetration by gases to sterilize interior surfaces of confined spaces, Appl. Microbiol. 12:27, 1964.

Gilbert, G. L., *et al.:* Effect of moisture on ethylene oxide sterilization, Appl. Microbiol. 12:496, 1964.

Ernst, R. R., and Shull, J. J.: Ethylene oxide gaseous sterilization I. Concentration and temperature effects, Appl. Microbiol. 10:337, 1962.

Lloyd, R. S.: Ethylene oxide sterilization of medical and surgical supplies, J. Hosp. Research 1:14, 1964.

CHAPTER 8

Airway Management

THE AIRWAY IN MAN plays an important part in maintaining itself by built-in safeguards which help to keep air flowing through it without impedance. Among these safeguards are the muscles of the upper airway, effective cough reflex, sighing, effective mucous membrane function and cilia. During disease states and unconsciousness, the upper airway may be ineffective in the exchange of gases and secretions may accumulate, thereby blocking the passage of vital gases. It is important that the respiratory therapist be familiar both with the normal function of the airway and with preventative measures to keep the airways open and functioning properly in times of stress. In recent years, much scientific research has gone into solving problems of airway obstruction; the outstanding work of Safar has made clear many of the factors involved. The following represents a summary of this work.

During complete airway obstruction in healthy persons, it has been proved that usually cyanosis will appear in 1 minute and asystole within 5–10 minutes. The rate of deoxygenation usually will vary with each person since it is dependent on individual lung volume, alveolar ventilation, metabolic rate and pulmonary and circulatory status. Irreversible brain damage may occur even before the action of the heart has stopped. Complete airway obstruction in the conscious person is usually recognized by the inability to see or hear air being moved by the lungs (chest excursions).

Partial obstruction usually results in hypoxia and hypercapnia and if not detected may lead to death. Partial obstruction is recognized by audible airflow, stridor and wheezing and, in some cases, retraction of the rib cage and respiratory muscles.

Because of the rapidity of the action required to correct airway obstruction before serious or irreversible damage occurs, the following steps, recommended by Nicholas and Rumer and by Safar, should be learned and practiced by the respiratory therapist:

117

1. A backward tilt of the head
2. Positive pressure inflation to upper airway, using mouth-to-mouth or bag-and-mask technique, with or without oxygen
3. Clearing of the pharynx
4. Forward displacement of the mandible
5. Insertion of a pharyngeal tube of proper size
6. Orotracheal intubation or cricothyreotomy under favorable conditions when the necessary equipment and facilities are available

BACKWARD TILT OF THE HEAD

In most unconscious patients, hypopharyngeal obstruction exists due to the relaxed base of the tongue which is pushed against the posterior pharyngeal wall of the upper airway. Positional obstruction most frequently occurs when the neck is flexed and almost always when the head is in the midposition. Such obstruction was recognized over 80 years ago by Esmarch and Heiberg, who recommended forward displacement of the mandible. The backward tilt of the head, however, is easier to perform and is used today in the unanesthetized patient.

Backward tilt of the head stretches the tissues between the larynx and

Fig. 55.—Reinflating ambu manual resuscitator. *A*, ambu valve; *B*, rubber bag with foam rubber inner lining; *C*, gas inlet.

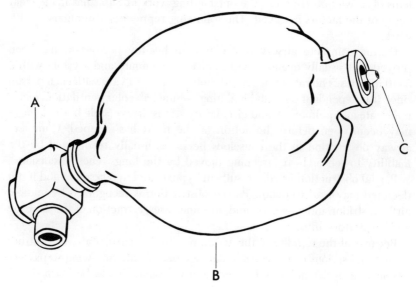

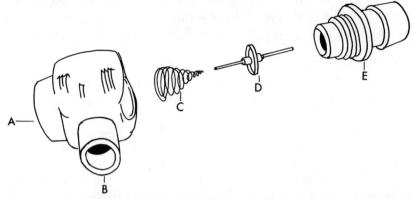

Fig. 56.—Nonrebreathing valve. *A*, exhalation port; *B*, endotracheal tube or mask adaptor; *C*, exhalation spring; *D*, valve disc; *E*, connection to self-inflating bag.

mandible, which lifts the base of the tongue off the posterior pharyngeal wall. The following steps are used in the backward tilt of the head:

1. Place the patient on his side or in the supine position. One of the therapist's or physician's hands is placed under the patient's neck.

2. Place the other hand on the patient's forehead.

3. Tilt the head back as far as possible; elevation of the shoulders may facilitate this maneuver.

4. The above steps are best done on a flat surface. Pillows under the head will flex the neck and should not be used.

POSITIVE PRESSURE

After the backward head tilt has been applied, positive pressure with bag (Figs. 55 and 56) and mask is used when ventilation remains inadequate. In applying positive pressure to the airway, the operator will get an idea as to how stiff the lungs are by the amount of pressure that is required for adequate expansion of the lungs.

CLEARING THE PHARYNX

If secretions or foreign matter are visible or audible in the upper airway, they should be removed by manual wiping or by suctioning. Usually, this is best achieved by turning the patient's head to the side and forcing the mouth open, using precaution not to break or damage the teeth. Large solid material is removed by manual wiping. Secretions or other liquids are removed by suctioning of the pharynx.

USE OF PHARYNGEAL TUBES

Pharyngeal tubes help to hold the base of the tongue forward and also help to prevent obstruction by the teeth and lips. With oropharyngeal tubes in place, the backward tilt of the head is used to insure a patent airway.

The Guedel type of oropharyngeal tube is most often used today. It is S-shaped and is manufactured in varying sizes. During insertion the following steps are recommended:

1. With the patient in the supine position, the mouth is forced open with the thumb and index fingers crossed or with the use of a tongue depressor.

2. The base of the tongue is pulled forward.

3. The tube is inserted and passed 2 or 3 inches inside the mouth and then rotated to insure that it is resting on the back of the tongue.

4. Check for proper positioning, gagging and laryngospasm.

5. If gagging, coughing or retching occur, the tube should be removed immediately.

Tracheal Intubation

Tracheal intubation is usually instituted when prior attempts to re-oxygenate the patient with airway support and bag-and-mask positive pressure breathing are unsuccessful.

Tracheal intubation may be instituted through the mouth or through the nose, although during emergency situations, orotracheal intubation is preferred because it can be carried out more rapidly.

It is the belief of the authors that all registered respiratory therapists should know how to intubate the trachea, even though in most emergency situations, reoxygenation of the patient can be achieved by using the bag and mask, with oxygen. An attempt by the respiratory therapist to intubate should be carried out as a last resort, when all simpler reoxygenating methods have failed and he is the most capable person present to perform the procedure.

EQUIPMENT

The equipment which should be at the site of the emergency should include the following items:

1. Curved as well as straight laryngoscope blades in varying sizes for adult and pediatric patients
2. Laryngoscope handle
3. Bite blocks
4. Adaptors of varying sizes
5. Topical anesthetic
6. Syringe
7. Rubber-shod clamps or Kelly clamps
8. Adhesive tape
9. Pharyngeal suction
10. Soft suction catheters of varying sizes
11. Cuffed orotracheal tubes of varying sizes
12. Water-soluble lubricant
13. Intubating forceps

GENERAL CONSIDERATIONS BEFORE OROTRACHEAL INTUBATION

Before any attempt to intubate the trachea is made, the anatomy of the patient's face and neck should be observed. The teeth should be inspected and steps taken to provide protection for them if necessary. Also to be observed are the degree of consciousness and the relaxation of the jaw and the throat muscles. The chief difficulties during intubation of the trachea are the responsiveness of the patient and the position of the patient's head.

PROCEDURE FOR OROTRACHEAL INTUBATION

1. The patient is placed in the supine position with the head tilted back while the operator supports the neck with his left hand and with his right hand supplies a gentle downward pressure on the patient's forehead. This position brings the axis of the trachea, pharynx and mouth into line.
2. The fingers of the operator open the patient's mouth and spread the lips apart to prevent trauma by the laryngoscope blade (using the cross-finger technique).
3. After he has moistened the blade with water, the operator grasps the laryngoscope in the left hand and introduces it into the right side of the patient's mouth and advances it forward and toward the center along the right side of the tongue (Fig. 57).
4. The blade is moved gently toward the epiglottis, keeping away from the posterior pharyngeal wall so as to prevent trauma (Fig. 58).
5. The laryngoscope blade is slipped beneath the tip of the epiglottis,

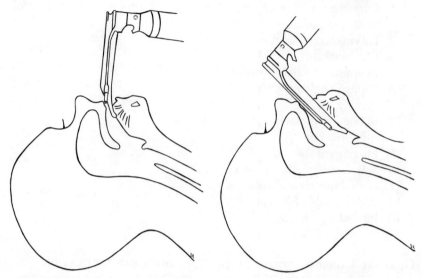

Fig. 57 (left).—The laryngoscope is introduced, and care is taken not to damage teeth or lacerate the mouth. It is guided over the dorsum of the tongue, forcing the tongue to the side of the mouth.

Fig. 58 (right).—Direct vision of epiglottis through the laryngoscope.

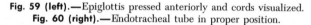

Fig. 59 (left).—Epiglottis pressed anteriorly and cords visualized.

Fig. 60 (right).—Endotracheal tube in proper position.

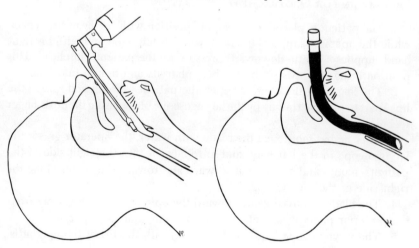

advanced a few millimeters, and exposure of the larynx is accomplished by an upward and forward elevation at a 45° angle from the face, which in turn causes elevation of the mandible (Fig. 59).

6. Never use the teeth to obtain leverage for exposing the glottis.

7. The endotracheal tube with cuff deflated is then passed beside the right side of the tongue and laryngoscope blade through the glottis opening and inserted 2–3 cm into the trachea in adults and 1–1.5 cm in infants and children.

8. After the tube is passed (Fig. 60), the operator should check both lungs for adequate expansion. Usually, the breath sounds of the left lung are checked first because the endotracheal tube may be inserted too far and may enter the right main stem bronchus.

9. The cuff is then inflated with air to insure a proper seal (Fig. 61), usually 2–6 cc. The tube is fixed firmly to a bite block (Fig. 62).

10. In nasotracheal intubation, a similar technique is used (Figs. 63 and 64).

GENERAL PRINCIPLES DURING TRACHEAL INTUBATION

1. Observe for normal and abnormal anatomy of the face and neck.

2. Test the laryngoscope light before attempting intubation.

3. Use suction as needed to withdraw mucus and other material from the pharynx.

Fig. 61 (left).—Cuffed endotracheal tube in place with cuff inflated.
Fig. 62 (right).—Endotracheal tube taped securely in place.

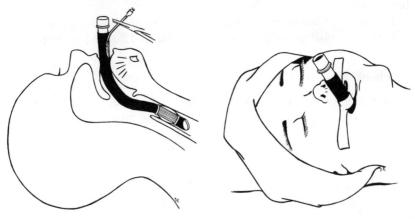

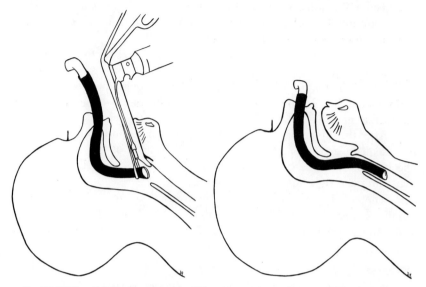

Fig. 63 (left).—If difficulty arises, Magill forceps may be used to grasp the tube and direct it into the larynx.

Fig. 64 (right).—Nasal intubation with endotracheal tube in proper position.

4. Cover or pad the teeth if necessary.

5. Choose the proper size endotracheal tube.

6. Check all necessary equipment prior to intubation.

Intubation with a curved blade is essentially the same process, with a few alterations which are listed below:

1. The laryngoscope blade is gently passed down over the center of the tongue toward the right side.

2. The tip of the epiglottis is not elevated by the blade; rather the tip of the curved blade rests between the epiglottis and the base of the tongue.

Tracheotomy

For the purposes of this book, tracheotomy is the term used to refer to the operative opening into the trachea through the 2d, 3d or 4th tracheal rings. The opening which is the result is termed "tracheostomy."

A tracheotomy is done either on an elective or on an emergency basis. The purposes of a tracheotomy are as follows:

1. To relieve obstruction of the upper airway

2. To provide more ready access to the lower airways

3. To facilitate suctioning of the airway
4. To facilitate prolonged artificial ventilation
5. To reduce anatomic dead space

The Operation of Tracheotomy

Emergency intubation is usually carried out prior to tracheotomy for the following reasons:

1. To restore normal pulmonary ventilation
2. To avoid a hasty operation without the necessary equipment and facilities
3. To avoid some of the common complications during tracheotomy, such as pneumothorax and excessive hemorrhaging

Figure 65 illustrates the equipment used for performing tracheotomy.

ORDERLY TRACHEOTOMY PROCEDURE

1. The patient is placed in a high semi-Fowler position with the neck hyperextended.

2. The entire neck from the submental region to the supraclavicular and anterior chest region is prepped anteriorly as well as laterally to the lateral borders of the sternomastoid muscles. The area is then draped.

3. The patient's face should be visible to allow close observation of clinical signs.

4. The area of incision and the tissue lying between it and the trachea are infiltrated with local anesthetic.

5. A horizontal skin incision is made in order to allow for the natural tension of skin folds.

6. The operator grips the subcutaneous tissue on either side of the midline with forceps, undermining bluntly upward and downward, for dissection along the midline. After each new cut, the trachea is carefully examined. A clamp is then passed between the trachea and the isthmus, spread, and other clamps are passed over the isthmus. The isthmus is separated between the clamp, dissected back from the midline and usually sutured with a 00–chrome-catgut suture.

7. At this point, the first tracheal ring is seen; the trachea is incised through any two rings below it. The 2d and 3d rings are preferable.

8. As soon as the trachea is entered, the several cartilages are grasped with an Allis clamp and a small portion of each is cut away on each side of the midline.

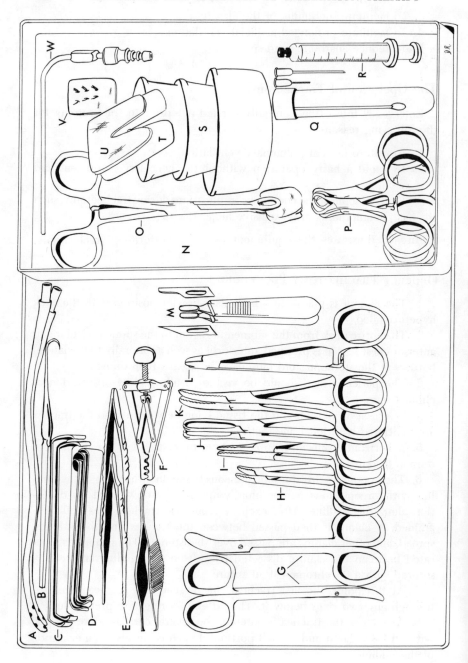

Fig. 65.—Instrument setup for emergency tracheotomy tray. **A,** rubber multiholed suction catheters, sizes #10–16; **B,** tracheal hook; **C,** right angle retractors (2); **D,** "S" retractors (3); **E,** regular plain forceps (2) and plastic toothed forceps (1); **F,** mastoid self-retaining retractor; **G,** dissecting and suture scissors; **H,** plastic curved hemostats (2); **I,** straight hemostats (2); **J,** Allis clamps (2); **K,** curved Kelly clamps (2); **L,** needle holder; **M,** knife handles (2) with #11 and #15 blades; **N,** oblong pan containing; **O,** sponge stick; **P,** towel clips (4); **Q,** culture tube; **R,** 5-cc syringe with #25- and #20-gauge needles; **S,** three small prep basins; **T,** rubber tracheotomy sponge; **U,** gauze tracheotomy sponge; **V,** sponge with French spring eye needles; **W,** mastoid metal suction tip.

9. The size of the opening should approximate the size of the tracheotomy tube. If an endotracheal tube is in place, it should not be withdrawn from the larynx until the tracheotomy tube is properly inserted and connected by appropriate adaptors and ventilation system.

10. During the first 48–72 hours, careful examination for proper placement of the tube should be practiced frequently. During this time, the dislodgment of the tube may lead to loss of the airway due to spasm and to swelling of the trachea and incised tissue layers.

TRACHEOSTOMY CARE

Good tracheostomy care depends on consideration of these basic requirements:

1. Airway patency
2. Asepsis
3. Maximal humidification of air
4. Avoidance of trauma to the tracheobronchial tree

TRACHEOTOMY TUBES IN CURRENT USE

Rubber.—Double cuffed (poliobulbar), sizes 28–38 with adaptors for ventilators without inner cannula (Fig. 66).

Fig. 66.—Rusch double cuff tracheotomy tube. A, built-in adaptor for syringe; B, pilot balloons; C, 15-mm adaptor; D, flange; E, proximal cuff; F, distal cuff.

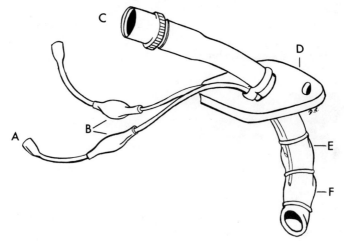

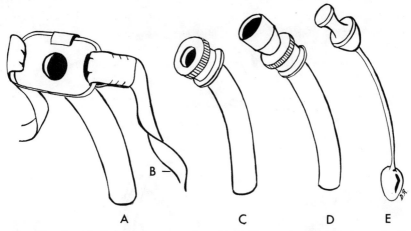

Fig. 67.—Special silver tracheotomy tube with Hollinger curve. **A,** outer cannula; **B,** toy tape to secure tube in place; **C,** inner cannula; **D,** inner cannula with built-in 15-mm adaptor; **E,** obturator.

Silver.—Sizes 00 to 8 with or without built-in 15-mm adaptors for ventilators, with inner cannula, with or without fenestration (Fig. 67).

Plastic.—These tubes have built-in 15-mm adaptors (Fig. 68).

TRACHEOSTOMY PRECAUTIONS

(*To be observed until discontinued by physician*)

1. Masks are to be worn by all personnel in the vicinity of the patient.

2. Aseptic technique (use of sterile gloves and equipment) is to be observed in caring for the tracheotomy tube and in suctioning.

HUMIDIFICATION

1. Adequate humidification reduces the need for tracheal suctioning. Inadequate humidification causes drying of secretions and hence may cause airway obstruction. Blockage of the lumen of the airway will make tracheobronchial toilet difficult. Inspired gases must be properly humidified at all times.

2. Methods of humidification:

    a) Tracheostomy mask (Fig. 69) with sterile heated nebulizer containing sterile distilled water, utilizing air or oxygen.

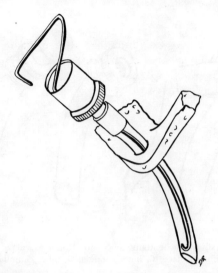

Fig. 68.—Silastic tracheotomy tube constructed of material which is essentially nonreactive to body tissue and fluid.

b) During controlled or assisted ventilation, a large inline nebulizer or humidifier is indicated. Medications may be given intermittently by incorporating a small nebulizer in the inspiratory line, usually every 4 hours or as indicated for 5–10 minutes.

Fig. 69.—Tracheotomy mask in place with large-bore corrugated tubing.

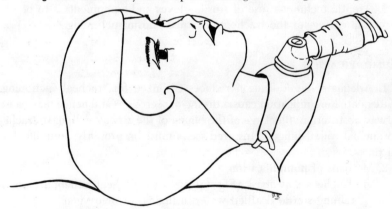

Dressings

A cut, 4 × 4 gauze square, not cotton filled, is changed when necessary to avoid skin irritation. The skin is cleansed with a sponge moistened with benzalkonium chloride (Zephiran) 1 : 750. Securing tapes are tied with a square knot at the side of the neck.

Changing of Tubes

Rubber and plastic tubes.—Since there is no inner cannula, blockage of the lumen by secretions must be considered. However, experience has shown that this is unlikely if there is proper humidification.

The entire tube is changed when necessary by the physician. The first change, which may be very difficult, should be performed by the responsible surgeon.

Silver.—Inner cannula is removed, cleaned and sterilized by the nurse at least every 8 hours.

PROCEDURE.—The trachea is suctioned, the inner cannula is unlocked and removed, cleaned with a tracheostomy brush and hydrogen peroxide or soap and water, and autoclaved. It is then allowed to cool, replaced and locked in place. Interchangeable cannulae, when available, may be used.

Outer cannulae are changed by a physician only.

Use of Cuffed Tubes

1. *Indications.*—Patients who require assisted ventilation or who are aspiration risks because of coma, abdominal distention, upper gastrointestinal bleeding or other causes.

2. *Possible complications.*—Aspiration of pharyngeal or gastric secretions when cuff is deflated; airway obstruction if cuff is displaced beyond the end of the tube; obstruction of the main stem bronchus by too long a tube; kinking of rubber tube; and pressure necrosis of the trachea.

3. *Deflation.*—To reduce the likelihood of pressure necrosis with a double-cuffed tube, the cuffs are alternately deflated every hour. To prevent aspiration, the pharynx must first be suctioned clear of secretions. The empty cuff is first inflated, then the full cuff is deflated. The person suctioning should be prepared to suction the trachea clear of any secretions that may escape as the cuff is deflated.

Single cuffs are deflated for a few moments every hour after the pharynx is thoroughly suctioned. The care just cited *must be observed.*

Suctioning

Suction in clinical medicine and surgery is widely practiced today. In the past, many methods were used in routine suctioning, involving ingenious principles (Brodie, 1941; Actkin, 1949; Carr, 1949). Although there are many all-purpose suction units available today, the criteria which would determine the most suitable apparatus for a particular purpose have received very little attention, judging from available designs (Fig. 70).

It is important that one know the size of the connecting tubing and suction catheters and the physical characteristics of the fluid to be aspirated,

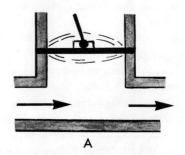

Fig. 70.—**A**, **B** and **C** demonstrate three types of pumps. **A** is a diaphragm pump, oilless; **B** is a piston pump; **C** is a rotary pump. **B** and **C** have friction surfaces which require lubrication.

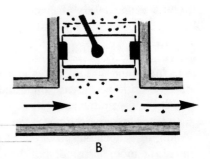

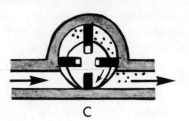

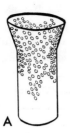 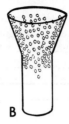 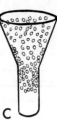

A   B   C

Fig. 71.—Flow of gases through a tube. **A,** large flow rate possible with very little resistance; **B,** in smaller tube, numbers of molecules are decreased, and more touch walls of the tube; **C,** increased turbulence due to increased resistance, and hence an increased pressure is needed to overcome frictional resistance.

as these factors will greatly influence the performance of the suction device.

Each clinical situation will present difficult problems that have to be mastered in order to extract the unwanted secretions, and, in doing so, care must be taken to see that harm to the patient both from trauma due to the suction catheter tip and from increased subatmospheric pressures does not result.

Physical characteristics affecting flow of fluid through tubes (Fig. 71) is an important factor during suctioning. Suction is created by the lowering of the pressure at one end of a tube that is directly attached to a negative pressure device, the basic suction unit. The distal end is open to the atmospheric air. A suction apparatus produces a negative pressure, which, when applied to a fluid or semisolid particle, will overcome resistance and induce a flow if the tube is large enough to accommodate the obstructing material. The resistance of the tube depends on the diameter and length of the tube being used. It is also, in the case of laminar flow, affected by viscosity and density of the fluid flowing through the tube. As the length of the tubing is increased, so is the resistance, thereby causing a new flow pattern of fluid through the tube, even though the maximal suction pressure of the apparatus is unchanged.

There are many other precautions and factors one should keep in mind while performing suctioning of the airways:

1. Suction from an open site most often involves the removal of blood. The tube bore should be as large as possible; narrow catheters and nozzles inevitably result in smaller flows.

2. Avoid the use of rigid suction catheters that could damage mucous membranes. The open end should be smooth and well rounded.

3. The suction unit should be regulated to the smallest possible pressure for adequate aspiration.

4. Never attach the suction tubing directly to the tracheotomy or endotracheal tube, as this makes the system a closed one, resulting in a biopsy of the trachea itself.

5. Never apply suction when inserting the catheter into an airway, as gases are removed from the lungs by this measure. Suction is applied only during the removal of the catheter from the airway.

6. Use sterile technique at all times; sterile gloves, catheters and masks are essential in this procedure.

In those patients who may require suctioning, either oropharyngeal, nasopharyngeal, endotracheal or tracheal, the proper care and technique are of utmost importance. Those patients with tracheostomies or who may have endotracheal or nasotracheal tubes in place should be on reverse precautions, and those persons providing care should wear masks, gown and don gloves during suctioning procedures. Before routine suctioning procedures for patients with and without tracheostomies, the operators should wash their hands in antiseptic solution. Separate sterile catheters for trachea and nasopharynx with "T" tubes should be provided for each patient. Catheters and all solutions should be changed at least every 8 hours. The proper suctioning technique cannot be emphasized too much. Many physicians, nurses and respiratory therapists prefer catheters with curved tips with one or two extra holes in order to decrease chance of blockage.

Rather than discuss routine nasopharyngeal suctioning, this section will be devoted to procedures for deep endotracheal suctioning.

The purpose of deep endotracheal suctioning is to aspirate secretions from the tracheal bronchial tree whenever the patient is unable to raise them by coughing.

ENDOTRACHEAL SUCTIONING

1. Deep endotracheal suctioning can be lifesaving in many instances but can also lead to cardiac arrest if not done properly. Deep suctioning should be attempted only by qualified persons.

2. Prolonged suctioning, suctioning with too large a catheter or failure to allow the patient time to ventilate between suction attempts can lead to hypoxia.

3. A supply of humidified oxygen should always be available for use in the event of respiratory distress during suctioning attempts.

4. A sterile catheter, sterile gloves and mask are required each time the procedure is attempted.

5. In the course of the procedure, it may be necessary to contaminate one hand. The operator must keep this in mind so that the hand which

remains sterile is the hand with which it is most convenient to handle the suction catheter.

6. The indications for and frequency of deep endotracheal suctioning should be specified in the doctor's order book (see Writing Orders for Inhalation Therapy in Glossary).

EQUIPMENT

1. Wall or portable suction unit with connecting tube
2. Sterile gloves
3. Sterile catheters of varying sizes
4. Sterile cups (disposable) for sterile water
5. Sterile pick-up forceps
6. Sterile water or saline for catheter and inner cannula cleaning
7. Hydrogen peroxide for cleaning inner cannula
8. Container for refuse

PROCEDURE

1. Wash hands thoroughly with antiseptic solution.
2. Assemble equipment.
3. Fill empty sterile disposable cups with sterile water or saline.
4. Fill bowl in container, which may already have sterile pipe cleaners and sterile tracheotomy sponges, with sterile water.
5. Open sterile equipment.
6. Aseptically, place sterile catheters of appropriate size in the container which already holds sterile "T" tubes and sterile 4 × 4 sponges.
7. Check for properly functioning suction equipment.
8. Open catheter and gloves.
9. Don gloves and remove catheter from sterile packet.
10. Protecting sterile catheter in palm of hand which is to remain sterile, pick up suction connecting tube with hand to be contaminated and attach to suction catheter.
11. Using the contaminated hand, apply gentle pressure on the flange of the tracheotomy tube to prevent its being dislodged (tubes with inner cannula), carefully unlock and remove inner cannula and place it in the bowl provided for its cleaning.
12. Approximate the length of catheter needed to enter the bronchus by measuring the distance from the orifice of the endotracheal or tracheotomy tube to the end of the xiphoid.
13. Moisten the catheter with sterile water.

14. With the suction off, introduce the catheter through the tube until the patient coughs. On the inspiration following the cough, advance the catheter into either main stem bronchus. To enter the left main stem bronchus turn the patient's head to the right (Fig. 72). The right main stem bronchus can be entered by turning the head to the left.

15. With a continuous twisting motion remove the catheter from the tube while applying intermittent suction with the "T" adaptor (Fig. 73). If signs of respiratory distress are noted, administer humidified oxygen to the patient. Also keep in mind the length of time to suction: each attempt should be no more than 15 seconds.

16. Rinse catheter with sterile water or saline.

17. Repeat suction as necessary to clear the airway, keeping in mind that too frequent suctioning may cause unnecessary trauma. Allow time for reoxygenation between suction attempts.

18. Detach catheter from suction and place in container for used equipment.

19. With sterile forceps in contaminated hand, pick up enough pipe cleaners to clean lumen of inner cannula.

Fig. 72.—When suctioning the trachea, insertion of the catheter is done without application of suction. The head of the infant is turned to the right to facilitate suctioning of the left bronchus.

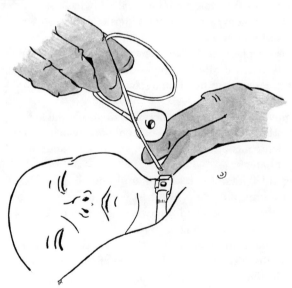

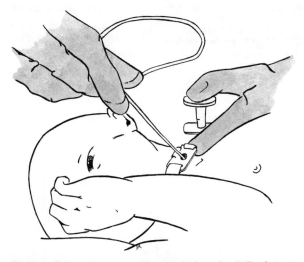

Fig. 73.—Suctioning procedure. Pressure is applied to the "T" adaptor intermittently while the catheter is rotated slowly and removed from the airway. (NOTE: suction should not last more than 15 seconds in order to prevent hypoxia from occurring.)

20. With hand which has been kept sterile for suctioning, remove inner cannula from bowl of sterile water.

21. Advance pipe cleaners through lumen of inner cannula. Small wire and gauze strips may be substituted for pipe cleaners to clean inner cannula.

22. Replace inner cannula in tracheotomy tube carefully and lock in place.

23. Change tracheostomy dressing as needed. Usually the first dressing change after a tracheotomy is done by the surgeon.

24. Apply humidified oxygen and make the patient comfortable.

25. If possible, allow enough time for the patient to relax before attempting further care.

Removal of secretions is one of the major practical problems in the total management of respiratory care.

REFERENCES

Hillard, E. K., and Rosen, M.: The use of suction in clinical medicine, Brit. J. Anaesth. 32:486, 1960.

Safar, P., *et al.: Respiratory Therapy* (Philadelphia: F. A. Davis Company, 1965).

Bendixen, H., *et al.: Respiratory Care* (St. Louis: C. V. Mosby Company, 1956).

Macintosh, R.; Mushin, W. W., and Epstein, H. C.: *Physics for the Anaesthetist* (2d ed.) (Oxford: Blackwells Scientific Publications, 1958).

Aitken, D.: A new surgical suction pump, Brit. M. J. 1:1094, 1949.

Brodie, E. L.: A thermal operated drainage pump, J. Urol. 45:507, 1941.

Elam, J. O., *et al.*: Head tilt method of oral resuscitation, J.A.M.A. 172:812, 1960.

Nicholas, T. H., and Rumer, G. H.: Emergency airway—A plan of action, J.A.M.A. 174:1930, 1960.

CHAPTER 9

Resuscitation

THE DEFINITION of resuscitation comes from the Latin "to restore to motion." It represents a combination of maneuvers which must take place to restore the *milieu intérieur*. Restoration of airway, artificial ventilation, administration of drugs, fluids and blood, manual systole and the use of external electric current, all may be required to perform the act of resuscitation. All this must take place in a very brief period, before biochemical death has become irreversible.

History

Prior to 1773 the act of resuscitation was performed by laymen. In this year in England under the auspices of the medical profession, the Royal Humane Society was organized to investigate and formulate rules for "authentic restoration of life."

The earliest recorded act of resuscitation that may be cited is found in I Kings 17:21–22

> And he stretched himself upon the child three times, and cried unto the LORD. . . . And the LORD heard the voice of Elijah; and the soul of the child came into him again, and he revived.

Resuscitative measures were first used on newborn infants or on patients suffering from violence, drowning or suffocation, the last related especially to mine accidents. With the discovery of anesthesia and the use of depressant drugs, the medical profession required increased knowledge of resuscitation. Another step forward was taken with the attempts to revive and maintain people with progressive respiratory paralyzing diseases. The field has been progressively expanded to its present state.

Early methods of resuscitation included warming, use of loud noises, such as shouting into the ears of the patient, and torture by burning, pulling of teeth and flagellation. Surprisingly, mouth-to-mouth insufflation combined with compression of the chest for expiration and pinching of the nostrils was in widespread use in Europe before A.D. 1530. This method was especially used for resuscitation of infants who failed to breathe at birth. Primarily the layman used this method because it was regarded as a very vulgar act by the medical profession.

In A.D. 1530, Paracelsus combined the use of fireside bellows with a catheter introduced into the mouth as an aid to resuscitation, and this may be regarded as the first usage of a practical mechanical device. (See Chapter 10.)

In the years following A.D. 1530, many attempts were made to modify resuscitative techniques. The instillation of tobacco smoke both into the rectum and into the mouth, rolling the patient either in or over a barrel, jackknifing of the patient's arms or legs rapidly, all were used with a modicum of success. During this time through the 18th Century, the use of mouth-to-mouth resuscitation became more widespread and was modified by various practices, such as cupping of the hands over the patient's mouth during resuscitation, and the use of snuff to make the patient sneeze periodically.

During this period of history the machine age was beginning, and attempts to adapt the machine to resuscitation are described in the following chapter on Mechanical Ventilation.

In approximately 1852, Ashley Cooper and Leroy of Paris are credited with the first logical attempts at manual respiration by means of alternate compression and relaxation of the chest and abdomen. Compression caused exhalation and passive relaxation caused inhalation for the next compression. For maintenance of the airway and also for better means of removing the water from the lungs of drowned persons, Marshall-Hall, in 1856, first utilized the prone position.

Over the next century many people devised varying modifications of this technique. Sylvester, Howard, Schafer, Nielsen, Thompson and Aferson were but a very few of those who developed varying modifications of the method. An excellent review of these methods is presented in the *Journal of the American Medical Association* (147:1444, 1951).

In the 1950s, as better means of scientific measurement became possible, Safar and Elam showed that positive pressure applied to the upper airway was a much better means of creating artificial ventilation than any of the other manual means. At about the same period of time, the development of the self-reinflating bag combined with a mask came into widespread use. Today, these are the techniques in most widespread usage.

In 1960, Kouwenhoven, Jude and Knickerbocker developed the technique of external manual compression of the chest to maintain circulation by alternate compression of the heart. Since that time, this technique has been universally accepted and thousands of lives have been saved.

Resuscitative Methods

At present, there are many variations in techniques of resuscitation that depend on a number of factors, such as the expense of equipment and the training of the individual performing the resuscitation, the equipment available at the time (see Fig. 74) and the differences in the cause of the respiratory and/or cardiac arrest. The method presented here is a general one utilizing a number of adaptations, but it should be remembered that it can be changed in a number of details.

Observe time:

1. Observe patient for lack of respiratory movement while feeling for peripheral pulses, such as carotid or femoral.
2. Place patient in supine or slight head-down position with firm thorax support.
3. Open patient's mouth to see if vomitus is present and clear the airway.
4. Place patient's head in extension and begin mouth-to-mouth resuscitation (Fig. 75). If suitable equipment such as a self-inflating bag and mask (with or without oxygen) is available, this should be substituted.
5. If an assistant is present, he should begin external manual systole (Fig. 76) by chest compression at a rate dependent on age, if not, alternate ventilation with compression and an attempt to obtain additional personnel and equipment.
6. Visually inspect the chest for inflation.
7. Palpate a peripheral pulse, preferably a femoral or carotid pulse for efficiency of cardiac action.
8. If equipment and an experienced individual are available insert endotracheal tube rapidly and continue ventilation with 100% oxygen.
9. Check pupillary size and reaction to light, being certain that both lungs are being ventilated.
10. Attach electrocardiogram to establish type of complex present. The two most common complexes in this situation are:
    a) ventricular fibrillation
    b) ventricular standstill

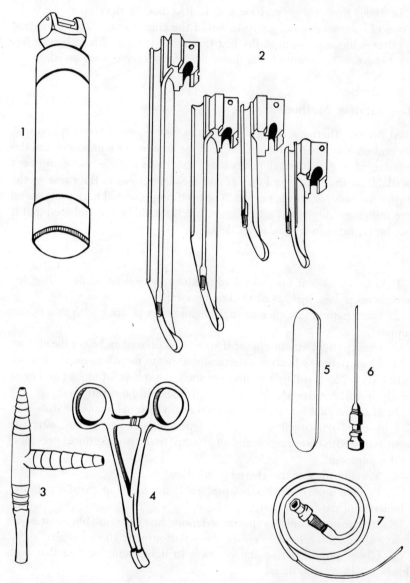

Fig. 74.—Mechanical aids for resuscitation. **1,** Miller laryngoscope handle with battery; **2,** Miller blades, sizes 3–0; **3,** "T" adaptor for suction apparatus; **4,** rubber-shod Kelly clamp; **5,** tongue depressor; **6,** spinal needle for percutaneous cardiac injection; **7,** #18-gauge polyethylene tubing for suctioning infant endotracheal tubes. (*Continued.*)

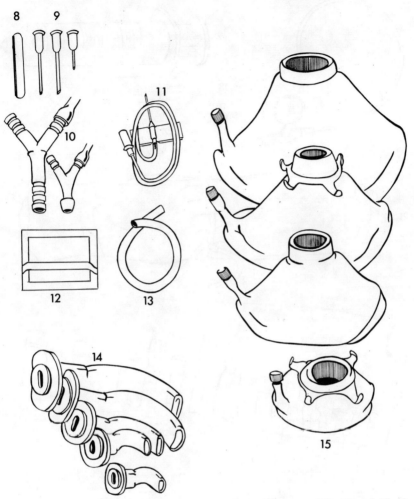

Fig. 74 (cont.).—**8,** file for opening ampules; **9,** needles, sizes #23, 20 and 25; **10,** Ayres "Y" tube; **11,** butterfly scalp vein needle; **12,** alcohol sponge; **13,** rubber tourniquet; **14,** oropharyngeal airways, from adult to pediatric sizes; **15,** anatomic rubber masks, varying from adult to pediatric sizes. (*Continued.*)

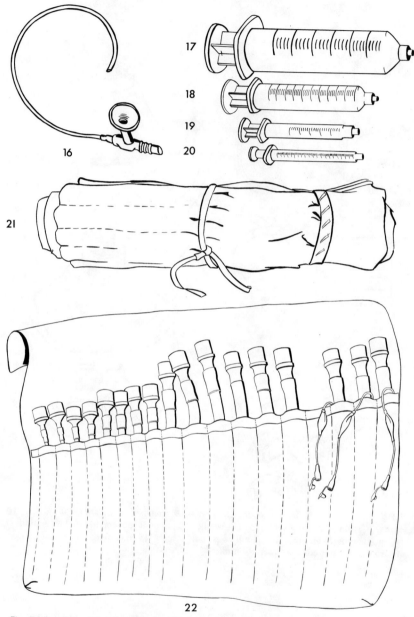

Fig. 74 (cont.).—16, infant regulated vacuum plastic suction catheter; **17,** plastic 30-ml luer lock syringe; **18,** plastic 10-ml luer lock syringe; **19,** plastic 2-ml luer lock syringe; **20,** plastic tuberculin syringe; **21,** endotracheal pouch (*closed*). **22,** endotracheal pouch (*open*), sizes varying from #2.5 to 9.0, including three cuffed tubes, sizes 7.5, 8.5 and 9.5. (*Continued.*)

144

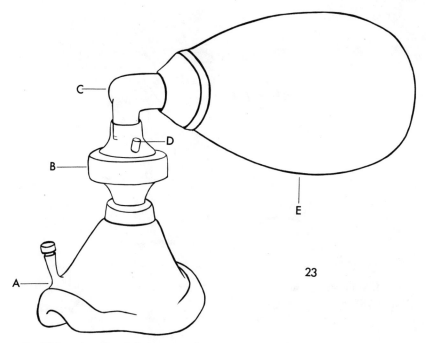

Fig. 74 (cont.).—23, reinflating manual resuscitator: *A*, mask; *B*, valve assembly; *C*, right angle adaptor; *D*, gas inlet; *E*, neoprene rubber bag.

Fig. 75.—Correct position and technique in facilitating mouth-to-mouth resuscitation is of vital importance. Note that the head and neck are hyperextended with the support of both hands, one on the forehead and the other under the spinal column. The operator's mouth is covering both mouth and nares of the infant to insure a proper seal in order to deliver an adequate tidal volume with each breath.

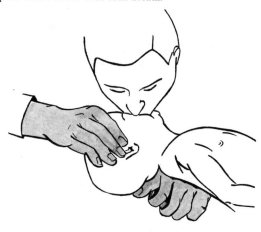

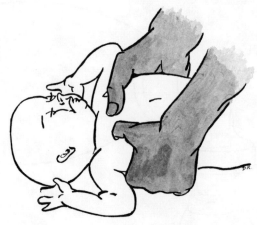

Fig. 76.—External cardiac massage applied with thumbs and the fingers giving support to the spinal column.

11. If standstill or asystole is present, the following drug therapy (Figs. 77 and 78) may be used:

a) sodium bicarbonate   c) calcium gluconate
b) adrenaline   d) dextrose 50%

Fig. 77.—Intracardiac injection of drugs for cardiac arrest. The needle is placed percutaneously at the sternal border of the 5th rib interspace. The syringe and needle are directed downward and medially.

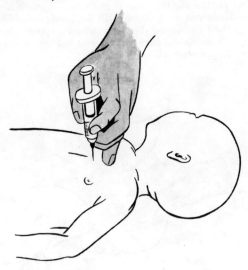

Agent	Concentration	Dose Under 10 lb	Dose Over 10 lb
Epinephrine	1/1000 (0.1%)	0.2 ml	0.25 ml/25 lb
Calcium gluconate	100 mg/ml (10%)	1 ml	1 ml/15 lb
Glucose	500 mg/ml (50%)	1 ml	1 ml/15 lb
Sodium bicarbonate	3.75 Gm/50 ml (44.6 mEq/50 ml)	3–4 ml	1 ml/3 lb
Tris(hydroxymethyl) aminomethane (THAM)	200 mg/ml (1.5 M)	3–4 ml	1 ml/3 lb
Isoproterenol (Isuprel)	1/5000	0.2 ml	0.1 ml/15 lb

The bicarbonate is given to reduce the acidemia present and to allow the adrenaline to be effective because adrenaline is not effective in acid media. Calcium gluconate is given to increase heart rate, and dextrose 50% for fuel.

If ventricular fibrillation is present:

a) Adrenaline may be given to produce a more coarse form of fibrillation

b) External defibrillation may be used.

Fig. 78.—Intracardiac injection via the substernal approach. The needle is placed percutaneously in the midline at the lower border of the sternum and directed inward toward the left lateral.

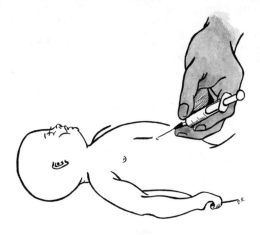

Since the voltage output of a child's heart and adult heart are not too far apart, dosages of electrical current in joules are difficult to specify. However, a schedule such as follows seems to work comparatively well. If no effect is obtained, the next dosages are raised.

	Initial Dose	*Second Dose*
Under 10 lb	15–30 Joules	Increases by
10–100 lb	60–90 Joules	50 joules
100–200 lb	90–125 Joules	

12. When the patient's systole again resumes, the blood pressure should be taken. Vasopressor drugs may be needed.

13. After the acute episode is over, a plan of management of causative factors is set up. The patient may be placed on automatic ventilation, which will be treated in another section. (See Chapter 10.)

REFERENCES

Elam, J. O.; Greene, D. G.; Brown, E. S., and Clements, J. A.: Oxygen and carbon dioxide exchange and energy cost of expired air resuscitation, J.A.M.A. 167:328, 1958.

Gordon, A. S.; Frye, C. W.; Gittelson, L.; Sadove, M. S., and Beattie, E. J., Jr.: Mouth-to-mouth versus manual artificial respiration for children and adults, J.A.M.A. 167:320, 1958.

Luckhardt, A. B.: Official "Edict" by the city of Zurich, Switzerland, 1766, A.D., on the methods of resuscitation to be employed on drowned or asphyxiated persons, Bull. Hist. Med. 6:171, 1938.

Safar, P.: Ventilatory efficacy of mouth-to-mouth artificial respiration, J.A.M.A. 167:335, 1958.

Safar, P.; Escarraga, L. A., and Elam, J. O.: Comparison of mouth-to-mouth and mouth-to-airway methods of artificial respiration with chest pressure arm-lift methods, New England J. Med. 258:671, 1958.

Safar, P.; Escarraga, L. A., and Chang, F.: Upper airway obstruction in the unconscious patient, J. Appl. Physiol. 14:760, 1959.

Baringer, J. R.; Salzman, E. W.; Jones, W. A., and Friedlich, A. L.: External cardiac massage, New England J. Med. 265:62, 1961.

Kouwenhoven, W. B.; Jude, J. R., and Knickerbocker, G. G.: Closed-chest cardiac massage, J.A.M.A. 173:1064, 1960.

Lown, B.; Amarasingham, R., and Neuman, J.: New method for terminating cardiac arrhythmias, J.A.M.A. 182:548, 1962.

CHAPTER 10

Mechanical Ventilation

Automatic Ventilation of The Lungs

History

THE HISTORY of the development of automatic ventilation is closely associated with the history of resuscitation. The concept of the ventilator is an old one, but the search was long indeed for an effective mechanical device that would provide a better and more constant method of revival than mouth-to-mouth resuscitation, that would free the operator for other procedures necessary to the patient and that would provide continuing respiratory care in a precise manner.

Paracelsus, who, in 1530, used fireplace bellows attached to a tube placed in the patient's mouth as a respiratory aid, is usually credited with the first use of mechanical means of ventilation. Anthony Fothergill, in 1740, criticized this method as being harmful to the lungs. In 1763, Smellie inserted a flexible metal tube via the mouth into the trachea. A glass bulb was placed in the middle of the tube to collect mucus from the lungs when suction was placed on the flexible tube. Positive pressure was administered to the lungs by blowing into the tube. In 1774, John Fothergill modified this technique by using a fireplace bellows attached to the flexible tube.

John Hunter, in 1775, devised for experiments in animals a double-acting bellows with a valve which allowed fresh air to be sucked into one bellows while exhaled air was collected in the other bellows. This was adapted for use in patients by the Royal Humane Society in 1782. Charles Kite, in 1786, modified the bellows so that it had two valves and a 500-cc capacity, which represents the first time a ventilator's inspiratory capacities had been related to normal adult tidal volumes. Both of these methods utilized tubes placed in the nostrils. Kite also recommended the use of pressure on the chest to aid expiration and pressure over the cricoid cartilage to prevent air from entering the stomach.

Gorcy, in 1789, suggested constant rebreathing of exhaled air as a source

149

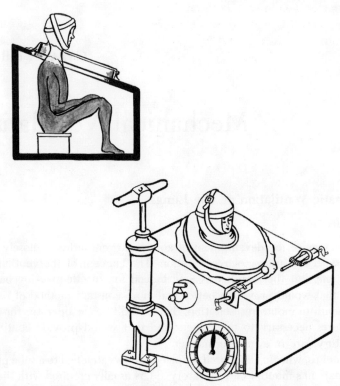

Fig. 79.—The earliest known body-enclosing iron lung was described by Alfred F. Jones of Lexington, Kentucky, in 1864. U.S. patent No. 44198 states, it "cured paralysis, neuralgia, rheumatism, seminal weakness, asthma, bronchitis, and dyspepsia. Also deafness . . . . When properly and judiciously applied many other diseases may be cured . . . ."

of stimulation to respiration. Hans Courtois, in 1790, developed the first piston and cylinder to replace the bellows, and the usefulness of this adaptation became widespread.

The status of mechanical ventilation then remained much the same until 1864. Over this period of time, much controversy developed on the use of mechanical devices to apply positive pressure to the airway. The problems encountered can well be imagined. Sterilization was practically nonexistent for mechanical devices. Proper methods of cannulation of the trachea had not yet been devised, and, due to overdistention of the lungs on the stomach, often as much harm as good was done.

Some of the reports from this era stated that constant supervision of the equipment was necessary in order to keep it in working order. Cost was also a factor, and many complaints were related to the time necessary for the equipment to arrive where it was needed. Few people knew how the equipment was to be used when it did arrive. Also, equipment which was powered by compressed air required cylinders which were constantly running out of gas. The physiology of the lung was poorly understood, and consequently many errors were made.

Another approach to the problem was attempted by the use of a barorespirator into which the patient was placed for the application of alternative positive and negative pressure. The method was considered safer than the piston and cylinder system, and airway maintenance was less crucial. In 1864, Jones devised the first of a long series of barorespirators (Fig. 79).

In 1876, Woillez devised the first workable barorespirator (Fig. 80). Breuillard, Braun, Eisenmenger, Davenport, Hammond, Lord, Severy, Steuart, Chillingworth and Schwake, as well as many, many more, devised various types of barorespirators (Figs. 81–90). It was not until 1928, however, that they were adapted for widespread use. In this year, the New York Consolidated Gas Company commissioned Drinker and Shaw of the Harvard School of Public Health to develop a method by which artificial respiration might be applied for an indefinite period (Fig. 91).

Fig. 80.—In 1876, Doctor Woillez of Paris built the first workable iron lung, which he called a "spirophore." It had the basic elements of modern respirators, including an adjustable rubber collar and a sliding bed. A unique feature was a rod which rested lightly on the patient's chest to give visual proof of actual lung expansion. In a brilliant lecture presented before the Academy of Medicine on June 20, Woillez showed a thorough understanding of the physiology and mechanics of artificial respiration. He refused to patent his invention. A colleague suggested placing spirophores all along the Seine for drowning rescues, but finances for this public service were lacking. (The illustration was reconstructed by Maxfield Parrish, Jr., for a legal battle years before a photograph was discovered.)

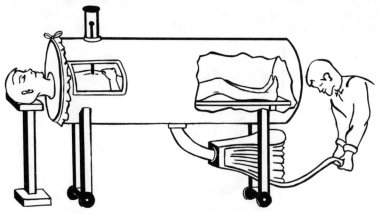

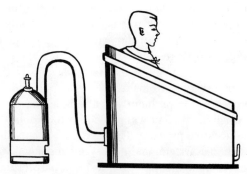

Fig. 81.—Dr. Charles Breuillard of Paris patented a "bath cabinet" type of respirator in 1887. For a source of vacuum, he recommended a "steam ejector fed by a steam boiler . . . heated by a spirit lamp." The patient himself was supposed to operate a valve, alternately connecting the cabinet with the vacuum for inhalation and with the atmosphere for exhalation. Breuillard also described a chest respirator (cuirass) to be operated in the same way, and a face mask.

The resultant respirator (Fig. 92) proved so successful that Dr. James L. Wilson of Children's Hospital in Boston had an entire room constructed as a respirator, which saved many lives in several poliomyelitis epidemics.

The J. H. Emerson Company of Cambridge, Massachusetts, made commercially available a practical barorespirator in 1931 (Fig. 93), and this allowed hospitals throughout the world to have a standard respirator for which parts could be replaced and exchanged between machines.

Fig. 82.—For "resuscitating asphyxiated children," Dr. Egon Braun of Vienna devised a small wooden box in which pressure and suction were created by the doctor's own breath (through the tube at the right). The infant was supported in a plaster mold, with nose and mouth pressed against an opening in the rubber closure. (This picture from the *Boston Medical and Surgical Journal* of 1889, is only a rough diagram.) Doctor Braun reported 50 consecutive successful cases.

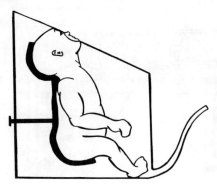

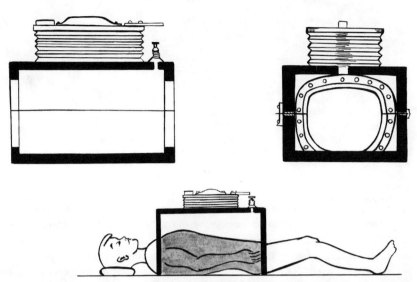

Fig. 83.—In 1901, Rudolf Eisenmenger of Piski, Hungary, patented a portable respirator which consisted of a "simple, two-part box" enclosing only the patient's chest and abdomen. Later, he became Medical Professor in Vienna and there continued to improve his invention. He stressed the importance of access to the patient's throat and limbs, of portability and of hand operation. (Motors were also mentioned.) There are reports of "extraordinary success" with Eisenmenger's respirators.

Fig. 84.—William Davenport of London clearly understood the mechanics of artificial respiration. His patent in 1905 mentions a box, a rubber collar and a simple bellows or piston pump. He lacked the sliding bed (of Woillez and modern iron lungs) but made several good suggestions, including the supplementary use of oxygen. He proposed several types, including a "collapsable form . . . to facilitate transit."

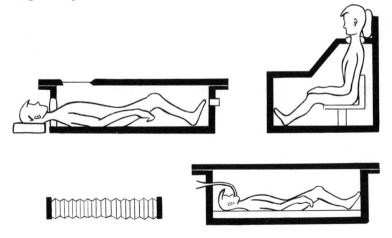

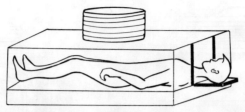

Fig. 85.—Dr. Charles Morgan Hammond of Memphis, Tennessee, built his first "artificial lung" in 1905 and a series of improved models throughout the next 20 years. He performed experiments and treated patients successfully, but his respirators were not produced commercially and remained unknown to the public for many years.

This, however, was not the final solution to the problem of ventilation. There were many problems associated with barorespirators. They were not applicable to all patients; they were difficult to move and impractical for use in immediate resuscitations. Sterilization was difficult if not impossible: It separated the patient from the nurse and physiotherapist, and specialized techniques for care had to be developed by both.

Fig. 86.—In 1908, Peter Lord of Worcester, Massachusetts, patented a respirator room. He pictured huge pistons to create the pressure changes and to supply fresh air. An enormous motor would have been needed and very heavy construction. However, the idea of a room is good because it makes nursing care easy.

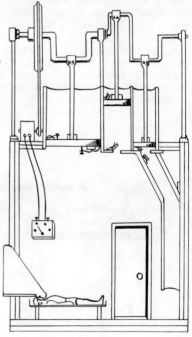

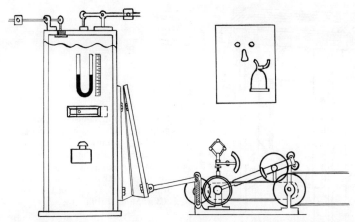

Fig. 87.—The patent granted to Melvin L. Severy of Boston, Massachusetts, in 1916 shows little concern for the patient's comfort but includes ingenious mechanical elements. In the model illustrated, the patient was obliged to stand, pressing his nose and mouth against a triangular aperture below two eye-windows. Severy also described variable speed pulleys and elaborate electromagnetic controls for regulating speeds and pressures. He suggested cams to produce various pressure curves. A cuirass respirator and mask resuscitator were mentioned also.

Fig. 88.—Dr. W. Steuart of South Africa built a simple respirator and demonstrated a working model to his colleagues (M. J. South Africa, 1918). He proposed plaster of paris to seal around the patient's shoulders and pelvis, but friends quickly suggested other more practical materials. Steuart was the first to think primarily of poliomyelitis. He even envisaged a ward piped with intermittent suction to which individual body casings could be attached.

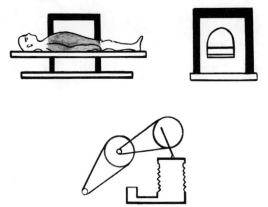

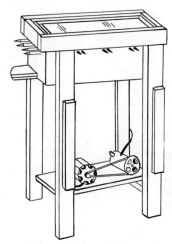

Fig. 89.—Felix P. Chillingworth and Ralph Hopkins of New Orleans, Louisiana, built a plethysmograph to study circulatory changes resulting from lung distention. They also used it as a dog respirator. ". . . pulmonary ventilation is accomplished by rhythmic changes in air pressure within the plethysmograph causing alternate distention and collapse of the lungs." (J. Lab. & Clin. Med., 1919.)

Many men were diligently at work on the problem of making a practical positive-pressure device which could be used to resuscitate and also to ventilate for prolonged periods. At the same time, better methods for cannulation of the airway, both by tracheotomy and by development of proper materials for endotracheal intubation, were being developed. Rapid

Fig. 90.—Wilhelm Schwake of Oranien-burg-Eden, Germany, patented a "pneumatic chamber" in 1926. He was concerned with portability and with exactly matching the patient's breathing depth and rhythm. He also stated that "negative pressure . . . upon the skin . . . draws out . . . the gaseous by-products." We would not consider this respirator practical for severely ill patients, but the picture is a great favorite.

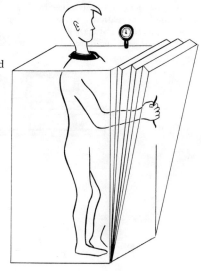

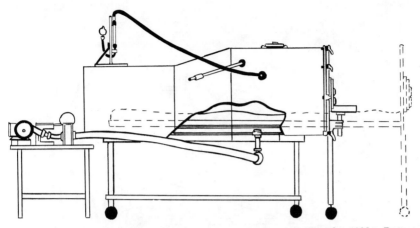

Fig. 91.—The first "iron lung" to receive widespread use was developed in 1928 in Boston and was patented by Philip Drinker and Dr. Louis Agassiz Shaw. It was cumbersome and inconvenient but saved a number of lives. It had a sliding bed with headwall attached and a rubber collar. Pressure changes were created by a rotary blower and an alternating valve. During a polio epidemic, the Consolidated Gas Company of New York paid for building large numbers of these respirators, and reports of their use spread quickly around the world.

Fig. 92.—In the early respirators, it was difficult to give complete nursing care and to change the patients' position frequently. This care was found to be of lifesaving importance, so Dr. James L. Wilson asked for a room in which several patients could be made to breathe simultaneously. A nurse could enter by the door and perform all procedures efficiently. The room pictured was built at the Children's Hospital in Boston, Massachusetts, and was used successfully during several polio epidemics.

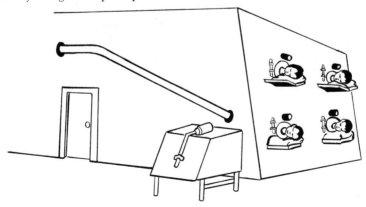

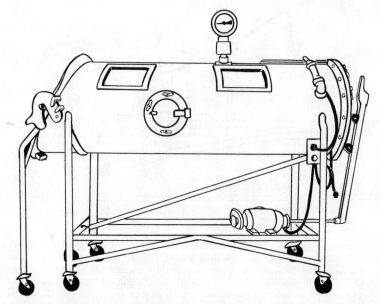

Fig. 93.—Because of a severe poliomyelitis epidemic in 1931, John Haven Emerson of Cambridge, Massachusetts, built a simplified respirator. It cost less than half as much as others but contained many improvements. It operated quietly, using a bellows to create the changes of pressure (as Woillez's did, but with a motor added). A wide range of speeds was instantly available. Opening and closing were rapid and convenient. It could be pumped by hand if electricity failed. The first Emerson "iron lung" is now preserved in a glass case in the United States National Museum (the Smithsonian Institution) as the prototype of respirators constructed since 1931 in America and Europe.

growth and development in the field of anesthesia helped point new directions for respiratory treatment and care.

One such positive pressure device to receive widespread use was the Pulmotor (Fig. 94), developed in 1911 by Drager, which utilized compressed air or oxygen for energy, and a balancing system of bellows and valves. Its operation was essentially automatic and depended on the pressure in the cylinder. This was applied to the patient via a mask placed over the nose and mouth. It was suggested with its use that a small catheter with a balloon be passed into the esophagus and the balloon be inflated to prevent the passage of air into the stomach.

Several other devices similar to the Pulmotor were developed about the same period. The E & J Resuscitator, the McKesson Resuscitator, and the Salvator are but a few. Yandell Henderson and H. W. Haggard developed, in 1922, a demand valve system assuring a constant percentage of oxygen

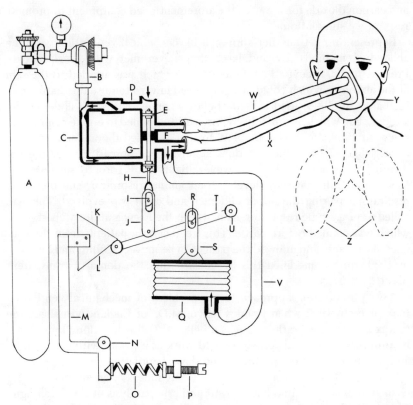

Fig. 94.—The Drager artificial breathing apparatus consists of pipes D and C which branch from pipe G in which an abutment, F, is fixed. Pipe D has a throttle valve. Pipe V branches off from pipe X near its point of connection with pipe G. Pipe V leads to a bellows, Q, the object of which is to move the pistons, E. A mixture of gases is driven to the lungs, Z. At the same time a portion of these gases is led to the bellows, Q, by way of pipe V. As the lungs fill, the flow of gases meets an increased resistance and the pressure increases in the bellows, Q, which now acts on the pistons, E, to change their position, resulting in a negative pressure which evacuates gases from the lungs and bellows. As long as the lungs are able to give air, the sucking action does not increase to such an extent as to decrease the pressure in the bellows. When, however, the lungs are exhausted, the action becomes stronger and the bellows contracts so as to draw the pistons into the first position. This operation is then repeated. If a faster rate is desired, the links S and J are provided with slots R and I, respectively, into which pins on the piston rod H and lever T project which later is pivoted to some fixed point by a pin, U. A second lever, K, is pivoted to a fixed point by pin L, one end of this lever, K, being acted upon by a spring, O, the tension of which may be regulated by a screw, P.

and carbon dioxide for use with the aforementioned equipment to promote respiratory stimulation.

Representing yet another approach to mechanical ventilation were the abdominal methods. By and large they never met with great success. Pressey, in 1894, devised an adhesive pad which was applied to the skin of the abdomen which could be compressed inward to raise the diaphragm. Hofbauer, in 1908, used a metal bellows connected to the abdomen by a rubber bag which alternately compressed and pulled to create respiration. Gann, in 1939, and Swan, in 1940, further modified the abdominal respirator. None of these modifications achieved widespread use for the abdominal approach. In 1937, however, Banting of Toronto suggested to Lieble and Hall that they develop their animal respirator, and the dome respirator covering the upper abdomen and chest was evolved. This was called a cuirass-type respirator, named after the French military chest piece which was donned before battle. This freed certain patients from the confines of the tank, and allowed the patient to be moved. Collins and Drinker, in 1939, further modified this by constructing the dome of transparent plastic.

A very interesting approach to the problem of mechanical ventilation took place in 1932 when Frank C. Eve, M.D., of England visualized the thorax as a cylinder rather than as a bellows. Following along these lines, he proposed that the diaphragm could work as a piston within a cylinder and that by moving the piston up and down ventilation would take place. He succeeded in saving a 2-year-old child by means of an antique rocking chair (Fig. 95). The child had a postdiphtheric paralysis of the diaphragm. This method has been continued over the years, particularly at times of poliomyelitis epidemics, and has evolved into electric "Eve Rocking Beds," which are still in use today.

While this work was being advanced, many men continued work on the principle of positive-pressure devices, known more commonly as the resuscitator.

In 1933, Goodner of Glendale, California, developed a piston-operated "resuscitator." The concept of volume ventilators did not come into prominence in inhalation therapy for almost 30 years after this. J. A. Heidbrink, in 1933, developed a "pulmonary ventilating apparatus" which could be regulated by the pressure developed in a patient's lung. Many mechanical types of positive pressure breathing machines were developed, some used and some abandoned, only to be "rediscovered" again as other changes in medicine, such as better airway management, occurred.

Adaptations to Emerson, E & J, Kreiselman, Torpin, Blanchard, Stephenson, M.S.A. Pneophore, all occurred during the 1930–1940 era.

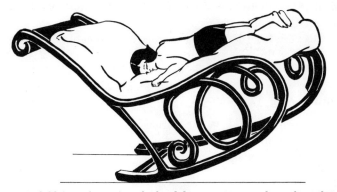

Fig. 95.—A child (convalescent) in the head-down position on the rocking chair, which was used when the diaphragm was paralyzed. The retaining strap for the buttocks is missing. (Frank C. Eves' patient with diphtheria—first usage of the rocking respirator.)

In 1942, V. Ray Bennett, as a consultant engineer to the U.S. Air Force, developed a demand valve oxygen administration device for use of crews of high-altitude aircraft. This valve allowed balanced pressure oxygen demand as needed at varying locations within the aircraft. Further refinement of this valve allowed the development of the concept of "intermittent positive pressure breathing," i.e., breathing in which the pressure is elevated in the inspiratory phase and is zero or negative during the expiratory phase. This system was later able to provide either "automatic" or nonautomatic patient-controlled respiratory units. V. Ray Bennett and Associates was incorporated in 1951, and the firm was purchased by the Puritan Compressed Gas Company in 1956. This company has further changed the unit and developed newer modifications, which will be discussed later in this chapter.

In 1952, Henry Seeler obtained a patent from the United States Patent Office for an intermittent positive-pressure breathing device, which was assigned to the United States Air Force. The machine utilized the principle of a slidable rod for gas flow direction, which had at its opposite ends a permanent magnet and an armature capable of relative rotation to vary the attractive force between the magnet and armature. This machine was never widely produced commercially, but was another great step forward in ventilator designs.

In order to obtain history on the widely produced Bird IPPB machine, correspondence with Mr. Bird yielded the following information: He describes the design of the Bird valve as directed toward pressure-suit regulation and early experience in de-icing the wings of aircraft.

He further credits Doctor Cournand with the adaptation of this equipment for medical application.

From this very brief look at the history of automatic ventilators, let us examine some of those in current use today.

Automatic Lung Ventilators

1. To augment or replace the patient's own respiratory effort when attached to the upper airway.
2. Mode of attachment:
   a) Nasotracheal tube
   b) Endotracheal tube
   c) Tracheal tube
3. To deliver an effective aerosol to the bronchial tree of the lungs to relieve airway obstruction due to spasm and retained secretions.

ASSISTORS AND CONTROLLERS

1. *Assistor.*—A ventilator which will inflate the lungs in response to an inspiratory effort initiated by the patient. Usually a sudden reduction to airway pressure is the signal to which the assistor responds.

2. *Controller.*—A ventilator which will cycle automatically on the totally apneic patient; a timing mechanism regulates its operation during all phases of the respiratory cycle.

3. *Assistor-controller.*—A ventilator that operates both as an assistor and controller. An assistor-controller can be triggered into the next phase at an earlier time; however, the patient has to generate signals.

CONTROL OF TIDAL VOLUMES

1. *Controlled-pressure devices.*—The maximal airway pressure adjusted by the operator to provide a suitable tidal volume. The volume is often altered by changes in lung compliance and compressed gases within the tubing.

2. *Controlled-volume ventilators.*—These devices deliver a predetermined volume of gas during each inspiratory phase. At a constant flow, the peak inspiratory pressure will increase as the lung compliance decreases.

Controlled-pressure and controlled-volume ventilators will deliver constant tidal volumes so long as there is no change in the patient's resistance to inflation, compressibility of gas in the system or leaking from the airway.

If airway resistance increases or if the compliance of the patient's lungs decreases, then more driving force will be required to produce the same tidal volume. Controlled-volume ventilators, such as the Engström, Mörch Piston, Air-Shields, Emerson or the Bennett MA-I will respond by delivering the inspired gases at a higher pressure.

Tidal volume losses from volume-limited type ventilators can be calculated by the use of Boyle's law, if the compressible volume and the peak pressures are known.

DS_{ToT} = total dead space in ml.

TV_1 = preset tidal volume (prior to compression) in ml.

P_x = pressure above ambient in cm of water.

TV_2 = delivered tidal volume in ml.

P_1 = ambient pressure in cm of water

V_1 = $(DS_{ToT} \times TV_1)$ = total volume to be compressed in ml.

P_2 = $(P_1 \times P_x)$ = pressure to which V_1 will be compressed in cm of water

V_2 = $(DS_{ToT} \times TV_2)$ = total volume after compression in ml.

Using Boyle's law

$$P_1 \cdot V_1 = P_2 \cdot V_2$$

And substituting we arrive at:

$$P_1 \cdot (DS_{ToT} \times TV_1) = (P_1 \times P_x)$$
$$(DS_{ToT} \times TV_2)$$

And solving for TV_2:

$$TV_2 = P_1 \frac{(DS_{ToT} + TV_1)}{P_1 + P_x} - DS_{ToT}$$

EXAMPLE: Calculate the delivered tidal volume in an Emerson Ventilator adjusted to 600 ml requiring a pressure of 20 cm of water above ambient to ventilate a patient. Assume the humidifier contains 1,400 ml of water, making a total dead space of 4,200 ml.

Positive pressure portion, including humidifier	4450
Connecting tubes and drains	1150
Total dead space	5600
Total dead space with 1,400 ml of water in humidifier	4200

$$TV_2 = P_1 \frac{(DS_{ToT} + TV_1)}{P_1 + P_x} - DS_{ToT}$$

$$TV_2 = 1033 \frac{(4200 + 600)}{1033 + 20} - 4200$$

$$TV_2 = 509 \text{ ml delivered volume to patient}$$

RESPIRATORY TRACT IMPEDANCES.—Obstruction may occur at any point in the upper airway. Secretions may decrease compliance by reducing the amount of lung participation in effective gas exchange. Thus, the patient with a wet lung will receive progressively smaller tidal volumes from a controlled-pressure ventilator as secretions accumulate. Since chest wall muscle tone is an important component of compliance, the ability of a patient to cooperate with the lung ventilator will determine the efficiency of ventilation.

HUMIDIFICATION.—The gas from the ventilator usually passes through a large main-line humidifier on the way to the patient. Large amounts of water may condense in the patient-supply tube from the humidifier; this is usually manifested by oscillating movements of the pressure gauge, or the condensation may be seen in the tube. The hose should be positioned in such a manner as to facilitate drainage. The hose should be drained of condensed water at least hourly and preferably halfhourly. The water as well as the gas temperature should be monitored; it should be near body temperature. The water level must be kept sufficiently high with sterile distilled water; it should cover at least half of the immersion heater.

Expiratory resistance.—Graded expiratory resistance can be produced by imposing a variable size orifice cap over the exhalation valve. This cap must never be put on so that it completely blocks exhalation. The pressure registered on the pressure gauge should fall to zero before the end of expiration.

INSPIRED OXYGEN CONCENTRATION.—With the average pressure-limited ventilator, the inspired oxygen concentration will vary on air admixture. As airway resistance increases, the oxygen concentration increases. Thus, oxygen concentrations should be analyzed and monitored closely, or the unit may be powered by compressed gas and oxygen titrated into the system as needed. Air-oxygen mixers are available commercially which give varying concentrations from 21 to 100% oxygen. Also to insure proper inspired oxygen concentrations, it is important to do arterial blood gas studies frequently.

Effective ventilation can rarely be achieved in adults if the respiratory rate exceeds 24 or 25 per minute at rest. An increase in spontaneous respiratory effort above this value may be caused by hypoxia or hypercapnia and usually requires prompt treatment.

Volume-Limited Ventilators

Volume-limited ventilators are represented by the Emerson Postoperative Ventilator, the Engström, Air-Shields, Bennett, and the Mörch I ventilators. The basic controls are those of stroke volume, duration of inspiration and duration of expiration. The Air-Shields and Bennett ventilators are capable of providing assisted ventilation. Transmission of the preset stroke volume from the ventilator to the lung depends on an airtight fit between the ventilator and the patient's airway. Only in the absence of a leak does the stroke volume from the ventilator equal the tidal volume. Leaks in the system are evident by a fall in the peak airway pressure as it is registered on the pressure gauge and by a fall in exhaled tidal volume.

Significant leaks lead to inadequate ventilation and should be promptly corrected. Small leaks may be created around the tracheotomy cuff purposely and can be compensated for by increasing the stroke volume. The Emerson ventilator is almost noiseless; an alarm, which goes off in case of accidental disconnection or if the power fails, is available commercially.

The Air-Shields ventilator produces a fog by use of a rapidly spinning disk. In the Emerson, Engström, and Bennett MA-I ventilators, the gas passes through a large reservoir containing hot sterile distilled water. The inspired gas should be 30° to 35° C at the trachea. When the motor is turned off during weaning periods, while the heater is left on, the first 5–6 breaths may be very hot. Do not connect to the patient until a few cycles have passed. The inspired gas may also become too hot when very small tidal volumes are used, especially for infants. Condensation in the tubing occurs with all ventilators and necessitates frequent emptying of water.

On these five volume-controlled ventilators, the inspired oxygen concentration can be varied between 21% (room air) and 100% by adjusting the oxygen flow to ventilator on the wall flowmeter.

The primary aim of artificial ventilation is to produce a certain required tidal volume or minute volume, which is the tidal volume times the rate per minute. The tidal volume delivered by a pressure-limited ventilator depends on several factors, the most important of which are:

1. Peak positive pressure setting on the ventilator
2. Rate of inspiratory gas flow from the ventilator
3. Resistance of the patient's lungs and chest wall to inflation

With a volume-limited ventilator, the tidal volume is predetermined by the ventilator, provided no significant leak is present between the ventilator and the patient. Here, the resistance of the patient's lungs and chest wall to inflation, as well as the rate of inspiratory gas flow and duration of inspiration, will determine the peak positive airway pressure required to introduce the tidal volume.

The resistance to inflation has two components: elastic resistance (Fig. 96) and frictional resistance (Fig. 97). An increased elastic resistance (low compliance) is seen with pulmonary disease; for example, atelectasis, pul-

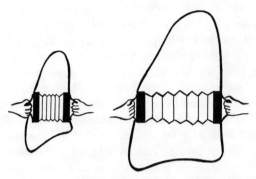

Fig. 96.—The compliance, or elastic recoil, of the lung may be compared to the stretching of a bellows. When lung tissue becomes more fibrous and less distensible, compliance decreases.

monary edema, pneumonia, fibrosis with obesity, abdominal distention and with spasm of the chest wall and abdominal muscles. In the average patient with normal lungs, 20 ± 5 cm H_2O pressure is required to produce a tidal volume of 1 L. In patients with severe lung disease, the pressure required may be three or four times as large.

Frictional resistance is primarily a resistance to gas flow through the conducting airway and bronchi. It is increased with bronchospasm, bronchial mucosal edema, obstruction of the airway from secretions and plugging or kinking of tubes. When frictional resistance is very high, it may be necessary to use a low-inspiratory flow rate to obtain a more even distribution of inspired gas to all areas of the lungs and to avoid a too rapid buildup of airway pressure (Figs. 97 and 101).

Fig. 97.—Frictional resistance. Internal diameter of bronchiole is decreased, thereby leading to frictional resistance to air flow.

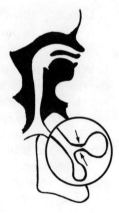

When pressure-limited ventilators are used, any increase in the resistance of the lungs to inflation leads to a fall in tidal volume. To guard against such changes, the exhaled tidal volume or minute volume is measured by attaching a ventilation meter or Wright respirometer during exhalation at the patient-machine interface.

PERIODIC DEEP LUNG INFLATIONS.—During prolonged ventilation, it is important that periodic deep lung inflations be given ("sighing") to prevent diffuse atelectasis and hypoxia.

Volume and frequency of artificial sighing required for prevention of atelectasis have not been established and probably vary between patients and among disease conditions. It is a general opinion that a volume three times the normal tidal volume has proved quite beneficial.

A self-inflating bag-mask unit as well as a 2–3 L capacity bag is desirable at the bedside of all patients requiring controlled ventilation. Care must be taken not to exceed critical peak inspiratory pressures during deep lung inflations lest rupture of the lung occur.

In patients who cannot cough, sighing should be combined with artificial coughing whenever secretions are audible. The use of chest physiotherapy is used in this situation.

MANAGEMENT OF PATIENTS UNDERGOING PROLONGED ARTIFICIAL VENTI-LATION.—Artificial ventilation is used for patients who suffer from respiratory insufficiency from any cause.

Controlled or assisted ventilation.—Controlled ventilation is used to replace the patient's own respiratory effort when a respirator is attached to the upper airway. The work of breathing is done in large part by the respirator at a predetermined frequency and tidal volume.

During assisted ventilation, the inspiratory phase of breathing is triggered by the patient's spontaneous effort, which in turn is boosted by the respirator, having been set at a predetermined volume or pressure. The frequency of respirators is triggered by the patient's respiratory efforts and needs.

Indications for artificial ventilation

1. When doses of relaxant medication are given in sufficient amounts for abdominal relaxation

2. Paralysis of the respiratory muscles

3. In chronic lung disease where there is increased carbon dioxide retention

4. When the work of breathing is increased due to severe lung pathology, severe asthma attacks or following extensive pulmonary secretions

5. When movements of the diaphragm are restricted due to abdominal surgery, distention, obesity or with tight binders around the thorax and abdomen

6. Metabolic acidosis, as may occur during diseases of the kidney and liver

7. When there is general obstruction of the airway from any cause

8. When there is severe shunting, 40% and above

When to start artificial ventilation

1. Signs of anoxia
   a) Restlessness
   b) Dyspnea
   c) Increased work of breathing
   d) Profused sweating
   e) Rise in blood pressure and pulse rate followed by a fall in both

2. Volume exchange
   a) Inadequate or decreased tidal volume
   b) Increased rate of breathing
   c) Increase in anatomic dead space
   d) Decreased vital capacities
   e) Increase in physiologic dead space

3. Hypoxia
   a) Never rely on cyanosis; when in doubt, blood gas determinations should be done
   b) When hypoxia develops, compensating circulating changes take place which tend to maintain the supply of oxygen to the brain

4. Carbon dioxide accumulation
   a) Hypercapnia is usually recognizable: by (1) skin becomes hot, flushed and moist (2) surgical wounds bleed freely, (3) rise in blood pressure (4) marked increase in secretions produced or accumulated and (5) cerebral congestion develops and the cerebrospinal fluid pressure increases

5. Hyperventilation
   a) Tendency toward hyperventilation when ventilating patient with hand resuscitator
   b) When using ventilators, there is a tendency to hypoventilate patients
   c) Hyperventilation in excess can lead to tetany, which is a twitching of facial muscles or limbs

Estimation of ventilation requirements

1. Frequent blood gas determinations
2. Monitoring of tidal volumes and taking end-expiratory CO_2 samples

3. Monitoring the inspired oxygen concentration
4. Use of nomograms (Figs. 98 and 99)

Maintenance of a clear airway

1. Frequent suctioning
   a) Endotracheal tube
   b) Tracheostomy tube
   c) Nasotracheal tube
2. Positioning
3. Patency of airway

TECHNIQUE IN ARTIFICIAL VENTILATION

During controlled ventilation, the patient must have a cuffed endotracheal or tracheotomy tube in place. The tube prevents gastric inflation and variable air leaks. These tubes also facilitate tracheobronchial suctioning and provide a patent airway with fairly constant resistance. Assisted respiration by mechanical means is not satisfactory via a mask when it is strapped in place without a knowledgeable attendant supporting the airway. Usually, the results are leakage of air, gastric insufflation and hypoventilation.

Tracheal tubes are usually tolerated well by patients in need of artificial ventilation, even when conscious, provided there is minimal or no movement of the head. Laryngeal obstruction very rarely occurs following intubation of several days duration, if cleanliness, optimal humidification and aseptic suctioning techniques are used.

If necessary, small amounts of opiates or "softening doses" of curare are given to make the patient tolerate the tracheal tube without bucking. Whenever artificial ventilation is required for short periods, an endotracheal tube should be inserted first. In some infants, soft plastic orotracheal or nasotracheal tubes have been used successfully for several weeks.

When using an orotracheal tube, a bite block is essential for securing the tube in place. These bite blocks can be made of rolled gauze and toy tape and placed between the teeth. The endotracheal tube must be firmly secured to the respirator with nonkinking, slip-proof connectors. To prevent leaks in the airway, air is inserted into the cuff of the endotracheal tube, using precaution not to insert too much as it may cause pressure necrosis over a period of time. In some instances, variable leaks are indicated. If the endotracheal tube has double cuffs, inflation of the cuffs should be done on an alternate basis every hour. When single cuffed tubes are used, they should be deflated 2–5 minutes every hour, if feasible.

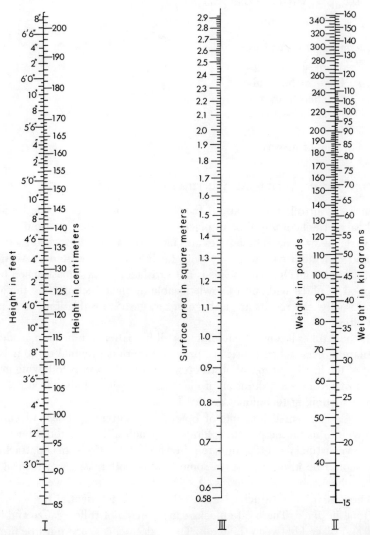

Fig. 98.—DuBois body surface chart (as prepared by Boothby and Sandford of the Mayo Clinic). Directions: to find body surface of a patient, locate the height in inches (or centimeters) on scale *I* and the weight in pounds (or kilograms) on scale *II* and place a straight edge (ruler) between these two points which will intersect scale *III* at the patient's surface area.

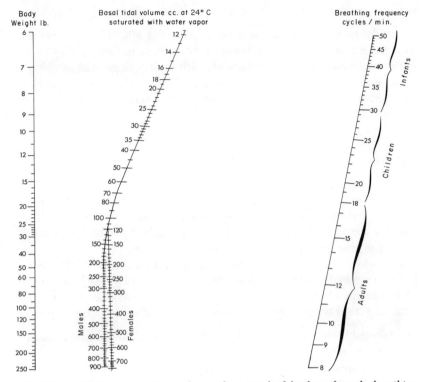

Body Weight lb.	Basal tidal volume cc. at 24° C saturated with water vapor		Breathing frequency cycles / min.

Fig. 99.—Radford nomogram for predicting the optimal tidal volume from the breathing frequency and body weight of the patient. Corrections to be applied as required: *daily activity,* add 10%; *fever,* add 5% for each degree F above 99° (rectal); *altitude,* add 5% for each 2,000 feet above sea level; *metabolic acidosis during anesthesia,* add 20%; *tracheotomy and endotracheal intubations,* subtract a volume equal to ½ the body weight; *added dead space with anesthesia apparatus,* add volume of apparatus and mask dead space.

Tracheotomy is indicated for respirator care when the need for a tracheal airway is anticipated for a prolonged period of time. Tracheotomies facilitate removal of secretions and reduce anatomic dead space, which may improve ventilation.

Tracheotomy should be performed in a well-oxygenated patient whose ventilation is assisted via a manual-inflating bag and mask or manual-inflating bag and endotracheal tube. Tracheotomy should not be used as an emergency reoxygenation procedure.

Cuffed tubes are preferred in adults to prevent air leakage, thereby providing constant tidal volume ventilation. The cuff also prevents aspiration of foreign matter. In small children, uncuffed tubes are used to minimize trauma because leakage is a minor problem due to the multiple gradation of tube sizes available.

Ventilators are becoming increasingly complex and difficult to operate. New models are continuously being introduced. It is, therefore, more important to have a good understanding of the physiologic and mechanical principles underlying mechanical ventilation rather than have a superficial knowledge of the mechanical peculiarities of the many different ventilators in use.

WEANING PATIENTS FROM RESPIRATOR SUPPORT

The patient should stay on controlled ventilation no longer than is necessary; weaning should start as soon as possible since the longer the period of controlled ventilation, the greater will be the weakness of the respiratory muscles due to prolonged inactivity. Also, psychologically this helps the patient in that he can see the progress he is making.

A good rule of thumb in weaning a patient from controlled ventilation is not to attempt weaning until the vital capacity is 10 ml/kg body weight. This corresponds to approximately twice the normal tidal volume. The following steps are usually used in weaning the patient from the respirator:

1. Assisted breathing for at least 15 minutes and, if possible, increased expiratory resistance.
2. Vital capacity 10 ml/kg body weight.
3. Blood gas determinations.
4. If blood gases are within normal range, the patient is allowed to breathe without the respirator for 3–4 minutes.
5. Every half hour gradually increase the period off the respirator if tolerated.
6. Adequately humidified oxygen is always provided when the patient is off the respirator.
7. Serial blood gases are drawn, analyzed and read.
8. Continue blood gas determinations until the patient is well along in the weaning process and until arterial blood gas studies indicate that adequate oxygenation is maintained while breathing room air.
9. Close observation of the vital signs.
10. During weaning period, the patient may require assisted ventilation during night hours.

THE MÖRCH PISTON RESPIRATOR (FIG. 100)

1. Motor-driven timed-cycled controller.
2. Exhibits characteristics of both controlled-pressure and controlled-volume ventilators.

3. An electric motor which drives a large-bore piston.

4. Frequency of respiratory cycle is regulated by a variable speed gear.

5. The stroke of the piston is determined by a variable crank.

6. Air is entrained through a filter into the cylinder with provision for enrichment with oxygen.

7. Air is expelled into the patient from the cylinder through an unheated, blowover humidifier and an automatic nonrebreathing valve.

8. The Mörch Piston ventilator was designed for attachment to a loose-fitting metal tracheotomy tube.

9. In use, the stroke of the piston is adjusted to provide adequate expansion of the lungs and to compensate for the deliberate leak which serves to sweep secretions accumulating around the tube upward through the larynx.

10. Variation in the resistance of the leak alters airway peak pressure reciprocally so that an increase of the leak will result in a lower airway

Fig. 100.—Schematic diagram of the Mörch Piston Respirator. *A*, variable crank; *B*, speed variator; *C*, electrical motor; *D*, nonrebreathing valve; *E*, metal tracheotomy tube without cuff; *F*, blowover humidifier (unheated); *G*, cylinder; *H*, piston; *I*, check valve; *J*, air-uptake filter.

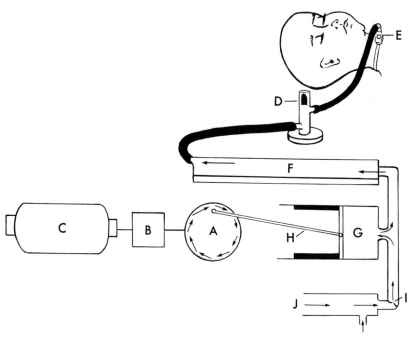

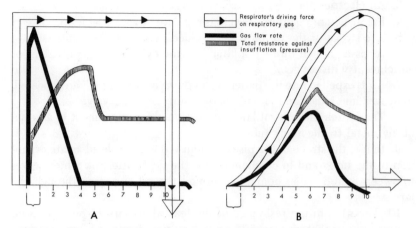

Fig. 101.—Example **A** illustrates the principal differences in characteristics between common types of respirators. Notice the harmful effect on intrapulmonary gas distribution because the respirator's driving force on respiratory gas starts abruptly, with a resulting high initial rate of gas flow which decreases when resistance increases. In example **B**, the driving force on respiratory gas gradually increases due to accelerating speed of the piston in the cylinder, thus causing the flow rate of the inspiratory gas to increase simultaneously with increasing resistance (increasing force generator). The effect on intrapulmonary gas distribution is even.

pressure and relatively less tidal volume will be lost. Conversely, a reduction in the size of the leak causes an increase in airway pressure which increases the flow rate through the leak and protects the patient from overexpansion.

11. No pressure-relief valve is included in the system, resulting in high-peak pressures being delivered in airway impedances.

THE ENGSTRÖM RESPIRATOR (FIG. 102)

1. A controlled volume, timed-cycled controller.

2. An electric motor-driven piston in a double-ended cylinder drives gases into a rigid plastic canister during the inspiratory phase.

3. A sliding-valve mechanism in the cylinder releases the pressure generated by the piston before the stroke is completed, so that the ratio of the inspiratory phase to total cycle duration is 0 : 33.

4. A bag enclosed in the plastic dome is compressed and a predetermined volume of gas is forced into the patient's airway through a warmed flowover humidifier.

5. During the exhalation phase, the dome is evacuated by the piston and cylinder and a measured amount of air, which can be enriched with oxygen, is drawn into the bag through an adjustable vent.

6. The airway pressure in the inspiratory line is indicated by both an aneroid manometer and a water manometer, which also acts as an adjustable pressure relief valve.

7. The expired gas can be vented through a respirometer, which measures the volume of the exhaled air, or it can be opened to a Venturi which is powered by the opposite side of the cylinder and which can produce negative airway pressure to promote circulation or compensate for narrow-lumened endotracheal or tracheotomy tubes.

8. Changes of airway resistance are easily detected on the water manometer by a rise in the inspiratory phase airway pressure; increased peak inspiratory pressure signals the need for tracheal aspiration.

9. A decrease in the exhaled tidal volume indicated on the spirometer warns of a leak in the airway or the connection to the airway.

Fig. 102.—Diagram of the Engström Respirator, Model 150. *1*, pressure regulator for the Venturi; *2*, selector switch; *3*, left compressor manometer; *4*, compressor cylinder; *5*, respirator bladder; *7*, adjusting screw for water manometer; *9*, Venturi recording negative airway pressure; *10*, dosage valve calibrator; *11*, regulator for insufflation rate; *12*, right compressor manometer; *14*, dosage valve for atmospheric air; *15*, pressure-relieving valve, also used for instantaneous emptying of respiration bladder; *16*, inlet stopcock for the rotameter unit; *17*, pressure-controlled expiration valve; *18*, additional inspiration valve, two positions (open and closed); *19*, precision manometer; *20*, rotameter unit; *21*, water manometer tube; *22*, vertically adjustable indicator; *23*, connection for manual operation; *24*, metal connection; *25*, condensed-water retainer; *27*, Y-piece (straight); *28*, tracheal tube with inflatable rubber cuff; *29*, respiratory frequency regulator (between 10 and 30 cycles per minute); *30*, three-way stopcock with three positions—to Venturi, to spirometer, for expanding lungs; *31*, spirometer measuring the expiratory volume; *32*, valve box containing the pressure-controlled expiratory valve; *33*, glass cylinder containing the water trap with water manometer and the respiration bladder; *41*, blocking tube for the water trap, reversible, with engraved instruction text; *44*, heating cushion to increase relative humidity of the inhaled gases.

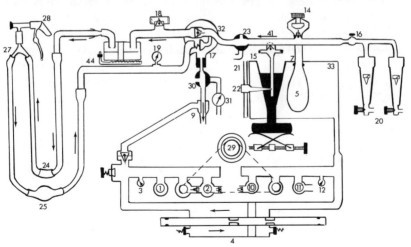

GENERAL COMMENTS.—The Engström Respirator is used to provide mechanical assistance in the absence of the patient's respiratory effort. The Engström Respirator Model 150 will deliver accurately the predetermined alveolar ventilation under a wide range of compliance and resistance changes without adjustment of the unit. Utilization of a primary or driving system and a secondary or patient-supply system allows this flexibility. The "increasing force generator" of this respirator indirectly provides an accelerating flow of the tidal volume to the alveoli. The slow initial flow, which constantly accelerates even against increasing frictional airway resistance, insures that alveoli behind the more stenosed bronchi receive as large a percentage of the predetermined volume as possible. The increasing force generator of the Engström Respirator provides gas flow in the patient's system which continuously accelerates, even as the pressure increases during the inspiratory time. The more stenosed bronchi, having been expanded as much as possible during the slow flow at the beginning of insufflation, will allow a more uniform inflation of the more inaccessible alveoli during the higher gas flow rate.

The Engström Respirator incorporates a waterlock which limits patient airway pressure to a predetermined safe level. During obstruction of the airway, the unit will indicate visibly and audibly that preset tidal volume is in part blown off. The Engström Respirator allows for spontaneous inspiration at any time and at any flow rate, without resistance, as required by the patient. The patient expiratory valve, which is operated pneumatically, allows the pressure in the alveoli behind the collapsed bronchi to recede in phase with the respirator pressure, thus precluding collapse of stenosed bronchi.

The Engström Respirator devotes two thirds of the total respiratory cycle to expiration. This is clinically an optimal ratio of inspiration to expiration and can be maintained because the inspiration, by accelerating flow technique, assures that the total insufflation can be accomplished in a designated time, regardless of patient compliance, airway resistance and the tidal volume required. The mean airway pressure is thus kept at the lowest possible range while still maintaining required alveolar ventilation.

There is a selective mean by which negative pressure can be used to support expiration. When in operation, the negative phase is initiated during the last half of the expiratory phase. When the negative-phase pressure is used, there is sufficient time before the start of the next active inspiration to allow the thorax to return to its normal position.

TECHNIQUE.—The technique is as follows:

1. Connect the patient-supply tubing to the flowover humidifier.
2. Fill the humidifier with sterile distilled water.

3. Fill the column in the waterlock of the overpressure aggregate.

4. Start the motor by means of an electrical switch.

5. Adjust the desired minute ventilation; the respiration gas is in most instances composed of liters of air per minute adjusted on the dosing valve and liters of oxygen per minute adjusted on the oxygen rotometer.

6. Adjust the respiratory frequency to the desired rate while the motor is running.

7. Adjust by means of the control the right manometer to $+55$ cm H_2O and adjust the deviation of the needle to the left of the same manometer as far as the red mark, by means of the control. Adjust the waterlock to read 35 cm H_2O. By this adjustment, an automatically ranging pressure of at least 20 cm H_2O will result in the overpressure aggregate, causing the rubber bag to collapse during each inspiration and delivering the respiration gas to the patient. If the air passages of the patient offer a greater resistance than 35 cm H_2O (the level to which the waterlock has been adjusted), the gas will partly bubble out through the waterlock.

8. If negative pressure in the airways is necessary, adjust the Venturi control to the desired negative pressure, which will be indicated on the manometer. The selector switch is adjusted to Venturi and the three-way stopcock is also adjusted to the Venturi position.

9. Check the unit by obstructing the "T" piece with your thumb.

10. Make connection to the patient's endotracheal or tracheotomy tube.

Adjustments

1. In the presence of spontaneous respirations by the patient adjust the supplementary inspiratory valve to closed position.

2. Check for leaks in the patient-supply system.

3. Check for total gas respiration per minute, which has been adjusted. (The total gas consumed should be equal to the input volume present on the rotometer and/or dosing valve.)

How to correct irregularities

1. If there is bubbling through the waterlock due to an increase in resistance for any reason:

Correction
a) Suction the patient with sterile catheter
b) Check the position of the tracheal tube
c) The connection for manual operation has been left in manual operation position; turn it to automatic ventilation
d) The three-way stopcock has been put into the position "danger"; turn the three-way stopcock to the position spirometer or Venturi

2. If the patient expires less per minute than the total minute ventilation which has been adjusted on the respirator:

Correction

a) The dosing valve has been filled with dust; clean dosing valve with alcohol and replace
b) The oxygen supply is exhausted; replace oxygen supply
c) Leaks may occur around the tracheotomy or endotracheal tube or anywhere in the inspiratory supply system
d) The plexiglass cover of the valve box is loose; tighten and recheck for leaks
e) The deviation to the left of the indicator of the manometer is adjusted incorrectly; adjust to red mark

EMERSON POSTOPERATIVE VENTILATOR (FIG. 103)

The Emerson Postoperative Ventilator is used to provide continuous mechanical assistance in the absence of the patient's respiratory effort. The respirator will deliver a predetermined volume of gas or gases during each inspiratory phase. At a constant flow, the inspiratory pressure will increase as the lung compliance decreases. *Example:* Flow 10 L per minute pressure 25 cm H_2O may increase to 30 cm H_2O at the same flow because of a decreasing compliance. A kettle is incorporated into the system to provide adequate humidification of the inspired air. This kettle is heated by a hot plate underneath to approximately 120° C. Supplementary oxygen, or oxygen and an anesthetic gas, may be administered through a hose connection located on the back of the ventilator, which leads to the accumulator or "trombone" just upstream from the piston chamber.

TECHNIQUE.—The technique is as follows:

1. Attach the power cord to an alternating current, 110-volt, 60-cycle electric outlet.

2. Put warm water in the humidifier kettle until its level shows at the middle of the gauge glass at the right.

3. Turn on the heater switch marked "pump," on the upper panel.

4. Turn on the motor switch marked "humidity," on the upper panel.

5. Adjust the tidal volume by turning the handwheel located low center on the front of the ventilator. Above this is a scale which shows the selected stroke volume. The amount of gas actually delivered to the patient's lungs will be somewhat less than the stroke volume selected because of loss through compression of dead space air. Measure tidal volume during exhalation with respirometer attached to tracheal tube.

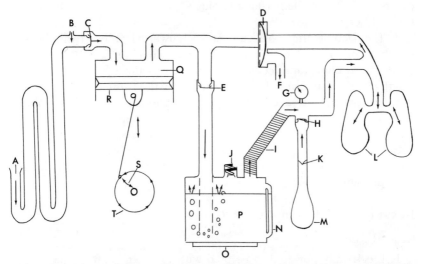

Fig. 103.—Schema of Emerson Postoperative Ventilator. *A,* air inlet; *B,* oxygen inlet; *C,* inlet check valve; *D,* diaphragm-controlled exhaust valve; *E,* outlet check valve; *F,* exhaled air; *G,* pressure gauge; *H,* check valve; *I,* copper wool; *J,* adjustable blowoff valve; *K,* valve opens on inhalation cycle only; *L,* patient's lungs; *M,* deep breather; *N,* humidifier; *O,* heater; *P,* water; *Q,* variable volume; *R,* piston; *S,* variable stroke; *T,* variable speed, each half revolution.

6. Respiratory rate is controlled by adjustments marked "inhale" and "exhale" on the front panel. When both are turned clockwise, the rate is more rapid. When only one of the adjustments is turned, the phase that it controls is lengthened or shortened. Thus, the respiratory pattern can be selected that will govern inhalation and exhalation. Usually, exhalation time is twice that of inhalation time, but this will vary with the patient being treated.

7. A trim screw, located between the inhalation and exhalation adjustments, permits speed compensation if the ventilator is operated on abnormal line voltages. Optional voltage regulators are available.

8. The tubing from the ventilator to the patient should not be allowed to sag and collect moisture. A trap jar in the inspiratory line is provided on the front of the ventilator which must be emptied from time to time.

9. The spirometer is mounted over the control panel on a frame made of stainless steel tubing. When the flexible hose of the spirometer is connected to the exhalation port of the ventilator, each exhaled breath advances the spirometer needle. This needle indicates approximate tidal volumes. Approximate minute volumes can be determined by noting the total

excursion of the needle during a minute's time. It can be used either continuously or intermittently.

10. The deep-breathing attachment is a blower which is activated periodically to provide a greatly increased tidal volume for several breaths. A control knob allows for a decrease or an increase in the sighing pressure. The length of time between sighs is determined by the width of a notch in the slowly revolving black and white disc. This is normally set for the minimum of two breaths, but may be adjusted to a larger percentage of the total 7-minute cycle if the setting screw is loosened. There is an on-and-off switch between the time and pressure adjustments, and there is a test button which permits manual operation of the "sigh" during treatment or for setting the peak pressure.

Bennett MA-I Respirator (Fig. 104)

General features:

1. Electrically powered to be used with 115-volt AC 60 cycle.
2. The unit is a controller, assistor or an assistor-controller.
3. Volume limiting.
4. Gas percentages may be regulated from room air to 100% oxygen.
5. Heated adjustable humidity can be delivered into the inspiratory line from a cascade nebulizer.
6. Bronchodilators and other aerosols can be administered from an inline 70-ml nebulizer.
7. There is a spirometer for monitoring exhaled volumes of gases.
8. Alarm system for monitoring system preset pressure limits.
9. Adjustable flow.
10. Thermometer in system to measure inspired gas temperature.
11. Automatic deep-breathing unit with adjustable sighing volumes and rate per hour.
12. Adjustable sensitivity.
13. Monitoring lights for assisted ventilation, as well as for indicating the deep breath (sigh).
14. Adjustable expiratory retard.
15. Built-in circuit breaker.
16. Negative-pressure control.
17. Oxygen-in-use monitoring light.

Assembly.—The assembly of the Bennett MA-I Respirator is carried out as follows (Fig. 105):

1. Assemble unit by attaching the mounting plate to the right side of the respirator with the four screws provided.

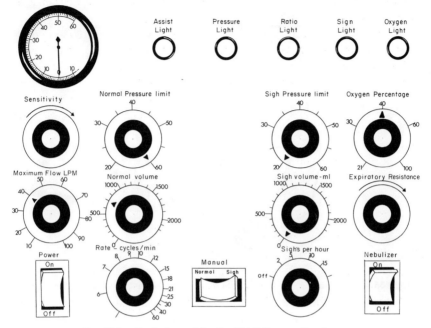

Fig. 104.—Control panel for the MA-I Bennett Respirator.

2. Insert the condenser tube into the mounting bracket. Tighten and mount the spirometer base on the tube.

3. Set the black hard rubber tube to the color-coded connector (black) underneath the spiromcter base and to the black spirometer connector.

4. Connect condenser and vial to the condenser tube.

5. Connect cascade humidifier to the heater assembly; secure in place by the two knobs.

6. Inside the door, connect main flow bacteria filter through the hole at the upper left, observing the flow direction listed on the filter. Secure in place.

7. Connect the angled connector to the filter outlet and to humidifier inlet. Fit the right-angle tube to the filter inlet to the outlet.

8. Screw the support arm into the top of the unit. Attach manifold assembly to the support arm. Insert bacteria filter to the white jet connector on manifold.

9. Connect main-line tube to the humidifier outlet and the manifold inlet.

10. If the optional negative-pressure attachment is supplied, detach if not to be used.

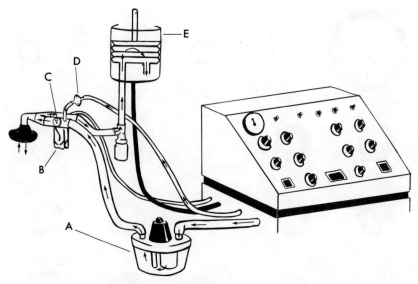

Fig. 105.—Schema of an MA-I Bennett Respirator readied for use. *A*, humidifier; *B*, nebulizer; *C*, thermometer; *D*, bacteria filter; *E*, spirometer.

TECHNIQUE.—The technique is as follows:

1. Switch on the electrical power unit.

2. Fill humidifier jar (Fig. 106) with sterile distilled water to the full mark and set temperature control to numeral 6. Allow a warm-up time of 5–10 minutes.

3. Place medication as ordered in nebulizer.

4. Adjust maximal flow control to 40 L per minute, or as necessary for adequate flow.

5. Set the normal pressure limit control in accordance with compliance/resistance changes.

6. Adjust the required tidal volume. The respirator is designed for use as a volume respirator with pressure variable and with pressure limits acting as a safety and warning feature.

7. Determine the frequency of respiration per minute.

8. Set sensitivity to "off" position by turning counterclockwise during controlled ventilation. During assisted ventilation, adjust as necessary by turning clockwise.

9. Adjust the number of sighs per minute as well as the volume of each sigh.

10. Set nebulizer switch at "off."

11. Adjust the pressure warning buzzer to desired level.

12. Adjust for desired oxygen concentration as determined by blood gas analysis.

13. Record the expired tidal volumes after correction for tubing compliance.

During a manual, assisted or controlled ventilation, the Bennett MA-I Respirator determines whether the breath will be to the normal volume

Fig. 106.—Cascade variable humidifier is used in line with IPPB units or ventilators in order to add substantial quantities of water vapor to the inspired gases. The gases enter the inlet (B) from IPPB unit and go through a one-way valve and depress the surface of the water beneath the tower (G). This causes the water within the reservoir to rise above the level of the small port in the side of the tower. Water flows through this port and "cascades" in a thin film across a grid. The resulting agitation creates a foam that provides a large interface or contact area, insuring rapid evaporation. A, water temperature control; B, inlet; C, cover; D, safety shut-off control; E, jar; F, cascade effect; G, tower; H, thermoswitch; I, thermowells; J, heater; K, outlet.

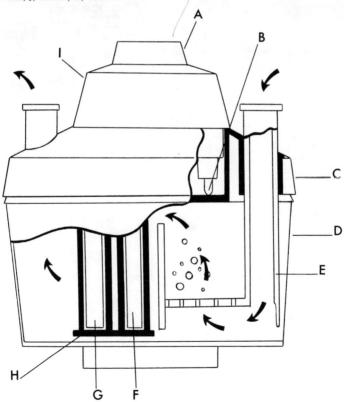

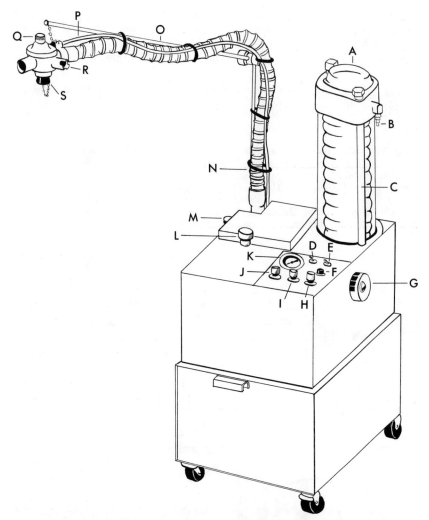

Fig. 107.—Operating features of the Air-Shields Respirator. *A,* microfilter; *B,* oxygen nipple adaptor; *C,* tidal volume indicator scale; *D,* "on-off" switch; *E,* control-assist control switch; *F,* assisted ventilation indicator lamp; *G,* adjustable flow control (volume 0–2,400 cc); *H,* expiratory time control; *I,* sensitivity control; *J,* inspiratory time control; *K,* pressure manometer; *L,* humidity chamber knob; *M,* humidity reservoir fill pipe; *N,* patient supply tubing; *O,* support arm; *P,* pressure relief small-bore tube; *Q,* expiratory resistance control; *R,* expiratory port; *S,* nebulizer attachment port.

and pressure limits. If it is to the sigh limits, the sigh indicator lights and will stay on until the next inspiration starts. If inspiration is begun by patient effort, the assist indicator lights to indicate this action. It is also possible for both assist and sigh indicators to light together, since the timed periodic sigh is triggered by normal rate, assist or normal sigh start.

During inspiration, the gases pass through the main flow bacteria filter and through the humidifier. If the nebulizer switch is on, a fraction of gas is diverted to the nebulizer.

AIR-SHIELDS RESPIRATOR (FIG. 107)

1. Controlled volume, timed-cycled assistor-controller.
2. Electrically driven motor.
3. Sensitivity adjustable at maximal setting requires displacement of 4 cc to activate assistor.
4. Bellows of 2,500 cc assures sufficient capacity to ventilate most patients.
5. Air cut-off plate allows delivery of 100% oxygen if desired.
6. Pressure-breathing monitor warns of power failure, accidental dislocation of connecting tubing to endotracheal or tracheotomy tubes.
7. Entrainment of room air through a microfilter.
8. Spinning disc blower over humidifier provides mist to inspired air.
9. Operator can vary expiratory resistance.
10. Inspired gases can be adjusted within the range of 21% up to 100% oxygen by adjusting the flow to the ventilator from a reducing valve that is back-pressure compensated.
11. Tidal volumes can be monitored.

REFERENCES

Rattenborg, C. C.: Basic Mechanics of Artificial Ventilation, in *Management of Life-Threatening Poliomyelitis*, Lassen, H. C. A. (ed.) (Edinburgh: E. & S. Livingstone, Ltd. 1956), p. 23.
Elam, J. O.; Kern, J. H., and Janney, C. D.: Performance of ventilators, effect of changes in lung-thorax compliance, Anesthesiology 19:56, 1958.
Mapleson, W. W.: The classification of respirators, Anesthesiology 16:512, 1961.
Engstrom, C. G., and Norlander, O. P.: A new method for analysis of respiratory work by measurements of the actual power as a function of gas flow, pressure and time, Acta anesth. scandinav. 6:49, 1962.
Sechzer, P. H.: *The Bird Respirator* (Houston, Tex.: D. H. White & Co., 1965).
Saklad, M., Wickliff, D.: Functional characteristics of artificial ventilators, Anesthesiology 28:716, 1967.
Pierce, E. C., and Vandam, L. D.: Intermittent positive pressure breathing, J. Am. So. Anesthes. 23:478, 1962.

Mead, J., and Whittenberger, J. L.: Physical properties of human lungs measured during spontaneous respiration, J. Appl. Physiol. 5:12, 1953.

Fenn, W.: Mechanics of respiration, Am. J. Med. 10:77, 1951.

Dittmer, D. S., and Grebe, R. M. (eds.): *Handbook of Respiration* (Part XI) (Philadelphia: W. B. Saunders Company, 1958), p. 137.

CHAPTER 11

Chest Physiotherapy

CHEST PHYSIOTHERAPY is used for the prevention of respiratory complications and for the improvement of pulmonary function in cases of acute or chronic pulmonary disease. The physiologic rationale is to teach proper relaxation in order to avoid muscle splinting; to train patients in the effective use of both normal and accessory respiratory muscles for the purposes of effective coughing and expansion of all parts of the lungs; and to aid in the removal of secretions by postural drainage and by manual assistance to coughing.

DIAPHRAGMATIC OR ABDOMINAL BREATHING

The first step in this method of removing secretions from the lungs and to provide adequate gas exchange is to teach the patient how to breathe deeply, using his diaphragm. The procedure for this is as follows:

1. Position the patient flat on his back with his head and neck in a neutral position and his knees flexed to permit the abdominal muscles to relax and allow maximal excursion of the diaphragm. (Once the patient has learned to breathe easily in this position, he should practice diaphragmatic breathing while lying prone on either side, or while sitting and standing.)

2. Teach him to inhale quietly through his nostrils, using his diaphragm to balloon the upper abdomen. (In learning this maneuver, the patient often finds it helpful to place one hand on his midabdomen.)

3. The patient is then instructed to exhale through his mouth while contracting his abdominal muscles.

4. Lateral expansion of the chest cage is best taught by applying counter pressure to the sides of the chest during inspiration, making the patient fully aware of his chest expansion.

5. Apical expansion is similarly brought to the patient's awareness by applying counter pressure just below the clavicles during inspiration.

POSTURAL DRAINAGE

In postural drainage, the patient assumes an "upside down" position so that the force of gravity, assisted by the natural ciliary activity of the smaller bronchial airways, will move secretions upward toward the main bronchi and the trachea. From this point the patient can cough them up.

Recently, it has been found that more effective drainage can be obtained if the patient is positioned according to the exact site of his disease. In bronchiectasis and chronic bronchitis, copious amounts of secretions are produced every day; therefore, it is necessary to let the patient assume the proper positions for 15–60 minutes, or as tolerated, several times daily.

For the great majority of patients receiving respirator support, and following surgery, less exaggerated positions need be assumed. Postural drainage is carried out in a head-down tilt of 10° to 20° with the patient in the lateral position, which favors drainage from the lower lobe of the upper lung. The straight lateral position is required for emptying the lateral segments; a more prone position favors removal of secretions from the posterior segment; a more supine position favors drainage of the middle lobe or the lingula, as well as the anterior segments of the lower lobe.

CUPPING

The technique is carried out with the operator's hand in a cupped position while the wrist is alternately flexed and extended (Fig. 108). The procedure is as follows:

1. The patient's chest wall over the involved area is cupped gently, usually for 1 or 2 minutes.

2. The air between the operator's hand and the chest wall is trapped, producing a characteristic hollow sound.

3. The percussive action produced by this dislodges plugs of mucus, allowing air in the lungs to penetrate behind the secretions and move them toward the main bronchi and trachea.

4. Cupping should not be attempted, however, if the patient is hemorrhaging or in severe pain.

5. Clapping is a similar procedure, but performed with the palm extended (Fig. 109).

VIBRATING

Vibrating is done only during the exhalation phase of breathing (Fig. 110). The technique is as follows:

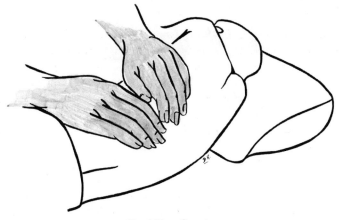

Fig. 108.—Cupping.

1. The patient is instructed to use diaphragmatic abdominal breathing, or, if he has not learned to do this, he is instructed to inhale through his nose and to exhale slowly and fully through the mouth.

2. The therapist places one hand on top of the other over the affected area or one hand on each side of the patient's rib cage, being careful to avoid the abdominal areas.

Fig. 109.—Clapping.

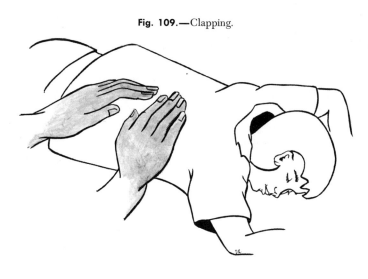

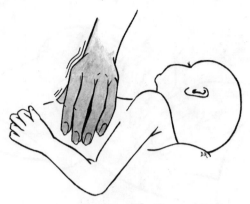

Fig. 110.—Vibration.

3. As the patient exhales, the therapist produces gentle vibratory movements which are transmitted to the patient's chest wall through the therapist's arms and hands. It is important for the therapist to use his shoulder muscles only, not those of the arms and hands, in this procedure to prevent damage to the ribs and internal organs.

4. After three or four vibrations, the patient is encouraged to cough using his abdominal muscles to increase the effectiveness of the cough.

THERAPY CYCLE

1. Tell the patient to commence diaphragmatic breathing slowly and deeply.

2. Position the patient according to the location of the involved area in the lung (Figs. 111–121), being certain that his spine is as straight as possible to permit optimal expansion of the rib cage.

3. Cup the chest wall for one to two minutes.

4. Have the patient inhale deeply; then, as he exhales, vibrate the chest wall during three or four exhalations.

5. Encourage him to cough using his abdominal muscles after a sufficient volume of air has been inhaled.

6. Allow him to rest for a minute or two; then repeat *steps* 3 through 6 for as long as is consistent with his condition and tolerance, which is usually 15–20 minutes.

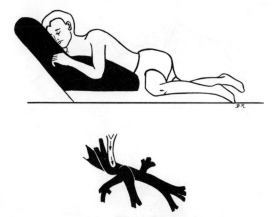

Fig. 111.—Position of patient for drainage of the left upper lobe and posterior segment of the lungs. Patient is positioned by making a quarter turn from prone-lying position, with right arm outstretched behind. Three pillows are used to raise the head and shoulders.

Fig. 112.—Position of patient for drainage of the lower lobes and posterior basal segments of the lungs. This method is useful when a frame is not available or space is limited. A sheet of foam rubber placed on the floor keeps the pillow clean and prevents its slipping. NOTE: The patient lies across the bed, with forearms resting on a pillow on the floor. The maintenance of an angle of 45° is essential to obtain maximal drainage. Common faults include: not being certain that the mattress covers the side of the bed; shoulder hunching; too perpendicular a position; the pillow too far from the bed, causing a hollow in the lumbar region and a flattening of the thorax.

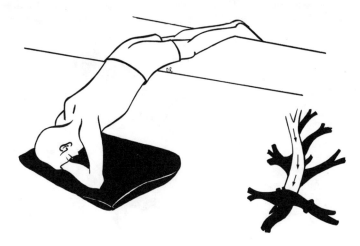

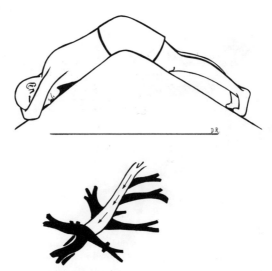

Fig. 113.—Position of patient for drainage of the lower lobes and posterior basal segments of the lungs. Patient is positioned over the frame, comfortably relaxed, with head slightly turned and resting on hands. The frame must be fixed at an angle of 90°. PRECAUTIONS: Be certain that the patient is secured in place by means of pillows at the head and on both sides of the mattress.

Fig. 114.—Position of patient for drainage of the lower lobes and posterior basal segments of the lungs. Patient is placed in prone position with two pillows under abdomen. This position should be used only when the positions shown in Figures 112 and 113 are too rigorous; for example, when the physical condition of the patient is critically hazardous to maintain life in the above position. The foot of the bed should be raised 18–20 inches.

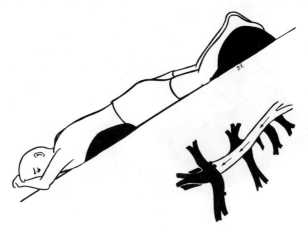

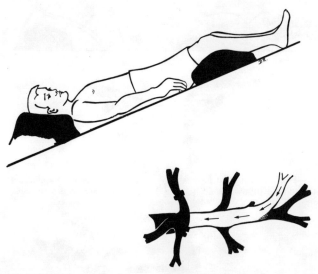

Fig. 115.—Position of patient for drainage of the lower lobes and the anterior basal segments of the lungs. Supine position with pillow under knees to assist relaxation of abdominal muscles. Foot of the bed should be raised 18–20 inches.

Fig. 116.—Position of patient for drainage of the left lower lobe and lateral basal segment of the lung. Side-lying position: pillow should be placed in waistline to keep spine straight. Shoulders must not rest on head pillow. Foot of bed should be raised 18–20 inches. PRECAUTION: A pillow should be wedged between the end of the mattress and the head bars of the bed to reduce slipping. It also acts as a pad for the patient's head.

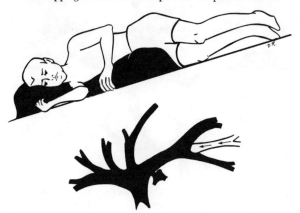

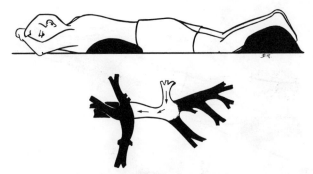

Fig. 117.—Position of patient for drainage of the lower lobes and apical segments of the lung. Prone position: pillow should be placed under abdomen to flatten back.

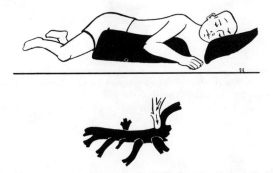

Fig. 118.—Position of patient for drainage of the right upper lobe and posterior segment of the lung. Quarter turn from prone-lying position with left arm outstretched and behind. The pillows should be placed so that the patient does not need to change position in order to expectorate.

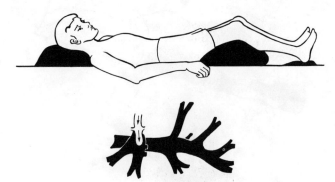

Fig. 119.—Position of patient for drainage of the upper lobes and anterior segments. Patient is placed in supine position with pillow under knees to assist relaxation.

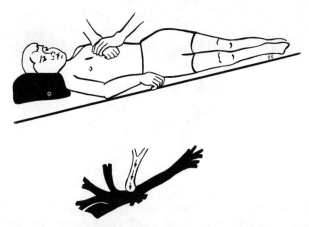

Fig. 120.—Position of patient for drainage of left upper and lingula lobes of the lungs. NOTE: Quarter turn from supine position, left side uppermost. The knees are bent to obtain relaxation of abdominal muscles. The foot of the bed is raised 12 inches. Vibrations are being given over affected area to facilitate removal of secretions.

Fig. 121.—Position of patient for drainage of apical lobes of the lung. The same as for lingula, but it follows that the right side is uppermost and the foot of the bed is raised 12 inches.

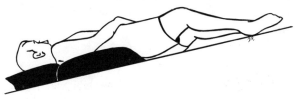

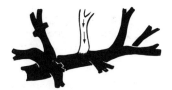

CHAPTER 12

Monitoring Devices

WHENEVER MAN AND MACHINE are placed in synergism with or without further combinations with drugs, there is an immediate need for knowledge of the progress of the event by a third party. This involves some means of data recovery and recording in order logically to make changes so that the system can be maintained. This is especially important in inhalation therapy procedures as machine and drugs are combined to maintain or improve the patient's condition.

The most readily available and adaptable forms of monitoring devices are vision, hearing and tactile sensation. The patient may be observed for changes in color of skin tone, motions of the body or any infrequent or unusual response. The machines may be observed for functional changes, mechanical failure or indicator variations. One may listen for changes in mechanical or pneumatic sounds in both patient and machine and be further aided by the use of certain simple instruments such as the stethoscope. Special attention is paid here to breath sounds which are obtained with a stethoscope (Fig. 122).

Breath Sounds

As a result of the turbulence (Fig. 123) produced by the movement of air through the bronchial tree, vibrations are produced. The rate of these vibrations must be within a certain range and intensity for sounds to be heard.

Sounds produced within the trachea vibrate at approximately 400 cycles per second, whereas sounds produced within a terminal bronchiole vibrate at 1,700 cycles per second.

The pitch of a sound depends on the length and diameter of the tube in which it is produced. If a tube is short and narrow, it will produce a high-pitch sound; on the contrary, if it is wide, it will produce a low-pitch

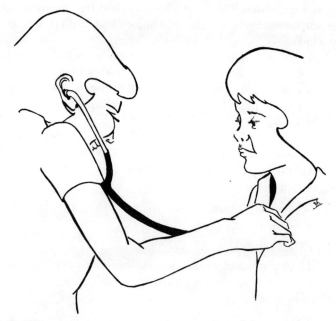

Fig. 122.—Auscultation of breath sounds over the chest with stethoscope.

Fig. 123.—Turbulence in airways during (**A**) expiration and (**B**) inspiration.

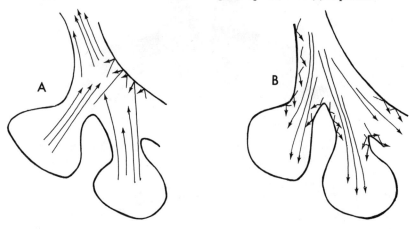

sound. Since each branch in the tracheobronchial tree is narrower than its predecessor, sounds become higher and higher, reaching a peak in the terminal bronchioles.

The "selector transmitter" properties of the alveoli dampen the high frequency vibrations, allowing those sounds with a frequency of 100–150 cycles per second to pass through the alveoli to the chest wall (Fig. 124). It is believed that the lungs lose this selective transmitter ability when they become diseased.

If the alveoli fill with inflammatory exudate, sounds are clearly felt and heard on the overlying chest wall. Auscultation of the lungs (Fig. 125) will detect the vibrations passing through the chest wall. Three observations must be made during auscultation:

1. Character of the breath sounds
2. Character of the vocal resonance
3. Presence or absence of other sounds

There are two types of breath sounds audible in certain parts of the

Fig. 124.—Vibrations produced by (**A**) heavy and (**B**) light percussion.

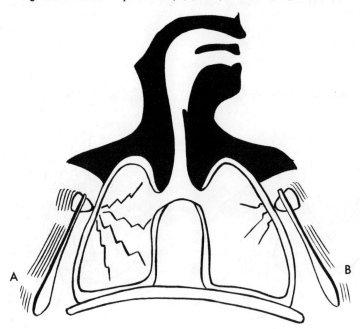

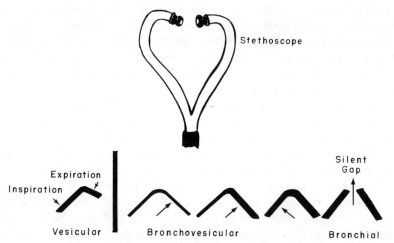

Fig. 125.—The breath sounds heard over the chest wall during auscultation result from the turbulence produced by the movement of air within the tracheobronchial tree.

chest in healthy normal lungs. The first is known as vesicular breathing and the second as bronchial breathing.

Normal breath sounds or vesicular breath sounds are heard over normal lung parenchyma; inspiratory sounds are very intense due to the turbulence produced by the current of air striking the borders of the bronchial bifurcations. They are heard during the whole inspiratory phase; the pitch is low and has a rustling sound.

Expiration follows the inspiratory sound without a pause; it only remains audible during the earlier part of expiration. It has a fainter sound because the exhaled air does not encounter any sharp bifurcations.

The normal breath sounds are heard throughout the entire chest, with the exception of the apex of the right lung where sounds are bronchovesicular because the bronchi are closer to the chest wall and are covered by a small amount of lung tissue. This type combines both vesicular and bronchial elements; in this case, it is usually the expiratory sound which has more of the bronchial character.

This occurs in other regions of the lung where anatomy favors its production, especially at the right apex fossa. In this same area, vocal fremitus and resonance may be increased and some degree of whispering may be heard.

This bronchovesicular sound is longer than a vesicular one; it is louder and higher in pitch. Bronchovesicular sounds are sometimes mistaken for bronchial sounds, but they can be differentiated easily because their end inspiration sound blends with the beginning of the expiratory sound.

If the underlying lung parenchyma is affected by disease which has altered its transmitter properties, bronchovesicular sounds are heard everywhere and will be an indication that some of the alveoli in the diseased area of the lung are still functioning normally (Fig. 126).

BRONCHIAL SOUNDS.—This type of sound is virtually identical with that which is normally heard in auscultation over the trachea, having almost the same intensity, pitch and duration. Bronchial sounds are produced when solidified parenchyma develops around a patent bronchus, making the lung lose its selector transmitter properties and allowing high pitch vibrations within the bronchial tree to be transmitted to the chest wall.

Inspiratory bronchial sounds have a hollow quality; it is moderately intense, becoming inaudible shortly before the end of inspiration. Expiratory bronchial sounds are more intense and the pitch is often higher; they are audible through most of the expiratory phase.

High-pitched bronchial breathing is heard when consolidation has occurred around a smaller tube as in pneumonia, where a perfect example of bronchial breathing may often be found. Here the character is aspirate

Fig. 126.—Patient with a pneumothorax showing the reflection of sound waves at fluid-air interfaces.

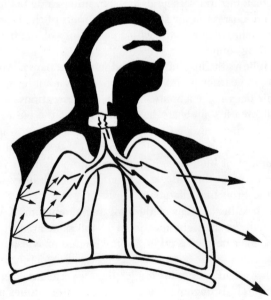

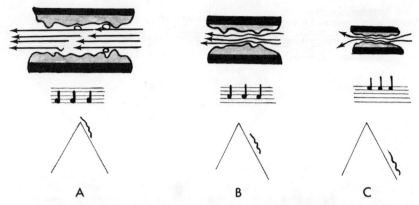

Fig. 127.—Rhonchi or dry sound produced during forced prolonged expiration as air passes through inflamed walls. Diagram demonstrates the relationship between the origin of rhonchi and their pitch. **A,** bronchus; **B,** bronchiole; **C,** terminal bronchiole.

rather than gutteral. This variety is often known as tubular breathing. Bronchial sounds differ from bronchovesicular sounds in that there is a gap between inspiration and expiration.

RHONCHI SOUNDS (FIG. 127).—These are dry sounds, like prolonged snoring or whistling, produced when the lumen of the tubes narrow because a partial obstruction has increased resistance to air flow. The cause of obstruction may be swelling of the mucosa or the presence of viscid secretions.

These sounds are only produced within the lumen of the tracheobronchial tree and are more pronounced in expiration due to the narrowing of the bronchi.

According to their pitch, there are three different types of rhonchi sounds:

1. *Sonorous rhonchous.*—This type originates in the large bronchus
2. *Medium pitch rhonchous.*—This type originates in the internal bronchi
3. *Sibilant rhonchous.*—This type originates in terminal bronchioles

Sibilant rhonchi are characteristic in chronic obstruction, emphysema or in an attack of bronchial asthma. Persistent rhonchi, localized in one part of the chest, are of particular importance because they may signify a growth, bronchostenosis or aspiration of a foreign body.

RALES (FIG. 128).—This type of sound is a short, uninterrupted, moist bubbling sound heard mostly during inspiration. According to their pitch and position, rales are classified or divided into four categories:

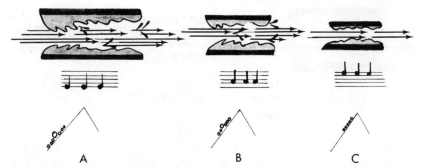

Fig. 128.—Rales or moist sound produced during forced prolonged inspiration as air passes through pus and inflamed walls. Diagram demonstrates the relationship between the origin of rales and their pitch. **A,** bronchus; **B,** bronchiole; **C,** terminal bronchiole.

1. *Coarse rales.*—This type is heard in the initial third of inspiration. They are very low in pitch, originating in the medium and large bronchi. When this type of rale is heard, it is a good indication that exudate is present in the bronchus.

2. *Medium-pitch rales.*—This type is heard during the middle third of inspiration, suggesting that small bronchi are involved.

3. *High-pitch rales.*—This sound is produced in the terminal part of inspiration and suggests the involvement of lung parenchyma.

These rales occur when the alveoli are filled with either serous fluid or inflammatory exudate. Rales are detected during the inspiratory phase because then the intrathoracic pressure is more negative, causing the bubbles of fluid within either bronchi or alveoli to burst. Medium and coarse rales are heard particularly in bronchitis and may also originate in pulmonary cavities.

Sometimes rales which have been heard on ordinary breathing may disappear after a cough, indicating that the secretions producing the rales have moved higher in the bronchial tree.

4. Posttussic rales: These cannot be detected in a normal inspiration, probably due to the small amount of disease involving the alveoli. This type of rale is easily heard at the beginning of inspiration following a cough.

CREPITATIONS.—Crackling interrupted sounds called crepitations are produced either in the alveoli or in the bronchioles and bronchi. They produce noise like the bursting of air bubbles and indicate the presence of fluid in the air cells or tubes. They are heard throughout inspiration as well as expiration. They are a good indication that there is fibrosis in the lung parenchyma or peribronchial tissue.

PLEURAL RUB.—These sounds are predominately heard during the latter part of inspiration and early part of expiration and are produced by the inflamed surface of the two pleural layers rubbing against each other during respiration. They are easily detected in the lower lobes where there is the greatest movement of the lungs.

SUCCUSSION SPLASH.—This type of sound is produced when the thoracic cage is shaken due to the presence in the pleural cavity of air or fluid.

If a bronchopleural fistula is present, there is a gurgling sound during inspiration, caused by air entering the pleural fluid through the fistula.

Tactile use may be made of the fingers and hands for palpation of the pulse and trachea, and the use of the palm on the chest to determine movements.

Devices

Of increasing interest and use are the mechanical devices used for monitoring. These will be briefly described.

The three most commonly used methods for recording data are the kymograph, the cathode ray tube and the magnetic tape system. These may be used in combination with one another; for instance, the cathode tube and the magnetic tape system. Let us briefly examine each of these systems:

THE KYMOGRAPH

In its early form, this device consisted of a smoked drum and stylus. As the smoked drum revolved, the stylus registered its impression by displacing the carbon on the paper. This system has evolved through various pen writers utilizing ink, burning of wax on paper, and photocopying directly from a cathode ray tube.

THE CATHODE RAY TUBE

This may be considered in its simplest form as a beam of electrons projected on a phosphorous screen, causing the screen to glow where it is intersected by the beam. There is retention of the image for a brief period before decay takes place. By the use of vertical and horizontal deflection plates and amplification, it is possible to sweep the beam and to change the size of the tracing (Fig. 129).

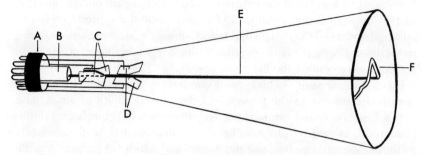

Fig. 129.—Oscilloscope. *A*, base of tube; *B*, electron gun; *C*, horizontal deflection plates; *D*, vertical deflection plates; *E*, beam of electrons; *F*, trace.

Magnetic Tape Systems

This data storage system is utilized in many industries, but probably to the greatest extent by commercial television. It consists of electrical impulses in some form of modulated carrier on the magnetic tape which may be recalled by suitable projection on a cathode tube or direct writer.

Fig. 130.—Diagrammatic representation of electronic acquisition, storage and recovery systems.

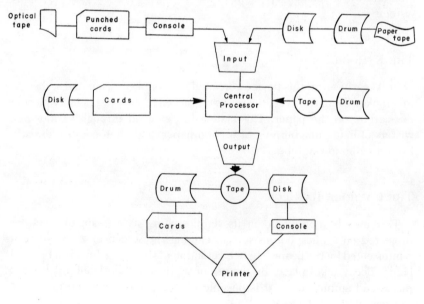

All of these systems are attached to sensors of varying types, depending on the type of parameter which is being monitored. Sensors for electrocardiogram, electroencephalogram, temperature, muscle, muscle activity and similar functions are activated by a change in electrical potential between two or more areas. This is then amplified and displayed (Fig. 130).

Pressure monitoring within a liquid system is best carried out by means of a transducer. The most common transducer in use today is the strain gauge. This is a sensor with combined mechanical and electrical circuitry. The electrical portion consists of a constant-voltage Wheatstone bridge circuit connected usually to a high-performance oscillographic galvanometer. The mechanical portion is a rugged, sterilizable manometer with a "flushing dome" containing the sensory membrane. In order to obtain satisfactory tracings, either hydraulic or electromagnetic damping is necessary to prevent prolonged oscillations of simple harmonic motions.

Simply being able to recover data is of very little value if it cannot be put to some practical use to benefit the patient. We have found in practice that the use of a typical written hospital record does not readily lend itself to very ill patients receiving multiple forms of inhalation therapy. As of this writing, the simplest and most utilizable form of presentation of data is a large display sheet which may be placed on the wall of a patient's room and the multiple parameters compared. It is sometimes difficult to find any correlation between data such as P_{CO_2} obtained 3 hours previous to a recording of P_{O_2} obtained 3 hours previous to a recording of P_{O_2} obtained at the present time. The display chart, therefore, should have time as its ordinate and the multiple parameters as the abscissa.

NOTE: Charts follow on pages 206–210

REFERENCES

Dornette, W. H. L.: The stethoscope, the anesthesiologist's best friend, Anesth. & Analg. 42:711, 1963.

Lambert, E. H.: Strain Gauges: Resistance Wire, in *Medical Physics* (vol. 2), Glasser, O. (ed). (Chicago: Year Book Publishers, Inc., 1950).

Severinghaus, J. W.: Methods of blood and gas carbon dioxide during anesthesia, Anesthesiology 21:717, 1960.

Cohen, D., and Hercus, V.: Controlled hypothermia in infants and children, Brit. M. J. 1:1435, 1959.

Stephen, C. R.: Postoperative temperature changes, Anesthesiology 22:795, 1961.

Burchfield, H. P., and Storrs, E. E.: *Biochemical Applications of Gas Chromatography* (New York: Academic Press, Inc., 1962).

Dornette, W. H. L., and Durbin, R. L.: Design and construction of an intensive care facility, Hosp. Management 91:35, 1961.

Data-Phone, the American Telephone and Telegraph Company.

NAME
AGE
SEX

WEIGHT (kg)
HEIGHT (cm)

Predicted M.V. _____ T.V. _____ V.C. _____

							RESPIRATION					VENTILATION		
TIME	TEMP	PULSE	BLOOD PRESS	R	TV	MV	Peak Insp Press	Insp Time	Exp Time	Sensitivity	Spont	Assist	Control

		BLOOD GAS ANALYSIS					BLOOD									URINE					
		P_{O_2}	P_{CO_2}	pH	CO₂ Cont.	O₂ Sat	HCT	WBC	Electrolytes			Sp Grav	AMT	Electrolytes			Osmolality				
									Na⁺	Ca⁺	K⁺			Na⁺	Cl⁻	K⁺					

	TREATMENT	I. V. FLUID		EEG (Interpretation)	EKG (Interpretation)
	Drugs and Amt (Antibiotics, Digitalis)	Amount	Type		

										SUCTIONING	

TREATMENT

HUMIDITY		INSPIRED GAS							SUCTIONING	
Type	% Conc	RM Air	O$_2$	L/Min	Conc	Other (Specify)	Deep Breaths (Sigh)	Oral	Endotracheal

THERAPY				
CHEST PHYSIOTHERAPY				
Type	How Often	Duration	Tracheal Installations	Comments

CHAPTER 13

Intermittent Positive Pressure Breathing

INTERMITTENT POSITIVE PRESSURE breathing (IPPB) combined with side arm or inline nebulization of a bronchodilator aerosol, as a specific form of therapy in chronic pulmonary disease, was first used in the treatment of coal miners with emphysema and fibrosis in 1947. Most early attempts of treating patients with respiratory diseases with intermittent positive pressure breathing were unsuccessful. It was not until 1954 that intermittent positive pressure breathing therapy came into extensive usage by physicians, nurses and technicians. By then, many newer devices were available commercially that offered more parameters to choose from in caring for the debilitated respiratory patient.

In normal healthy lungs, clearing of the respiratory tract is accomplished by coughing and the normal ciliary action. Alveoli are usually kept opened by periodic sighs. According to Safar *et al.*, when disease interferes with the normal protective mechanisms of the tracheobronchial tree, intermittent positive pressure breathing is used extensively to accomplish the following:

1. To prevent and to correct atelectasis by periodic deep breaths
2. Topical mechanical bronchodilation effect
3. To improve distribution and disposition of aerosols
4. To facilitate clearing of bronchial secretions
5. To prevent and counteract pulmonary edema
6. To decrease the cost of breathing
7. To regulate inspiratory and expiratory gas flow patterns

The effects of IPPB produced by mechanical devices demand considerable knowledge and understanding the over-all mechanics of breathing, the physical characteristics of ventilators and the pressure-flow volume relationship of the ventilator and the pulmonary system.

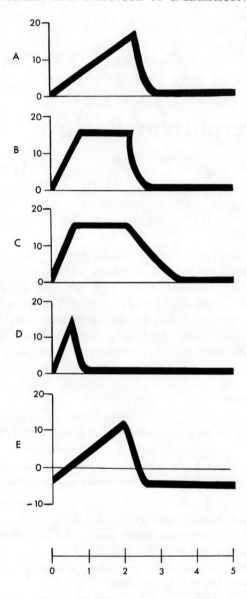

Fig. 131.—Diagrams illustrating the principle of "mean pressure in the lungs" during mechanical ventilation. In each instance, the total respiratory phase lasts 5 seconds, the tidal volume is 800 ml and the compliance is 0.05 L/cm H_2O; hence the pressure applied is 16 cm H_2O. The airway resistance is measured at 2 cm H_2O (liter per second). Changes in

During intermittent positive pressure breathing therapy as well as during controlled ventilation, circulatory response may vary, depending on physical status of the subject and the presence or absence of drugs with cardiovascular actions. In a healthy, conscious man, increase in intrathoracic pressure, impairment of venous return and reduction in cardiac output proportional to the mean positive pressure applied may occur. Compensatory peripheral vasoconstriction occurs and systemic venous distensibility is probably reduced. Peripheral venous pressure quickly rises with a consequent restoration of the venous gradient and cardiac output. Changes in systemic blood pressure are absent or minimal. There is a decrease in the volume of blood in the thorax, but, due to the increase in intrathoracic pressure, a net rise in venous pressure is found, despite the decrease in venous return. When IPPB is properly administered, mean pressure should be considerably below peak inspiratory pressure. If IPPB is given during circulatory failure, precaution should be taken because of the likelihood of circulatory collapse.

Cournand *et al.* recognized early the importance of the pressure pattern applied. The mean pressure (Fig. 131) is of the greatest significance in determining the degree of circulatory embarrassment. In the past, the arithmetic pressure was thought to be of great significance, but Mushin *et al.* proved that it was "not the arithmetical mean between the highest and lowest pressures in the respiratory cycle," but the mean of an infinite number of instantaneous readings of the pressure within the lung during one respiratory cycle that was important. Thus, five different pressure patterns can be obtained, all with the same peak pressure, rate of respiration and the same tidal volume, but with mean pressures varying from -0.2 to $+7.5$ cm of water.

---

other variables produced a wide range of mean pressures. **A,** slow inflation (flow rate of inflating gases is 24 L per minute). Expiration is passive. The resistance of the apparatus is measured as 2 cm H_2O (liter per second). The mean pressure is 3.8 cm H_2O. **B,** rapid inflation (flow rate is 96 L per minute) at the start of the respiratory phase. The lungs are held inflated for some period of time, making the inspiratory phase last 2 seconds. Passive exhalation, mean pressure is 6.2 cm H_2O. **C,** the inspiratory phase here is the same as in **B,** but expiration is impeded by an apparatus resistance of 10 cm H_2O (liter per second). The mean pressure is 7.5 cm H_2O. **D,** inflation is rapid (flow rate of inflating gases is 96 cm H_2O), followed by passive exhalation immediately. The mean pressure is 1.4 cm H_2O. **E,** inflation is slow (flow rate of inflating gases is 24 L per minute) and again occupies 2 seconds. During the expiratory phase, a constant negative pressure ($-$ 4 cm H_2O) is introduced. Expiration is passive. The mean pressure is 0.2 cm H_2O.

Low mean pressure can be achieved by using the following suggestions:

1. Inspiratory time should be equal to, or preferably shorter than, expiratory time.

2. On attainment of peak airway pressure, exhalation should commence promptly, avoiding a plateau period.

3. Rapid return to atmospheric pressure on completion of inspiration should be allowed by avoiding expiratory pressure.

4. Flow rates should be rapid in normal lungs. In patients with obstructive and restrictive diseases, the required low flow rates should be used when necessary.

5. Use of slight negative pressure (1–2 cm) during expiration is recommended, except in patients with severe obstructive diseases of the lungs.

NEGATIVE PRESSURE.—The application of slight negative expiratory pressure (1–2 cm) can increase venous return to the heart and effectively lower the peak positive pressure necessary for adequate alveolar ventilation; but, despite this, the mean peak pressure at some critical area remains above atmospheric pressure in many instances. Negative pressure may be indicated for use in patients requiring controlled ventilation who have circulatory disturbances without obstructive or restrictive lung diseases. Application of negative expiratory pressure in obstructive and/or restrictive disease may enhance the collapse of the small air passages and hinder expiration. It seems that emphasis should be placed on other factors that will lead to a low mean positive pressure and to restoration of cardiovascular effectiveness.

MECHANICS OF BREATHING

To understand fully the pressure-volume effects of controlled ventilation, one must first understand the normal mechanics of breathing. During each ventilatory cycle, the muscles of respiration must, by their energy, supply pressure sufficient to overcome the elastic and nonelastic "resistances" of the lungs and thorax. During controlled breathing, the force, pressure, is applied externally by the ventilator. The elastic "cost" in a normal adult male at resting midposition is about 10 cm of water per liter of volume change, divided nearly equally between lungs and thorax so that the change in pleural pressure is about 5 cm of water per liter. (The compliance of the total respiratory system, which is the inverse of the elastic resistance or stretch ability is in this case 0.1 L/cm of water and of the lungs and thorax about 0.2 L/cm of water each.)

In quiet inspiration by an adult with a tidal volume of 0.6 L and a maximal flow rate of 0.5 L per second, the elastic resistance of the lungs will normally be 6 cm of water, and the flow-resistance pressure will be 1 cm of water. The total pressure curve would be somewhat less and not the sum of the two values, because the flow and volume do not correspond in time: Maximal flow will occur at approximately mid-inspiratory position, and the maximum of the sum of elastic and flow-resistive pressures occurs at some point beyond that volume but always before the end of inspiration when the elastic pressure is maximal.

During quiet expiration, the "stored" elastic pressure is more than sufficient to overcome nonelastic resistance and to complete expiration in time for the next phase of the cycle. The energy used normally during the expiratory phase is provided by inspiratory muscles as they relax and allow the elastic forces to conform to their innate pressures.

The values for compliance and airway resistance vary in normal lungs but also vary considerably in patients with pulmonary disease. For example, in severe bronchitis, airway resistance may increase to 18 cm of water per liter per second. Also, compliance will change in response to accumulation of secretions, positional body changes, splinting of the chest, administration of drugs, and several other factors. These changes will occur from moment to moment.

MECHANICAL VENTILATORS

It is convenient at this point to consider a few fundamental principles of mechanical ventilators in order to understand more fully their clinical performances and application. The following description is abridged from Mapleson.

The majority of mechanical ventilators in common use today can be classified either as flow generators or pressure generators. Flow generators are designed to deliver either a constant flow of gases throughout the inspiratory phase or a preset pattern of the sine wave flow. (Fig. 133 is an example of the sine wave flow pattern, which is steadily increased flow up to maximal rate near mid-inspiration followed by a gradual decrease in flow during end-inspiration.)

FLOW GENERATOR: CONSTANT FLOW INSPIRATORY PHASE.—The pattern of gas flow during inspiratory phase as produced by a constant flow generator is shown in Figure 132,A. As the inspiratory phase begins, the flow rises to a constant value and remains at this point for the duration of the phase. Constant flow brings about an increasing volume in the lungs (B). Because the force or pressure in the alveoli of the lungs is commensurate with the volume forced into them, the increased pressure there is uniform (C). The constant flow also brings about a difference in pressure across the

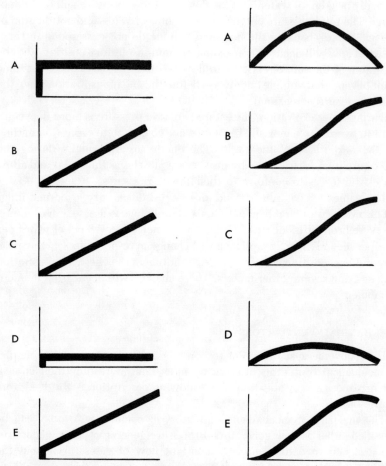

Fig. 132 (left).—Flow pattern of gases during the inspiratory phase: flow, volume and pressure patterns with constant flow ventilator. **A,** flow pattern of gases into the lungs; **B,** volume in the lungs; **C,** pressure in alveoli; **D,** pressure difference across airway resistance; **E,** pressure at the mouth.

Fig. 133 (right).—Inspiratory phase: flow, volume and pressure curves produced when using a sine wave flow ventilator. **A,** flow into the lungs; **B,** volume in the lungs; **C,** pressure in alveoli; **D,** pressure difference across airway resistance; **E,** pressure at mouth.

resistance of the airways (D). The combination of pressure in the alveoli and the pressure difference across the airway accounts for the peak pressure at the mouth (E). At the start of the inspiratory phase, there is an immediate rise because of the pressure difference across the airway resistance. Hence, a continual rise occurs because of the increasing pressure in the alveoli.

FLOW GENERATOR: SINE WAVE FLOW INSPIRATORY PHASE.—As with the constant flow generator, the starting point is the flow pattern produced by the ventilator; in this instance a half sine wave flow pattern as shown in Figure 133. The flow increases from zero to a point in the middle of the inspiratory phase, and then it decreases and returns to the starting point of zero (A). At first, the rate of increase of volume in the lungs is slow, then in the middle of the inspiratory phase it is rapid, and at the end it again becomes slow (B). There is a similarity in the pattern of pressure in the alveoli (C). The pattern of flow is always similar to the pressure difference across the airway resistance (D). The pressure at the mouth (E) is the sum of the pressure in the alveoli plus the pressure difference across the airway.

PRESSURE GENERATOR: CONSTANT-PRESSURE INSPIRATORY PHASE.—When the inspiratory phase begins and there is no volume or pressure in the lungs, the difference in pressure between the alveoli and the source is equal to the source pressure. The sum of the source pressure is applied across the total of the resistances of the airways and apparatus, and a rising initial flow is produced (Fig. 134,A).

This increasing flow brings about an immediate rise in the volume in the lungs (Fig. 134,B) and in the alveolar pressure (C). This produces a rapid fall in the pressure difference across the combined airway, apparatus resistance (D) and the flow through it into the lungs (E). Therefore, the rate of increase of volume in the lungs (B) and pressure in the alveoli (C) also constantly decreases throughout the inspiratory phase. Ultimately, if the inspiratory phase continues long enough, the alveolar pressure becomes equal to the generated pressure; there is no instant pressure difference across the airway and apparatus resistance, no flow, and a static volume occurs in the lungs, determined by the generated pressure and the total compliance of the lungs in this case. This condition can be allowed to occur only if the generated pressure is within the normal range of inflation pressures. When one says that an inspiratory phase longer than 1.5 seconds provides little useful increase in tidal air, one has in mind this type of ventilator in which a relatively low pressure is generated and the series resistance is small. It is also now possible to determine the pressure waveforms at the mouth. This will always be at some level between the pressure in the

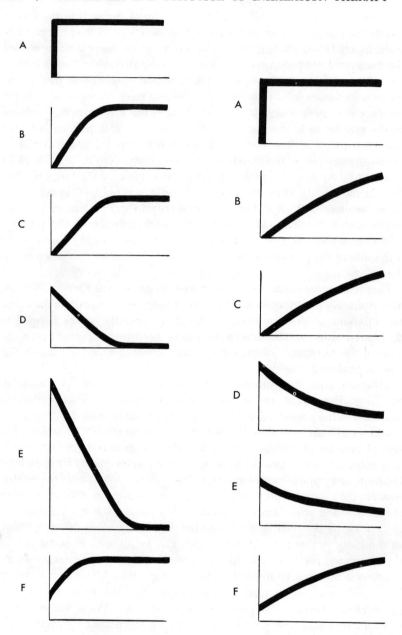

Fig. 134 (left).—Inspiratory phase: flow, volume and pressure patterns produced by a constant-pressure ventilator with apparatus resistance equal to patient's airway resistance.

alveoli and the constant pressure of the source. The precise point is determined by the ratio of the airway resistance to the apparatus resistance. The apparatus resistance (Figure 134,D) has been taken equal to the patient's airway resistance because the same flow occurs through both resistances, the pressure difference will remain the same across each and the pressure at the mouth will remain halfway between the pressure in the alveoli and the pressure at the source.

In drawing the graphs, it was assumed that the conditions are generally typical of ventilators in which the steady pressure arises from a second-stage reducing valve or a weighted concertina bag. When the constant pressure arises from an injector or a pressure transformer, the source pressure and the apparatus resistance are usually appreciably higher. This leads to flow and volume patterns similar to those of Figure 134.

In Figure 135, the constant pressure of the source is assumed to be 50% higher than in Figure 134, and the apparatus resistance is assumed to be nine times the apparatus resistance. Figure 135 is the intermediate obtained with a low constant pressure and low apparatus resistance and between those obtained with a constant flow. One can expect this because a source of very high constant pressure in series with a very high resistance is one of the arrangements for producing a constant flow.

FLOW GENERATOR: CONSTANT FLOW EXPIRATORY PHASE.—The patterns of flow, volume and pressure produced by a ventilator which serves as a constant flow generator during the expiratory phase are shown in Figure 136. They are the reverse of the patterns produced by constant flow during the inspiratory phase (Fig. 132).

The constant flow (Fig. 136,A) brings about a constant pressure difference across the airway resistance (D). The constant flow and constant pressure are in the opposite direction to that in the inspiratory phase and are ultimately shown below the lines of zero flow or pressure. The constant flow produces a steady decrease in the volume in the lungs (B) and, there-

A, pressure produced by the ventilator; B, volume in the lungs; C, pressure in the alveoli; D, pressure difference across sum of airway and apparatus resistance; E, flow into lungs; F, pressure at mouth.
Fig. 135 (right).—Inspiratory phase: flow, volume and pressure patterns with a constant-pressure ventilator with apparatus resistance equal to nine times the patient's airway resistance. A, pressure generated by ventilator; B, volume in the lungs; C, pressure in alveoli; D, pressure difference across sum of airway and apparatus resistance; E, flow into the lungs; F, pressure at mouth.

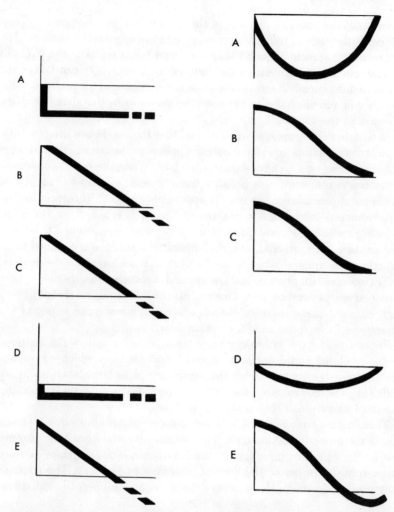

Fig. 136 (left).—Expiratory phase: flow, volume and pressure patterns produced by a constant-flow ventilator. A, flow from the lungs; B, volume in the lungs; C, pressure in alveoli; D, pressure difference across airway resistance; E, pressure at the mouth.

Fig. 137 (right).—Expiratory phase: flow, volume and pressure patterns produced by a sine wave flow ventilator. A, flow from the lungs; B, volume in the lungs; C, pressure in alveoli; D, pressure difference across airway resistance; E, pressure at the mouth.

fore, in the alveolar pressure (C). During this phase, the pressure at the mouth (E) is less than the pressure in the alveoli (C) judging by the amount of pressure difference across the airway resistance (D).

The *solid lines* end when the volume in the lungs has fallen to the normal expiratory level. The *dotted lines* indicate what happens if the constant expiratory flow continues beyond this point.

FLOW GENERATOR: SINE WAVE FLOW EXPIRATORY PHASE.—The patterns produced by a sine wave flow are shown (Fig. 137). Similar to those of the constant flow generator, the flow (A) and the pressure difference curves (B) appear below the zero lines because the direction of flow and pressure gradient is the reverse of that in the inspiratory phase. Similar to the sine wave flow in the inspiratory phase, the flow is first slow, then fast, then slow again; it produces a similar variation in pressure difference across the airway resistance (D) and in the rate of decline of volume in the lungs (B) and alveolar pressure (C). The pressure at the mouth (E) is less than the pressure in the alveoli (C) the amount of the pressure difference across the airway resistance (D).

The volume in the lungs and the alveolar and mouth pressures are here shown as becoming zero at the end of the phase, at the moment that the flow falls to zero. Evidently, this will be true only if at the start of the phase, the volume in the lungs is equal to the volume drawn out by the half cycle of the sine wave flow.

PRESSURE GENERATOR: CONSTANT PRESSURE EXPIRATORY PHASE.—Here may be seen the patterns that occur with a ventilator which "generates" constant atmospheric pressure and in which the apparatus resistance is equal to half the patient's airway resistance. The curves represent what happens when a patient expires freely to the atmosphere.

The starting point is the baseline zero pressure generated by the ventilator (Fig. 138,A). At the beginning of the expiratory phase, there is some volume in the lungs (B) and pressure in the alveoli (C). This pressure is resistance (D), resulting in a high initial flow (E). The pressure difference across the combined resistance (D) and flow (E) produced by it are shown as negative because the direction of both is the reverse of that in the inspiratory phase (see Fig. 134). The high flow produces a rapid fall in the volume in the lungs and the alveolar pressure and, therefore, in the pressure difference across the flow itself: all four decline toward zero. The time normally allowed for expiration is sufficient for all four curves to reach zero before the end of the expiratory phase. However, since the same flow occurs through the generator and airway resistance, the pressure at the mouth (F) is equal to one third of that in the alveoli.

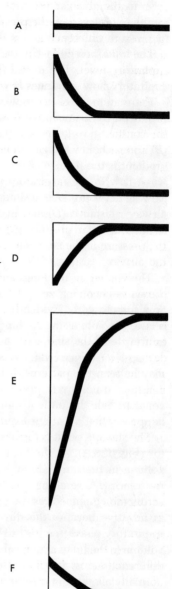

Fig. 138.—Flow, volume and pressure patterns with a constant atmospheric pressure generator with apparatus resistance equal to half the patient's airway resistance, patient exhaling freely to atmosphere. **A,** pressure produced by ventilator; **B,** volume in the lungs; **C,** pressure in alveoli; **D,** pressure difference across sum of airway and ventilator resistance; **E,** flow from the lungs; **F,** pressure at mouth.

The apparatus resistance between the expiratory outlet and the mouth has been taken to equal half the airway resistance. It is one third of the total resistance between the zero pressure generated at the expiratory outlet and the pressure in the alveoli. Because the same flow occurs through the apparatus resistance and the airway resistance, the pressure at the mouth (Fig. 139,*F*) is always equal to one third of that in the alveoli (*E*).

The way in which the patterns are changed when there is a substantial apparatus resistance and the constant pressure generated by the ventilator is negative.

The constant, negative pressure generated by the ventilator (Fig. 139,*A*) is combined with the pressure in the alveoli (*C*) at the beginning of the phase to give an increased pressure difference across the airway and apparatus resistance (*D*). Because of the eightfold increase in apparatus resistance, the initial flow (*E*) is less than before, so that initially the volume in the lungs (*B*) and the alveolar pressure (*C*) fall more slowly than before, as does the pressure difference across the combined airway and apparatus resistance (*D*) and the flow (*E*).

All four curves decline, but more gradually than in Figure 138. The pressure in the lungs declines toward the negative pressure that is generated by the ventilator, although the expiratory phase may end before that limit is reached. The *dotted lines* show how the changes continue if a longer expiratory phase is allowed than in Figure 138. Since the alveolar pressure declines toward a negative value, the volume in the lungs declines toward a value below the normal resting expiratory level which is shown as negative (*C*).

Since the apparatus resistance is much greater than the patient's airway resistance, the pressure at the mouth (Fig. 139,*F*) is much closer to that in the alveoli than when the apparatus resistance was low.

In comparison, it can be seen that although the negative pressure produces a more complete emptying of the lungs by the end of the phase, the increased apparatus resistance slows down the emptying initially. If an injector is added to a ventilator in an attempt to reduce the mean alveolar pressure by introducing a negative pressure phase, some additional apparatus resistance is introduced at the same time. If the negative pressure is used sparingly and the patient's airway resistance is normal, it is possible for the effect of the increased resistance to predominate, nullifying the effect of the negative pressure and resulting in an increase of mean pressure.

The change from the expiratory to the inspiratory phase and from the inspiratory to the expiratory phase may be as follows:

1. Time cycled, occurring after a predetermined period of time.

2. Pressure cycled, occurring when a pressure which is closely related, but not necessarily equal, to that in the lungs falls to some critical value.

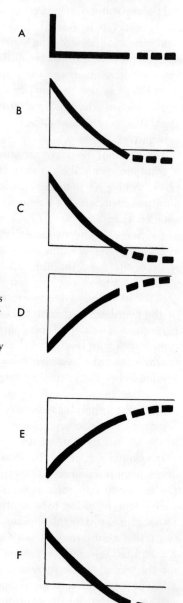

Fig. 139.—Expiratory phase: flow, volume and pressure patterns with a constant negative-pressure ventilator with apparatus resistance equal to four times the patient's airway resistance. **A,** pressure produced by ventilator; **B,** volume in the lung; **C,** pressure in alveoli; **D,** pressure difference across sum of airway and apparatus resistance; **E,** flow from lungs; **F,** pressure at mouth.

3. Volume cycled, occurring when preset volume has been introduced into the lungs.

4. Patient cycled, occurring when the patient initiates the inspiratory effort.

These ventilators in which the change is regulated by a combination of some of the above factors are referred to as mixed cycled.

It is important to remember that ventilators will function as classified under ideal situations but during adverse changes in compliance will perform with features that are characteristic of other ventilators.

Intermittent Positive-Pressure Breathing Devices

Pressure-Limited Ventilators

A pressure-limited ventilator requires a line pressure of incoming gas, oxygen or air, of approximately 50 pounds per square inch, which is about three atmospheres. Piped-in oxygen or compressed air outlets deliver such a pressure as does the one stage of a two-stage pressure regulator connected to a full oxygen tank under 2,000 pounds of pressure. The ventilator modifies the flow and pressure of the gas and delivers it to the patient intermittently with a flow rate and pressure which can be adjusted within certain limits. A Bird Mark VII (Fig. 140) ventilator has been chosen as a representative of the pressure-limited ventilators.

The basic controls are: peak positive pressure; air mix valve; duration of apnea (expiratory pause); sensitivity of the "patient-triggering" device; and the inspiratory flow rate.

During controlled ventilation, the respiratory rate is determined by the rate control, which is the black knob at the bottom of the front panel. To increase the rate or shorten the duration of apnea, turn the knob counterclockwise. The rate of automatic cycling can be determined by observing the rise and fall of the chest wall or by observing the movements of the sliding arm inside the back of the ventilator. When the arm engages with the central diaphragm, inspiration starts. During assisted ventilation, the inspiration is initiated by the patient's own inspiratory effort, creating a negative pressure which is transmitted to the ventilator. The smaller numbers on the sensitivity control correspond to the greatest sensitivity.

An excessive rapid inspiratory effort, producing a marked negative pressure of more than 1–2 cm in the airway and lungs, is harmful. Usually, a resetting of pressure, tidal volume, and rate is needed to correct the underlying inadequate ventilation. When assisted ventilation is used, the ventilator should be set to cycle at approximately 10 per minute in order to

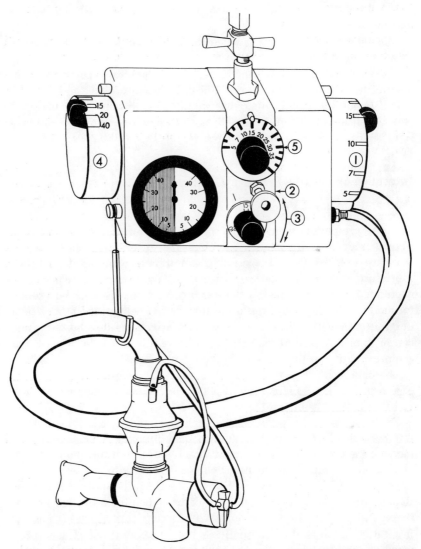

Fig. 140.—The Bird Mark VII intermittent positive-pressure breathing apparatus with mainstream micronebulizer mouthpiece, one-way exhalation valve and visible two-channel breathing tube. *1*, inspiratory pressure limit switch; *2*, air mix switch for varying concentrations of oxygen; *3*, apnea switch; *4*, sensitivity switch; *5*, inspiratory time flow rate switch.

prevent asphyxia should the patient become unable by his own effort to initiate assisted ventilation.

Once inspiration has started, it will continue until the pressure, which has been preset on the pressure control, has been built up in the airway. Gas flow then stops, the exhalation valve opens and exhalation takes place passively. During inspiration, the exhalation valve is kept shut by the pressure transmitted to the valve via a thin plastic tube from the ventilator. The high pressure oxygen in this line also operates the small micronebulizer. Pressure and flow in the line stop simultaneously with the end of inspiration, and the valve opens.

For a given preset pressure, the duration of inspiration is determined by the ventilator flow rate control, which is the large black dial at the top of the front panel. The higher the flow rate, the faster pressure in the airway builds up and the faster the peak preset pressure is reached; therefore, the shorter the inspiratory phase, and vice versa. Duration of inspiration should not normally exceed 3 seconds; a leak in the system reduces the effective flow rate to the airway and thus prolongs inspiration. With a large leak, the flow rate may be too small to allow build-up to airway pressure to the preset pressure on the ventilator. The result is a sustained "inspiration" with a continuous positive airway pressure and potential reduction in venous return. The three most common causes of serious leaks are:

1. A loose inline nebulizer reservoir jar
2. A large leak around the tracheostomy cuff; a small leak is often deliberate
3. A leaky exhalation valve, which is rare

The tidal volume delivered by a pressure-limited IPPB device depends on several factors; the most important are:

1. Peak positive-pressure setting on the respirator, which determines the peak airway pressure generated
2. Rate of inspiratory gas flow from the respirator
3. Resistance of the patient's lung and chest wall inflation

Humidification.—The gas from the respirator usually passes through a main-line humidifier on the way to the patient. A flow rate of at least 6–10 L of air or oxygen is necessary to create a mist or fog inside the chamber of the nebulizer. The mist is picked up by the gas from the main line and carried into the lungs.

Inspired oxygen concentration.—With the average pressure-limited respirator, such as the Bird or Bennett, the following inspired oxygen concentrations will be achieved when oxygen and compressed air are used in the following combination:

1. Air mix control not in operation (push in), 100% oxygen
2. Air mix control in operation (pull out), nebulizer or humidifier operated with compressed air at 8 L per minute, 61% oxygen
3. Respirator operated by compressed air, nebulizer or humidifier powered by oxygen at 8 L per minute, 57% oxygen
4. Entire system by compressed air, 21% oxygen

The above figures will vary due to increases or decreases in lung or chest wall compliance or both and also due to the type and length of the inspiratory phase.

Medications.—Place the prescribed medication in nebulizer. A treatment usually is 15 minutes, if tolerated, and usually given as frequently as every 2 hours in extreme conditions.

Equipment.—The Bennett PR–2 respirator (Fig. 141).

Preparation for treatment.—This is carried out as follows:

1. Attach nebulizer manifold to support arm. Attach the end of the main tube assembly with tubes of equal lengths to connector below peak flow control. Connect white nebulizer tube to white connector underneath unit. Connect clear exhalation valve tube to silver connector underneath unit. Connect large red negative tube to red connector on Venturi assembly.

2. Connect the other end of the main tube to one end of the nebulizer manifold. Slip Bennett Twin Nebulizer into nebulizer manifold. Connect white nebulizer tube into nebulizer. Slip manifold and fit exhalation manifold into the adaptor. Screw the negative-pressure cap to the top of the exhalation manifold.

3. Attach flex tube and mouthpiece or mask to the exhalation manifold as desired.

4. When dead space is important, use the minimal dead space manifold by substituting it for the standard exhalation manifold.

5. After attaching high-pressure hose to the filter housing, connect to wall outlet of piped oxygen for air system.

6. If cylinder oxygen is used, attach high-pressure hose to Bennett high-pressure regulator (50 PSI).

7. Secure and put prescribed medication in the Bennett Twin Nebulizer, being certain that the nebulizer is in the upright position.

8. As a starting point, set the positive-pressure limit control at 15.

9. Set the sensitivity to the normal position by turning the control knob all the way to the right. This control determines the amount of effort the patient must exert to trigger the unit during each successive inspiration.

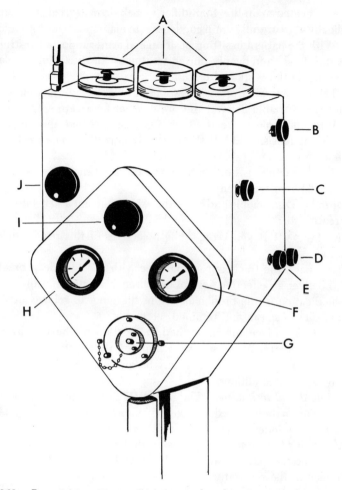

Fig. 141.—Bennett intermittent positive-pressure breathing apparatus. *A*, pistons; *B*, sensitivity adjustment; *C*, air dilutor; *D*, nebulization (inspiration); *E*, nebulization (continuous); *F*, control pressure gauge; *G*, Bennett valve; *H*, system pressure gauge; *I*, pressure control knob; *J*, automatic cycle rate.

10. Set dilution control for prescribed oxygen concentration. Push dilution control all the way in to "stop" position. This setting provides an oxygen mixture of approximately 40% oxygen from the Bennett valve when flow is unrestricted. However, oxygen flow through the nebulizer increases oxygen concentration, and the efficiency of the Venturi decreases at low flows, which also increases oxygen concentration. For 100% oxygen concentration, pull dilution control all the way out to "stop" position.

11. If a heated main-line humidifier or nebulizer is used with the unit, periodically and carefully drain condensate in main tube back into reservoir.

12. With the patient in sitting position and arms supported, instruct him to breathe slowly and deeply during treatment. Instruct him to relax and let the unit do the work of breathing.

13. The Bennett valve opens in response to slight inspiratory effort. Then an automatic variable flow, at the pressure set for treatment, inflates the lungs. When flow has decreased to a very small volume, the valve closes.

14. The patient should breathe in slowly until the lungs are full, relax for a few seconds and exhale completely.

15. Some practice by both patient and therapist should be required for the most effective treatment.

Cleaning.—Disassemble and clean the exhalation unit and nebulizer after each treatment.

BIRD MARK VII RESPIRATOR.—The objectives of this respirator are as follows:

1. To expand the tracheobronchial tree with periodic deep breaths.

2. To deliver an effective aerosol of a bronchodilator, mucolytic or enzyme medication to the bronchial tree of the lungs to relieve airway obstruction due to spasm and retained secretions.

Medications.—Place the prescribed medication in the nebulizer. The length of the treatment is usually 15 minutes, if tolerated. Medication is usually given four times daily but may be given as frequently as every 2 hours in extreme conditions.

Equipment and technique.—The Mark VII Respirator is complete with supply tubing, nebulizer, exhalation valve and mouthpiece (Fig. 140). If oxygen from cylinders is used, a special 50-PSI regulator must be used.

Preparation for treatment.—This is carried out as follows:

1. Connect the patient supply tube, nebulizer, exhalation valve and mouthpiece to the respirator.

2. Secure and put prescribed medication in the nebulizer and position the nebulizer so that the intravenous adaptor is upright.

3. Connect the respirator to the gas source, for example, compressed air or oxygen.

4. As a starting point, set the position of the pressure limit control knob at 15.

5. Set the sensitivity control on the number 15. This control determines the amount of effort the patient must exert to trigger the unit during each successive inspiration. If the patient is unable to start the inspiratory cycle at this setting, the control indicator should be turned counterclockwise to a lower number setting, which decreases the effort required to start

inspiration. Thus, the lower the number on the scale, the greater the sensitivity of the respirator; at one point below (the setting 5), the respirator will autocycle. The indicator then should be turned to a higher number in a clockwise direction.

6. Turn the inspiratory flow rate control to a starting point of 15. The flow control regulates the rate or the velocity of flow of gas into the patient's lungs. If the rate of flow appears to be too slow or too fast, readjust the flow control to a point where the patient is comfortable. Keep in mind that the time of expiration should be twice that of inspiration, normally a ratio of 1 : 2 and in some instances 1 : 3. The patient should be in the sitting position with his shoulders and the remainder of his body relaxed (Fig. 142).

7. The air mixture dilutor should be checked to be certain that the safety clip is in place. This insures low oxygen concentration; 40% is the lowest limit when the unit is powered by any oxygen source. The concentration will vary according to the resistance in the airway.

The clip is removed and the dilutor is pushed when 100% oxygen is required. The flow rate must be increased when the change is made from 40% to 100% oxygen to compensate for the 60% room air that is no longer being drawn in by the Venturi system.

Fig. 142.—Patient receiving intermittent positive-pressure breathing therapy.

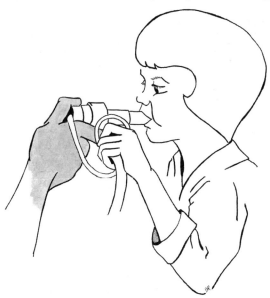

8. Be certain that the automatic cycle control, which is directly under the air mixture control, is turned off. The "off" position is in the clockwise direction. (This control is used in conditions in which a patient fails to ventilate on his own and has either an endotracheal or tracheostomy tube in place. Turning the knob counterclockwise increases the rate of controlled ventilation.)

9. The patient is instructed in the procedure.

10. In adults, a mouthpiece is usually the most convenient method for giving the treatment. A nose clip is used to keep the patient from losing part of the tidal volume through his nose during inspiration. He should be instructed to close his mouth around the mouthpiece because a closed system is essential to the proper functioning of any positive-pressure unit.

11. Allow the patient to become accustomed to the feeling of having his lungs mechanically inflated while breathing at his normal tidal volume. When he has become accustomed to breathing with the respirator, he should be instructed to produce a maximal expiration and follow this by a deep inspiration, which is held for several seconds. Frequent rest periods should be allowed during the treatment to avoid fatigue. The deep expiration followed by a deep inspiration held for several seconds should be done six times during the course of a 15-minute treatment.

12. A mask can be substituted for the nose clip and mouthpiece because a good seal is very important; there must be no leaks about the mask.

Cleaning.—The procedure is as follows:

1. The exhalation valve assembly should be taken apart and cleaned after each treatment.

2. The nebulizer should be taken apart and cleaned.

3. After cleaning the exhalation valve, nebulizer, and the patient-supply tubing, they should be properly stored in the patient area.

REFERENCES

Miller, W. F.: Intermittent positive pressure breathing, Minnesota Med. 47:272, 1964.
Cournand, A.; Motley, H. L.; Werko, L., and Richards, D. W., Jr.: Physiological studies of the effects of intermittent positive pressure breathing on cardiac output in man, Am. J. Physiol. 152:162, 1948.
Emmanuel, G. E.; Smith, W. M., and Briscoe, W. A.: The effect of intermittent positive pressure breathing and voluntary hyperventilation upon the distribution of ventilation and pulmonary blood flow to the lung in chronic obstructive lung disease, J. Clin. Invest. 45:1221, 1966.
Fairley, H. B., and Hunter, D. D.: The performance of ventilators used in the treatment of respiratory insufficiency, Canad. M. A. J. 90:1397, 1964.
Mushin, W. W.; Rendell-Baker, L., and Thompson, P. W.: *Automatic Ventilation of the Lung* (Springfield, Ill.: Charles C Thomas, Publisher, 1959).

Wu, N.; Miller, W. F.; Cade, R., and Richurg, P.: Intermittent positive pressure breathing in patients with chronic bronchopulmonary disease, Am. Rev. Tuberc. 71:693, 1955.

Elam, J. O., *et al.:* Performance of ventilators, effect of changes in lung thorax compliance, Anesthesiology 19:56, 1956.

Kamat, S. R.; Dulfano, M. J., and Segal, M. S.: The effects of intermittent positive pressure breathing (IPPB/I) with compressed air in patients with severe chronic nonspecific obstructive pulmonary disease, Am. Rev. Resp. Dis. 86:360, 1962.

Sheldon, G. P.: Asthma, chronic bronchitis and emphysema—The use of IPPB with inspiratory flow rate control, California Med. 98:216, 1963.

CHAPTER 14

Pharmacology of Inhalation Therapy

Introduction to Drug Usage in Inhalation Therapy

THE ADMINISTRATION of aerosolized drugs is one of the respiratory therapist's primary responsibilities in giving care to patients in respiratory distress. Because drugs have the potential to help or harm the patient, respiratory therapists must have sufficient knowledge about each drug administered. Only by knowing the essentials of what each drug does and why, will he or she know why the patient must receive the prescribed drug, the amount prescribed, dosage form prescribed, the proper route of administration and the proper time of administration.

In addition, the therapists must know the chemical, generic and brand names of the drugs being administered. He or she must also be acquainted with the indications, contraindications and associated problems of administration. The chemical name of the drug tells the therapist what the drug is and how it is molecularly structured; the generic name is used as a substitute for, and often is derived from, the chemical name. The brand name is the manufacturers' means of identifying their drug.

Drugs are manufactured and used in three basic physical forms—solid, liquid and gaseous. Many drugs in current use have more than one form, especially in solids and liquids.

SOLID FORMS.—Drugs in this category are administered in three ways— oral, topical and suppository. Tablets are examples of solid forms, appearing in varying sizes, weights and shapes and may be molded or compressed, containing medicinal substances in pure or diluted form. Topical forms are those used externally and are not absorbed by the system. Most important topical forms include ointments and creams, which usually serve as vehicles for drugs and as protective agents for skin. Molded, medicated masses melting at body temperature or dissolving in body cavities constitute the suppository form of drugs.

LIQUID FORMS.—The three general classifications of liquid drugs are solutions, suspensions and emulsions. *Solutions* are preparations containing one or more drugs usually dissolved in water, which are then subdivided into four types of solutions: Syrups, elixirs, tinctures and injectables. *Suspensions* are preparations of finely divided insoluble drugs intended for suspension in some suitable liquid vehicle prior to use or are already in suspension in a liquid vehicle. *Emulsions* are aqueous preparations containing fats or oils suspended with the aid of an emulsifying agent.

Since active ingredients of suspensions and emulsions are insoluble, they must be shaken well before administration so that active ingredients may be distributed evenly through the liquid material.

GASEOUS FORMS.—Gaseous medications are of considerable importance in inhalation therapy, and, because of the nature of these medications in most instances, the only route by which they can be used is through inhalation. Such forms of medication are divided into two main categories of use—therapeutic and anesthetic.

Therapeutic.—Oxygen is the most important of the therapeutic gases and has numerous uses. One of the most important indications is to help alleviate anoxia associated with acute respiratory difficulties.

Carbon dioxide-oxygen mixtures are frequently administered to counteract respiratory depression, asphyxia, carbon monoxide poisoning and, sometimes, to alleviate hiccoughs.

Anesthetic.—Numerous gases or volatile liquids in gaseous form are used in surgery for anesthetic qualities. Choice of particular ones will often depend on factors other than the anesthetic effect it may cause; for example, age and condition of patient and type of surgery being performed. Among the most widely used anesthetics are nitrous oxide, cyclopropane, ethyl ether, vinyl ether and halothane.

AEROSOLS.—An aerosol by definition is a suspension of particulate matter in a liquid or compressed gas form that is expelled from a container. Three types of aerosol forms are used in inhalation therapy:

1. Solution: Any liquid sprayed or aerosolized as a mist
EXAMPLE: Isoproterenol HCl in a nebulizer

2. Powder: Any powder dispersed through propellant within a container
3. Emulsion: Any drug forming a foam when aerosolized or sprayed

To be effective, any drug must be tailored to meet the needs of the particular patient being treated. Let us look into four of the factors which influence drug action. The authors have divided them into biologic and physiologic, psychologic, time, and external factors.

BIOLOGIC AND PHYSIOLOGIC FACTORS

Each individual is made up genetically different and, therefore, will react differently when drugs are administered. Drugs will react differently according to the time given. For example, if phenobarbital is administered in the evening, the total effect could be maximal depression and could result in maximal sedation; but if the same volume and dilution is given in the morning, some patients will exhibit light sedation. Many factors could be attributed to the above-mentioned conditions. The state of an individual's body metabolism and general health condition may play an important role in drug absorption, as may the amount of food in the stomach and the rate of digestion of the food. Drugs given to pregnant women may have untold effects on the fetus as well as on the mother.

If some drugs are absorbed and the liver is malfunctioning, it could result in a major problem if not corrected. The rate of drug absorption will vary among individuals as well as among age groups. Young children are a real problem. Some of their enzymes which are needed to break down certain drugs are not fully developed; because of this factor, the drugs can be quite dangerous in some instances. It is obvious that the individual's body weight and size also play important roles in the rate of absorption.

The amount of absorption and the rapidity of effect will depend on how the drug is administered, the total amount of the drug given, conditions of absorptive surface area, solubility of the drug in water and tissue fluids and the adequacy of the circulation of blood. Drugs that are injected will take effect most quickly.

PSYCHOLOGIC FACTORS

Some patients may have acquired tolerance to a certain drug and, therefore, need a dose above the usual maximum to achieve the required effect. This, of course, may or may not have anything to do with habituation, a condition wherein one becomes accustomed to, but not seriously dependent on, a drug. Addiction is closely related to habituation, in that it can be defined as a condition of the mind or body which requires continuation of drugs and without which serious physical or mental derangement could result.

On the other hand, an individual may exhibit a placebo response, which is a reaction, psychologic in nature, whereby the patient shows improvement in response to an inert drug.

Time Factors

Time and duration of drug administration are very important concepts. For any drug to be effective, it must be given at a set time interval, either before or after meals. Drugs given orally are usually more effective when administered an hour or two before meals.

Some drugs, such as sedatives, are most effective when administered in the evening hours rather than in the morning.

External Factors

By far the most important of the external factors in drug administration is one involving iatrogenic-induced diseases. An example would be the use of a contaminated needle or syringe used to administer a drug by injection. A film may be left on an instrument or device due to improper cleaning or sterilization, which may mix with the drug and cause a decrease in the desired effects or reactions. Incompatibilities to a drug's reaction due to mixing of two or more drugs inside or outside the body may occur and should be kept in mind when mixing drugs in a container or syringe.

Pharmacology

All methods of ventilatory care for patients with respiratory diseases will be inadequate unless the airway is patent or unobstructed to a degree. If this were always the case, our role in respiratory care would be quite easy. But this is not so. In most instances, the airway is obstructed due to one or more of the following reasons: Constriction of bronchiolar smooth muscle, mucosal congestion or inflammation, tissue edema of the bronchi, blocking of the air spaces by mucus, edema fluid, exudate or foreign particles, cohesion of mucosal surfaces by surface tension forces, infiltration, compression or fibrosis of bronchioles or collapse or blockage of bronchioles due to loss of the normal pull of alveolar elastic fibers on bronchiolar walls or to loss of supporting tissues of the bronchial walls.

Bronchiolar obstruction is a general term used to denote a decrease in the lumen of the bronchioles. Since bronchiolar constriction of smooth muscle is different from bronchial obstruction, we should not use the two terms synonymously, although they have been used interchangeably in the past. Careless use of terminology usually leads to careless thinking. For instance, one might be confronted with a problem of airway obstruction and think only of a smooth muscle relaxant to relieve the obstruction.

Bronchodilator drugs are usually sympathomimetic agents that actively enlarge the inside diameter or lumen of the bronchioles by their effects on bronchiolar smooth muscles. These drugs may be given locally or systemically. In respiratory care, the method of choice is by aerosols. Often, if the desired effects are not evident after aerosol administration, the systemic route is used as well. The use of aerosols achieves a high concentration of the drug locally with minimal systemic absorption and few undesired side effects.

One disadvantage of the aerosol route is that the drug is propelled only where the inspired gas goes and does not reach the plugged areas of the lungs. With modern nebulizers and new respiratory techniques, this is less of a problem than it was 5 years ago. On the other hand, a bronchodilator drug given systemically reaches all bronchioles through their systemic bronchial arterial circulation, regardless of airway occlusion. Systemic administration has the disadvantage that the concentration of the drug is lower than that achieved locally by aerosol inhalation. Often, when a bronchodilator drug is given both by aerosol and systemic routes, the two reinforce each other and this reinforcement is called synergistic action.

Antibiotics are of important value in the total management of obstructive pulmonary disease in which airway obstruction is due in part to exudates or to inflammatory swelling of bronchiolar mucosa; this method of therapy is most effective if one knows what types of microorganisms are present. Many broad-spectrum antibiotic agents are used, however, as an emergency treatment for certain patients with severe pulmonary insufficiency before bacteriologic studies can be completed or even instituted. Antibiotics should be administered systemically and not by aerosol.

Enzymes are of significant importance when given by the aerosol route to alter the physical properties of sputum. Their action is the breakdown of protein and mucin to simpler compounds. Rational therapy with specific enzymes requires knowledge of the chemical composition of sputum in the patient being treated.

Other important factors to be determined in enzyme therapy are optimal concentration, proper chemical environment and time necessary for effective splitting of the chemical bond of sputum.

Detergents, wetting agents and surface tension reducers are agents used to combat the cohesive forces between mucus or sputum and the surfaces in the tracheobronchial tree. The detergents of considerable use in the past are used less frequently today.

Expectorants, iodides, ammonium chloride, ipecac and other drugs were used for generations and to an extent are still used to increase bronchial secretions.

The rationale of their use is the belief that viscid sputum is difficult to move upward by ciliary action or by coughing; however, if thinner or liquefied by a watery solution, it can be dislodged, mobilized and coughed up.

The effective administration of the classifications of drugs mentioned in this section depends on the particle size, its deposition on the bronchiolar mucosa and other physical factors, such as age, body weight and size, metabolic state, pathologic state and time of administration. These factors will depend on the rate and the amount of the drug absorbed. Older patients may have a decreased rate of absorption due to a lesser efficient enzyme system, and, therefore, larger concentrations of the drug may be necessary for effective results.

Other factors influencing drug reaction are dose response and biologic variations, idiosyncrasy, dose tolerance, habituation, addiction and placebo response. In all instances, the average dose should be used as a guideline, and the drug should be titrated to each individual patient's need. After the initial dose, the patient should be observed closely for drug reaction and possible side effects. Some patients will have an unusual physical response to a drug, more often immediately after the drug is administered. Idiosyncrasy or a placebo response may occur, as may physiologic variations, especially in patients with asthma and emphysema. These usually are either an overreaction or a placebo response.

The latter part of this section will give a better insight into some of the above factors, such as actions of drugs, dose form, site and manner of administration, concentration, duration and drug reactions.

Drugs Used in Inhalation Therapy

Federal regulations concerning drug concentrations and administration are very strict. This section conforms with these regulations in every instance.

ALEVAIRE (TYLOXAPOL)—BREON LABS., INC.—Alevaire, a mucolytic detergent, is a sterile aqueous solution for aerosol use, containing the detergent Superinone (brand of tyloxapol) 0.125%, with 2% sodium bicarbonate and 5% glcerin.

Alevaire is particularly recommended for aerosol use because it does not cause irritation and is chemically inert. It wets, thins and loosens viscid respiratory secretions, thereby facilitating their removal by physiologic processes such as ciliary action, bronchiolar peristalsis and coughing. Superinone is effective in lowering surface tensions; sodium bicarbonate creates an alkaline medium to help liquefy mucus; glycerin assists in the stabilization of the aerosol droplet. Alevaire is recommended for the treatment of patients with diseases and disorders of the lung, accompanied or complicated by the presence of excessive or thickened bronchopulmonary secretions. Such secretions may be present in laryngotracheobronchitis and laryngitis, bronchitis and bronchiolitis, bronchial pneumonia, asthma, emphysema and allergic bronchopneumonia, neonatal asphyxia due to mucus obstruction or inhalation of amniotic fluid, atelectasis, diaphragmatic paralysis due to poliomyelitis or encephalitis, bronchiectasis and pulmonary abscess. Alevaire is also useful in troublesome secretions which accompany general anesthesia, thoracic surgical procedures, tracheotomy, inhalation of noxious gases or dust and aspiration of material, such as foreign bodies, gastric contents or amniotic fluid.

Side effects.—Alevaire is usually well tolerated and does not produce irritation or discomfort, except for occasional nausea. No serious reactions have been reported following its administration.

Precautions.—Alevaire should not be diluted. The solution does not have a preservative, and, therefore, the remaining portion should be discarded within 72 hours after the bottle is opened.

Administration and dosage.—Alevaire is administered undiluted by a nebulizer which is attached to an air compressor or oxygen tank; a copious fine mist is delivered into a tent, incubator or breathing mask and may be administered intermittently or continuously.

For the seriously ill: Continuous therapy, 500 ml for 12–24 hours.

For lesser illnesses: Intermittent therapy of $\frac{1}{2}$–$1\frac{1}{2}$ hours of nebulization three to four times daily.

How supplied.—Alevaire is supplied in bottles of 60 and 500 ml.

NOTE: The above claims and dosage recommendations are taken from the manufacturer's literature only and thus cannot be accepted uncritically.

AEROLONE COMPOUND (CYCLOPENTAMINE AND ISOPROTERONOL HYDROCHLORIDE)—ELI LILLY & CO.—Aerolone Compound, a bronchodilator, is a combination of bronchodilators. Each 100 ml contains Clopane hydrochloride, 0.5 Gm, and isoproterenol hydrochloride, 0.25 Gm, with propylene glycol, ascorbic acid, coloring and purified water. Sodium hydroxide is added during manufacture to adjust the pH.

Action and uses.—Aerolone Compound is effective in preventing and relieving the symptoms of asthma. It affords almost complete relief in mild and moderate attacks and is of value in status asthmaticus.

Administration and dosage.—For use by aerosol only. The technique is the same as that for administering epinephrine 1:100. A nebulizer which produces a fine mist is necessary. The mist is inhaled through the mouth, and the breath is held in momentarily. Usually, six to twelve inhalations will bring adequate relief. Mild cases may require only one treatment per day, whereas very severe cases may need the medication every 15 minutes for 3 minutes each time.

Side effects.—Side effects depend on absorption into the blood. Rarely, insomnia, nervousness, vertigo, tachycardia and palpitations may occur, and, if so, dosage and frequency should be reduced.

Precautions.—Aerolone Compound should be used with caution in patients with serious cardiac disease, hypertension or hyperthyroidism.

How supplied.—Solution number 50 is supplied in one fluid oz bottles.

NOTE: The above claims and dosage recommendations are taken from the manufacturer's literature only and thus cannot be accepted uncritically.

BRONKOSOL—BREON LABS., INC.—Bronkosol, a bronchodilator, contains Dilabron (brand of isoetharine) HCl 1.0%; phenylephrine HCl 0.25%; and thenyldiamine HCl 0.10% in an aqueous glycerin solution containing saccharin sodium, with sodium chloride, sodium citrate, sodium bisulfite 0.3%, methylparaben 0.03% and propylparaben 0.014%, as preservatives. Bronkosol is an antiasthmatic solution for use in a conventional nebulizer.

Action and uses.—By depositing its active ingredients as a fine aerosol mist in the bronchi and bronchioles, Bronkospray provides rapid, highly effective and relatively long-acting symptomatic relief from bronchial asthma, with minimal side effects. It may be used to control an attack and/or prophylactically. Also valuable in other conditions in which bronchospasm may be a complicating factor, such as emphysema, bronchitis and other bronchopulmonary disorders. The combination of the bronchodilating bronchovasoconstrictor decongestant action of phenylephrine and the bronchodilating histamine antagonistic actions of phenyldiamine produces a synergistic relaxation of bronchiolar musculature and shrinkage of edematous bronchiolar mucosa. Bronkosol also aids expulsion of tenacious secretions and significantly increases vital capacity. Because of the synergistic combination of its active ingredients, an excellent therapeutic effect is claimed with smaller doses than would be necessary if each active ingredient were administered separately. Consequently, Bronkosol has a wide margin of safety.

Administration of dosage.—Oral inhalation. Can be administered by hand nebulizer, oxygen aerosolization or intermittent positive-pressure breathing (IPPB). (See table on p. 242.)

Usually, treatment need not be repeated more often than every 4 hours, although in severe cases more frequent administration may be necessary.

Precautions.—Bronkosol is relatively free from side effects, but, as with other sympathomimetic amines, too frequent use may cause tachycardia, palpitations, nausea, headache, changes in blood pressure, anxiety, tension, restlessness, insomnia, tremor, weakness, dizziness and excitement. As a

Method of Administration	Usual Dose	Range	Usual Dilution
Hand nebulizer	3–4 inhalations	3–7 inhalations	Undiluted
Oxygen aerosolization°	0.5 ml	0.25–0.5 ml	1:3 with saline
IPPB†	0.5 ml	0.5–1 ml	1:3 with saline

° Administered with oxygen flow adjusted to 4–6 L per minute when using a side-arm nebulizer or in main-line nebulizers, where flow rate is not adjustable over a period of 15–20 minutes. May be administered simultaneously with other therapeutic agents such as antibiotics or wetting agents.

† Usually an inspiratory flow rate of 15 L per minute at a cycling pressure of 15 cm H_2O is recommended. It may be necessary, according to patient and type of IPPB apparatus, to adjust flow rate to 6–30 L per minute; cycling pressure to 10–15 cm H_2O and further dilution, according to needs of the patient.

result, patients should follow dosage instructions exactly because of the possibility of excessive tachycardia. Bronkosol should not be administered concomitantly with epinephrine or other sympathomimetic amines. It may, however, be alternated with these agents. With the above side effects in mind, dosage must be carefully adjusted in patients with hyperthyroidism, hypertension, acute coronary disease, cardiac asthma, limited cardiac reserve and in individuals sensitive to sympathomimetic amines. The nebulizer should be kept away from extreme heat. *Do not incinerate.*

BRONKOTABS—BREON LABS., INC.—Each Bronkotab, a sympathomimetic amine, contains ephedrine sulfate, 24 mg; cylceryl guaiacolate, 100 mg; theophylline, 100 mg; phenobarbital, 8 mg (may be habit forming); and thenyldiamine HCl, 10 mg.

Action and uses.—Bronkotabs' multiple actions help relieve respiratory distress by decongestion and bronchodilatory action. Bronkotabs allegedly prevent and relieve symptoms of bronchial asthma, asthmatic bronchitis, chronic bronchitis with emphysema and emphysematous bronchospasm. They are also valuable in bronchospastic conditions associated with hay fever, allergic rhinitis and nonseasonal upper respiratory allergies.

Administration and dosage.—Bronkotabs may be administered by giving 1 tablet every 3 or 4 hours, not to exceed five times daily.

Children over age 6: One-half adult dose. The dosage should be adjusted to the severity of the condition and response of the individual patient.

Side effects.—With Bronkotabs therapy, sympathomimetic side effects are minimal, and there are none of the dangers or side effects associated with steroid therapy.

Precautions.—Frequent or prolonged use of Bronkotabs may cause nervousness, restlessness or insomnia. It is recommended that Bronkotabs be used with caution in the presence of hypertension, heart disease or hyperthyroidism. As drowsiness may occur, patients must be cautioned not to drive or operate machinery when receiving Bronkotab therapy.

How supplied.—Bronkotabs are supplied in bottles of 100 and 1,000 tablets.

NOTE: The above claims and dosage recommendations are taken from the manufacturer's literature only and thus cannot be accepted uncritically.

DORNAVAC (PANCREATIC DORNASE)—MERCK, SHARP & DOHME.— Dornavac is the enzyme deoxyribonuclease extracted from beef pancreas and lyophilized for increased stability. Pancreatic dornase rapidly degrades deoxyribonucleoprotein and deoxyribonucleic acid.

Actions and uses.—Dornavac is alleged to start on contact to reduce tenacity and viscosity of mucopurulent secretions in sinusitis, purulent bronchitis, bronchiectasis, abscesses, atelectasis, emphysema, unresolved pneumonia, chronic bronchial asthma and tracheitis sicca. Dornavac is alleged to provide valuable adjunctive therapy in the management of purulent urinary infections, also to loosen tenacious bronchial secretions in cystic fibrosis of the pancreas and to facilitate the obtaining of specimens for cytologic study in bronchogenic carcinoma. Clinical improvement often begins within 30 minutes after aerosol therapy. Dornavac has no enzymatic effect on living tissue and usually is well tolerated; local irritation is infrequent.

Administration and dosage.—An expensive medication not to be wasted with large volume mask therapy but with pressure nebulization giving one to three micra-size droplets. For the treatment of bronchopulmonary infections, the suggested dosage is 50,000–100,000 units administered as an aerosol one to four times daily for a period of 1–7 days until improvement occurs. Treatment may be repeated after an interval of a few days or when clinical symptoms indicate further need for therapy. The usual dosage in sinusitis is 50,000–100,000 units one to four times a week, administered by inhalation or irrigation. The recommended dosage for tracheitis sicca is 100,000 units daily for 2–9 days. The suggested dosage for cystic fibrosis of the pancreas is 50,000–100,000 units two to three times a day for a week or more. For use as an adjunct in obtaining specimens of bronchial secretions and cellular debris for cytologic study, the proposed dose is 100,000 units given as a single dose prior to bronchoscopy, or treatment may be continued over a period of days.

Precautions.—From the results of clinical investigation in a large number of patients, it would appear that the reactions due to sensitivity occur only rarely. The possibility of sensitivity to beef protein should nevertheless be borne in mind. To avoid bronchospasm, give Dornavac with Isuprel: e.g., 0.1 ml of Isuprel 1:200 plus 0.3 ml of propylene glycol and 1.6 ml of $\frac{1}{8}\%$

(0.125%) Neo-Synephrine. Dornavac should not be administered by the parenteral route.

How supplied.—Dornavac, which is a white powder, is supplied in a vial with vacuum-tight closure, each vial containing 100,000 units of pancreatic deoxyribonuclease, together with one 2 ml vial of sterile diluent.

NOTE: The above claims and dosage recommendations are taken from the manufacturer's literature only and thus cannot be accepted uncritically.

ISUPREL (ISOPROTERENOL HYDROCHLORIDE)—WINTHROP LABS.—Isuprel is a sympathomimetic amine. The Mistometer is a complete nebulizing unit (15 ml) containing Isuprel HCl 1:400, inert propellants (dichlorodifluoromethane and dichlorotetrafluoroethane), flavor, alcohol 33% and ascorbic acid 0.1%. It delivers 300 single oral inhalations (125 mg per dose). For use with conventional nebulizers: Solution 1:200 in a buffered aqueous vehicle containing sodium chloride, sodium citrate and glycerin with chlorobutanol 0.5% and sodium bisulfite 0.3% as preservatives; solution 1:100 in a buffered aqueous vehicle containing sodium chloride, sodium citrate, citric acid and saccharin with chlorobutanol 0.5% and sodium bisulfite 0.3% as preservatives.

Actions and uses.—A vasodilator, it is quick acting with bronchodilation in four to five breaths; it reaches peak in about 5 minutes, relaxes bronchial spasm, shrinks swollen mucous membranes, diminishes mucous secretions and facilitates expectoration of pulmonary secretions. It is frequently effective when epinephrine and other drugs fail and usually has a wide margin of safety. It is used for symptomatic treatment of bronchial spasm in asthma, emphysema and bronchitis.

Administration and dosage.—When using the Mistometer, a single inhalation generally will control an acute attack; a full minute should elapse if a second inhalation is required. Oral inhalation by a hand nebulizer is for adults and children, three to seven inhalations of 1:100 solution and five to fifteen inhalations of 1:200 solution, or by oxygen aerosolization 4 L of oxygen per minute for 15–20 minutes with up to 0.5 ml of 1:200 solution per treatment not more often than every 4 hours, except in severe cases. This drug is not to be used with epinephrine but may be alternated. Adjust dosage carefully in patients with acute coronary disease, hypertension, hypothyroidism, cardiac asthma or limited cardiac reserve and in persons sensitive to sympathomimetic amines.

Side effects.—Isuprel is usually well tolerated; however, occasionally, tachycardia, palpitation, nausea and headache may occur, especially with excessive use. Adjust dosage carefully in patients with hyperthyroidism, acute coronary disease, cardiac asthma or limited cardiac reserve and in persons sensitive to sympathomimetic amines.

Precautions.—Do not administer epinephrine with Isuprel, as both drugs are direct cardiac stimulants and combined effects may induce serious arrhythmia; they may be alternated, if desired, provided an interval of at least 4 hours has elapsed.

How supplied.—Isuprel is supplied in a Mistometer, 15 ml. For inhalation, solutions are 1:200 and 1:100. Solution 1:200 is supplied in bottles of 10 and 50 ml. Solution 1:100 is supplied in bottles of 10 ml.

NOTE: The above claims and dosage recommendations are taken from the manufacturer's literature only and thus cannot be accepted uncritically.

MUCOMYST (ACETYLCYSTEINE)—MEAD JOHNSON LABORATORIES.— Mucomyst, a mucolytic chemical, is alleged to be an effective mucolytic agent. It has been claimed to be very effective for the mucolysis of viscid secretions and is used as an adjuvant therapy in bronchopulmonary disorders when mucolysis is desirable. Studies in man and animals have shown acetylcysteine to possess a wide margin of safety. It may be administered in the hospital, in the physician's office or in the home. Acetylcysteine is the nonproprietary name for the N-acetyl derivative of the naturally occurring amino acid, L-cysteine. Chemically, it is N-acetyl-L-cysteine.

Actions and uses.—To liquefy and help remove viscid or inspissated mucous secretions in conditions such as:

Chronic bronchopulmonary disease
Acute bronchopulmonary diseases (pneumonia, bronchitis, tracheobronchitis)
Pulmonary complication of cystic fibrosis
Tracheostomy care
Anesthesia
Pulmonary complications associated with surgery
Atelectasis due to mucous obstruction
Posttraumatic chest conditions
Diagnostic bronchial studies (bronchograms, bronchospirometry, bronchial wedge catheterization)

Administration and dosage.—Mucomyst (acetylcysteine) may be administered by nebulization, intratracheal instillation or direct application. It is used with a face mask, mouthpiece or tracheal tube; 1–10 ml may be nebulized every 2–6 hours; however, for most patients, 3–5 ml of the 20% solution three to four times daily is used. It may be given in lesser percentages by diluting with water or saline and also may be mixed with a bronchodilator. Any unused portion of a vial should be refrigerated and used within 48 hours.

Side effects.—Untoward effects are rare; however, a few cases of stomatitis, nausea and occasional rhinorrhea have been reported. Certain highly sensitive patients, particularly asthmatics, may experience varying degrees of bronchospasm associated with the use of any aerosol; when encountered with the use of acetylcysteine, it may be alleviated by the use of a bronchodilator. No ophthalmologic irritation, evidence of sensitization or delayed reactions have been encountered even after prolonged administration with a closed tent.

Precautions.—After administration of acetylcysteine, the liquefied secretions (often in increased volume) must be removed. If cough is inadequate to clear the airway, mechanical suction is indicated. In case of a large blockage due to a foreign body or local accumulation of secretions, endotracheal aspiration with or without bronchoscopy should be used. Asthmatic patients under treatment with the mucolytic agent should be watched carefully. If bronchospasm occurs, this modification should be discontinued immediately.

Contraindications.—There are no known contraindications to proper use of this mucolytic agent.

How supplied.—Mucomyst is supplied in sterile 20% solution in plastic-stoppered glass vials of 10 ml in packages of three vials.

NOTE: The above claims and dosage recommendations are taken from the manufacturer's literature only and thus cannot be accepted uncritically.

TERGEMIST (SODIUM ETHASULFATE)—ABBOTT LABORATORIES.—Tergemist is a mucolytic detergent aerosol which is an aqueous solution of the detergent sodium ethasulfate (2-ethylhexyl sulfate) 0.125%, with potassium iodide 0.1%.

Actions and uses.—Tergemist is claimed to be of particular value in the therapy of various types of chronic pulmonary diseases characterized by thick tenacious sputum. Detergent in action, Tergemist wets, thins and loosens mucus which can then be coughed up. It is indicated in such conditions as bronchitis, laryngotracheobronchitis, asthma, atelectasis, pulmonary abscess and bronchiectasis.

Precaution.—Unused portions must be refrigerated and discarded 72 hours after opening. There is a theoretical possibility that sensitization to iodide or the detergent may occur. Should symptoms of hypersensitivity appear, treatment should be withdrawn. It may be contraindicated in thyroid disease.

How supplied.—Tergemist is supplied in bottles of 40, 250 and 500 ml.

NOTE: The above claims and dosage recommendations are taken from the manufacturer's literature only and thus cannot be accepted uncritically.

VAPONEFRIN SOLUTION (RACEMIC EPINEPHRINE)—USV PHARMACEUTICALS CORP.—Vaponefrin solution, a sympathomimetic amine, is a 2.2% solution of bioassayed racemic epinephrine as hydrochloride, equivalent in potency to 2.25% U.S.P. epinephrine base, with 0.5% chlorobutanol as a preservative.

Actions and uses.—Vaponefrin relaxes bronchial smooth muscles by acting on the muscle and reduces bronchial edema by vasoconstriction. It also produces prompt bronchodilation for effective relief of bronchial asthma, emphysema, chronic bronchitis or other respiratory disease in which relief of bronchospasm of mucosal congestion is indicated. Vaponefrin inhalation is notably free from side effects and can be administered to both adults and children.

Administration and dosage.—The solution is used in specially designed Vaponefrin standard- or pocket-size nebulizers or other suitable instruments. The Vaponefrin nebulizers are constructed to deliver particles in the range of 0.5–3 μ for deposition in the bronchi and bronchioles. Pour at least eight drops of Vaponefrin solution into the nebulizer; usually three to six inhalations will provide relief within 1–5 minutes. This dosage may be repeated four to six times daily, or as required. Four to ten drops in 4.5 ml volume for IPPB or four drops with eighty drops of water or with one hundred drops of 20% ethyl alcohol. For hand nebulization, use four to ten drops in 1–2-ml volumes.

Side effects.—When used in excessive dosage, epinephrine may cause bronchial irritation, nervousness, restlessness or insomnia, tachycardia and hypertension.

Precautions.—Vaponefrin solution is for oral inhalation only. It is very stable; however, once opened, storage of the bottle in a refrigerator is recommended. Excessive exposure to air or heat may cause some decomposition, and its use is not recommended if brown in color or a precipitation occurs.

Contraindications.—Because of possible circulatory effects, epinephrine should be used with caution in patients with high blood pressure, heart disease, diabetes or thyroid disease.

How supplied.—Vaponefrin comes supplied as a complete aerosol unit with separate standard- or pocket-size nebulizers and parts. Vaponefrin solution: Vials of 7.5, 15 and 30 ml.

NOTE: The above claims and dosage recommendations are taken from the manufacturer's literature only and thus cannot be accepted uncritically.

REFERENCES

Rodman, M. J., and Smith, D. W.: *Pharmacology and Drug Therapy in Nursing* (Philadelphia: J. B. Lippincott Company, 1968).

Horgan, P. D.: Caring for the drug-poisoned patient, R.N. 25:62, 1962.

Friend, D. G.: Pharmacology of muscle relaxants, Clin. Pharmacol. & Therap. 5:871, 1964.

Himwich, H. E.: The physiology of alcohol, J.A.M.A. 163:545, 1957.

Bresnick, E., *et al.*: Evaluation of therapeutic substances for relief of bronchospasm. V. Adrenergic agents, J. Clin. Invest. 28:1182, 1949.

Gay, L. N., and Long, J. W.: Clinical evaluation of isopropyl epinephrine in management of bronchial asthma, J.A.M.A. 139:452, 1949.

Kay, C. F.: Current status of therapy for congestive heart failure. Report to the Council on Drugs, J.A.M.A. 164:657, 1957.

CHAPTER 15

Pulmonary Function Testing

CLINICAL LUNG FUNCTION study had its beginning around 280 B.C., when experimental physiologists named Erasistratus and, later, Galen experimented with the diaphragm. Not only did they prove that the diaphragm was a muscle of respiration, but they also established the origin and functions of the phrenic nerve and the intercostal and accessory muscles of respiration. Around 1500, da Vinci observed the function of the thoracic cage and its relationship to ventilation. Vesalius (1514–1564) described collapse of the lungs, which was the result of a puncture of the pleural lining of the lung.

Ultimate need for fresh air was recognized by Galen, who postulated that fresh air, when in contact with blood in the left heart and arteries, produced the "vital spirit." He concluded that the communication between the pulmonary artery and the pulmonary vein were invisible pores of the two sides of the heart. The true function of the lung was yet to be discovered. Ibn-al-Nafis (1210–1288) experimented and proved that the barrier to the passage of blood was imposed by the interventricular septum and that blood passes from the pulmonary artery through the lung to the pulmonary vein. The experimental work by Harvey (1578–1657), dealing with the circulation of the blood through the lung, and by Malpighi (1628–1694), on the proximity of the capillaries to the smallest air sacs, prepared the way for a better clinical understanding of pulmonary function.

Barelli, in 1679, measured the maximum inspiratory volume of air in man for the first time. Hutchinson, in 1846, defined vital capacity while using his crudely designed spirometer. He also related vital capacity to the height of the subject, so that "for every inch of height (from five feet to six feet) eight additional inches of air at 60° F. are given out by forced expiration." He further demonstrated that the vital capacity is reduced by aging, obesity and respiratory disease. Davy, in the early 1800s, was the first man to measure residual volume, using the dilution method (hydrogen gas).

Between 1800 and early 1900, man and machine gradually replaced the older techniques of study by introducing the concepts of dynamic evaluation of the lung volumes for vital capacity.

Kory and Hamilton contributed considerably to this new approach by reporting results from the Stead-Wells spirometer. This design consisted of a light, plastic-noncounterweighted bell and a minimal dead space. This device proved superior to the common metal bell-type spirometer used for the dynamic lung volume measurements as a function of time. Even with improvement of design and technique, there existed still much confusion in dynamic lung volume measurements. To clear up this confusion, Wright developed a manometer through which the patient was instructed to exhale as fast and deep as he could. A needle on the dial of the Wright peak flowmeter moved to the maximal velocity or peak expiratory flow rate attained for a period of at least 0.1 second.

Ventilatory capacity is the maximal ability to move a gas rapidly in and out of the lungs. This ability is influenced by airway resistance, vital capacity and a number of other physiologic parameters; the actual measurements are also influenced by procedural factors and by the characteristics of the measuring devices.

Many tests are available today for measuring the degree of pulmonary insufficiency. These tests range from simple, such as instructing a patient with his mouth wide open to blow out a match held at increasing distances from his face, to very complex examinations requiring complicated equipment. Test of pulmonary function accurately portrays the nature and extent of impairment of ventilation.

These tests do not always indicate the cause of any impairment; instead the data obtained in these tests are quite useful in reaching a correct estimate of the efficiency of respiratory function in patients with respiratory abnormalities and in evaluating at various stages the therapy rendered these patients.

The terms used in pulmonary function testing can be confusing. In 1950, agreement on standard terminology between British and American clinicians and physiologists was achieved. These accepted terms in pulmonary function testing are given in Table 3 (pp. 252–253).

Measurement of the degree of expiratory airway obstruction is the most valuable clinical laboratory aid in the diagnosis of chronic obstructive lung diseases and in the estimation of their severity. Usually, during the testing procedure, the average subject needs one or two practice attempts in order to attain a reproducible level of performance. The testing measurements, therefore, will require a total of at least five determinations. The resulting measurement is influenced to a great degree by the personality and patience of the clinician. The clinician should be skilled in his procedures and should be aware of the patient's performance at all times.

The effects of abnormal air trapping is best observed if the time-volume relationship is measured during forced expiration. Often when the vital capacity is measured without the forced component, the values may be normal even in patients with chronic obstructive lung disease.

An even more striking reduction from the normal value in the forced expiratory volume is often seen when the volume exhaled in the first second (FEV 1.0) is compared with the test result predicted for a healthy individual of the same sex, age, weight and height.

To determine maximal voluntary ventilation, the patient is instructed to inhale and exhale through the spirometer tube as rapidly as possible for 12–15 seconds, choosing a tidal volume greater than his normal resting volume. The degree of the volume of air that this patient can move in a given period of time depends on the effects of airway obstruction and muscular fatigue. This measurement can be found by using either an open circuit or rebreathing equipment.

The forced expiratory volume is the quantity of gas which is expelled from the lung over a timed period when the subject makes a maximal expiratory effort from a position of full inspiration. The time interval which is adopted is usually 1 second when the index is called the FEV. Longer and shorter timed periods are used, but the volumes which can be expired over times of between 0.5 and 3 seconds are highly correlated; consequently, little additional information is obtained by making measurements at more than one time interval.

The forced expiratory volume is recorded either on the kymograph of the spirometer used for registration of the maximal voluntary ventilation or by a timing device attached to the spirometer. The kymograph should have a paper speed of at least 2.0 cm (sec).

Forced expiratory flow ($FEF_{200-1200}$), formerly called maximal expiratory flow rate (MEFR), is the average rate of flow for a specified portion of the forced expiratory volume, usually between 200 and 1,200 ml.

Forced mid-expiratory flow ($FMF_{20-75\%}$), formerly called maximal mid-expiratory flow rate, is the average rate of flow during the middle half of the forced expiratory volume.

The standard laboratory instrument used for most tests of ventilatory function is a recording spirometer (see Fig. 154), which is capable of measuring all categories of lung volumes and of time-volume relationships.

A relatively simple and inexpensive bellows device is shown in Figure

TABLE 3.—TERMINOLOGY OF LUNG VOLUME AND VENTILATORY MEASUREMENTS

STANDARIZED TERM	SYMBOL	DEFINITION	PREVIOUSLY USED TERMS
Lung volumes°			
Inspiratory reserve volume	IRV	Maximal volume of gas that can be inspired from end tidal inspiration	Complemental air Complementary air
Tidal volume	TV	Volume of gas inspired or expired during each respiratory cycle	Tidal air
Expiratory reserve volume	ERV	Maximal volume of gas that can be expired from resting expiratory level	Supplemental air Reserve air
Residual volume	RV	Volume of gas remaining in the lungs at the end of a maximal expiration	Residual air (RA) Residual capacity
Lung capacities †			
Total lung capacity	TLC	Amount of gas contained in the lungs at the end of a maximal inspiration	Total lung capacity
Vital capacity‡	VC	Maximal amount of gas that can be expelled from the lungs following a maximal inspiration	Vital capacity
Inspiratory capacity	IC	Maximal amount of gas that can be inspired from the resting expiratory level	Complemental air Complementary air
Functional residual capacity	FRC	Amount of gas remaining in the lungs at the resting end-expiratory level	Functional residual air Midcapacity Equilibrium capacity Normal capacity
Ventilatory measurements‡			
Forced vital capacity	FVC	The vital capacity performed with expiration as forceful as possible	Timed vital capacity Fast vital capacity Fast maximal expiratory capacity
Forced expiratory volume (qualified by subscript indicating the time interval in seconds from the beginning of expiration to the volume measured)	FEV_T	Volume of gas exhaled over a given time interval during the performance of a forced vital capacity (e.g., $FEV_{1.0}$ is the forced expiratory volume of 1 second)	Timed vital capacity Fast expiratory capacity Forced expiratory capacity Maximum expiratory volume

(Continued)

TABLE 3.—TERMINOLOGY OF LUNG VOLUME AND VENTILATORY MEASUREMENTS (cont.)

Standardized Term	Symbol	Definition	Previously Used Terms
Percentage forced expiratory volume (in T seconds)	$FEV_{T\%}$	FEV_T expressed as percentage of the forced vital capacity (i.e., $FEV_T/F_{VC} \times 100$)	Timed vital capacity Timed expiratory capacity % timed vital capacity §
Forced expiratory flow‖	$FEF_{V_1-V_2}$ $FEF_{V_1-V_2\%}$	The average rate of flow for a specified volume segment of the forced expiratory spirogram (e.g., $FEF_{200-1200}$ and $FEF_{0-25\%}$)	Maximal expiratory flow rate (MEFR)
Forced midexpiratory flow ¶	FMF	The average rate of flow during the middle two quarters of the volume segment of the forced expiratory spirogram (i.e., from 25–75% of the volume or $FEF_{25-75\%}$)	Maximal midexpiratory flow (MMF)
Maximal voluntary ventilation °°	MVV	Amount of air which a subject can breathe with voluntary maximal ventilatory effort per unit of time	Maximum breathing capacity (MBC) Maximal breathing capacity Maximum ventilatory capacity

° The term "volumes" refers to one of the four nonoverlapping primary compartments of the total lung capacity.

† The term "capacities" refers to one of the four measurements which are the sum of two or more of the primary "volumes."

‡ For measurements made when maximal inspiration follows maximal expiration, terms such as inspiratory vital capacity (IVC), forced inspiratory vital capacity (FIVC) and forced inspiration flow (FIF) should be used. The term maximal inspiratory flow rate (MIFR) has been used to refer to a specified portion of a forced inspiration.

§ The volume of forced expiration in a specified time has also been related to vital capacity. e.g., FEV_T, VC × 100, rather than as a percentage of the forced total capacity.

‖ The subscript $_V$ represents a particular volume-defined point on the forced expiratory spirogram (FES). V_1 represents the first such point, V_2 the second. Thus, in the expression $FEF_{200-1200}$, the 200 represents the 200 ml point on the FES and 1200 the 1200 ml point.

The subscripts V_1–$V_n\%$ represent volume points defined as percentages of the FVC. Thus, $FEF_{0-25\%}$ represents the rate of flow during the first 25% of the volume expired during the FVC.

¶ For the middle half of the volume of the FVC (forced midexpiratory flow), the symbol $FEF_{25-75\%}$ is also used.

°° When frequency is not controlled, the term used is maximal voluntary ventilation, free (MVV_F), but the frequency adopted by the subject may also be noted (thus MVV_{F40}, MVV_{F60}). When the frequency is controlled, the F subscript is omitted but the frequency actually used is indicated by a subscript (thus, MVV_{40}, MVV_{60}). Since the maximal breathing capacity may be assessed in several ways other than voluntary effort, such as after exercise and CO_2 inhalation, the term MBC should be reversed to indicate a maximal value for a given subject.

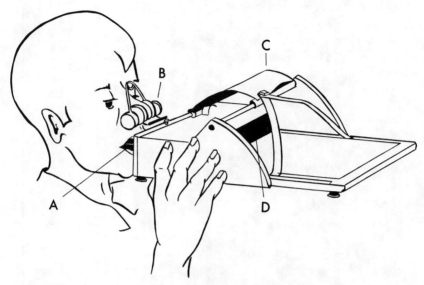

Fig. 143.—Vitalor, a bellows device which records a spirogram over a 6-second interval. A, mouthpiece; B, nose clip; C, spirogram scale; D, bellows mechanism.

143, which records a spirogram over a 6-second interval from which the FVC and FEV_1 can readily be determined. This bellows device may give a false low value for the forced vital capacity if severe airway obstruction is present, since only the volume exhaled in 6 seconds is recorded.

It is obvious that tests of ventilation fail to give information about respiratory gas exchange, except by implication. In managing patients with pulmonary disease, it is necessary to evaluate pulmonary function completely by means of all the tests of ventilation and gas exchange commonly used in cardiopulmonary function laboratories.

A method of screening pulmonary function that has been found to be effective involves the following steps:

1. Careful analysis of the patient's history
2. Careful physical examination of the heart and lungs
3. Study of serial chest x-rays
4. An effective record system of reporting and calculating measured data
5. Prolonged forced expiration

Study of x-rays.—The physiologic pattern that accompanies many pulmonary or cardiovascular conditions is suggested to the careful observer who comprehensively studies chest films. Serial chest x-rays can signify that the physiologic state is worsening or improving.

Record system.—In developing an effective record system, care must be used to avoid awkward and time-consuming data systems. The facts included should be all-inclusive and should provide as much meaningful data as possible.

History.—Special attention should be paid to disease or other factors which might reduce the ventilation of a lobe or of one or both lungs by affecting the ribs, diaphragm, pleurae, parenchyma or tracheobronchial tree. The presence or absence of dyspnea related to daily activities may be indication of breathing capacity.

Physical examination.—The following may offer clues to altered pulmonary function which may be discovered in the physical examination:

1. Pulse (cardiac disease)
2. Rales, wheezes (location of disease)
3. Labored breathing at rest or after mild exercise
4. Contour and mobility of chest, clubbing of nails of extremities

CLINICAL PULMONARY PHYSIOLOGY

The objective of clinical pulmonary physiology is to detect signs of restrictive and/or obstructive pulmonary disease.

Pulmonary respiration involves three fundamental processes, each going on simultaneously. There is the process of ventilation, in which the lung acts as a bellows in moving air in and out; the process of diffusion, in which oxygen and carbon dioxide pass across the alveolar capillary membrane; and the process of circulation or pulmonary capillary blood flow, the adequacy of which is essential for proper gaseous exchange.

The diffusion coefficient for carbon dioxide is twenty times greater than that for oxygen. This diffusion is dependent on a normal central nervous system mechanism to regulate it. In the lungs, there are approximately 1,000,000 bronchi, and about 750,000,000 alveoli. The upper airway down to and including the bronchioles does not participate in gaseous exchange. Rather, it is a passage that serves as a conducting airway for gases to flow to and from the alveoli where exchange does take place.

The volume of air present within the mouth, pharynx, trachea and larger bronchi not participating in gaseous exchange is called the anatomic dead space (Fig. 145). The space is approximately 150 cc in healthy adult males and 100 cc in healthy adult females and will usually vary with the height, weight and age of the individual.

(A)

PULMONARY FUNCTION REPORT A

| DATE |
| CLINIC OR |
| DIVISION ← |
| RECORD NO. |
| PT'S NAME |
| PARENT |
| ADDRESS ← |

| DATE OF TEST | SERIAL NUMBER |

STUDIED BY_____ REFERRED BY_____

REFERRAL DIAGNOSIS_____

PULMONARY
FUNCTION DIAGNOSIS_____

AGE (YR.) _____ WT (KG.) _____   CODE #

HT., (CM.) _____ S. A. (M²) _____

LUNG VOLUMES	Pre-dicted	Observed	% Pre-dicted	After 0.5% Isoprot'nol	% Pre-dicted	DISTRIBUTION OF VENTILATION	Pre-dicted	Ob-served
VITAL CAPACITY (VC) (L)						ALV. GAS UNIFORMITY (%) (% N_2 750-1250 ml)	< 1.5	
INSPIRATORY CAP. (IC) (L)								
EXPIRATORY RESERVE VOLUME (ERV) (L)						N_2 ELIMINATION RATE (%) (% N_2 after 7' breathing O_2)	< 2.5	
RESIDUAL VOLUME (RV) (L)						DISTRIBUTION OF GAS TO BLOOD	Pre-dicted	Ob-served
TOTAL LUNG CAP. (TLC) (L)								
RESIDUAL VOL./TLC (%)						WASTED VENTILATION (VD) (L) (physiological dead space)		
FUNCT. RESID. CAP. (FRC) 1. N_2 WASHOUT (L)						WASTED VENT./TIDAL VOL. (%)	< 40	
2. THORACIC GAS VOL.* (L) (plethysmograph)						EFFECTIVE MIN. VENT. (L/min) (alv. vent. calc. from wasted vent.)		
						ART.-"ALV." CO_2 DIFF. (mmHg)	< 4	
MECHANICS OF BREATHING						VENTILATION	Before Test	Air
FORCED EXPIR. VOL. (FEV₁) (L)						RESPIRATORY RATE (breaths/min) (f)		
% EXPIR. IN 1 SEC. (%)	> 79					TIDAL VOLUME (VT) (L)		
MAX. EXPIR. FLOW RATE (MEFR) (L/min)	400-500**					MINUTE VOLUME (VE) (L/min)		
MAX. INSPIR. FLOW RATE (MIFR) (L/min)	300-500**					EXPIRED PCO_2 (mmHg)		
PEAK FLOW RATE (L/min)						"ALV." PCO_2 (mmHg) ART. PCO_2 (mmHg) (by gas rebreath.)	Predicted 38-42	
						DIFFUSION	Pre-dicted +	Ob-served
AIRWAY RESISTANCE (RA) (cm H_2O/L/sec)						PULM. DIFFUSING CAP. (DCO) (ml/min/mmHg)		
LUNG COMPLIANCE (CL) (L/cm H_2O)						PULM. CAPILLARY BLOOD VOL. (VC) (ml)		
COMPLIANCE/PRED. FRC (L/cm H_2O)	0.04-0.07					MEMBRANE DIFFUSING CAPACITY (DM) (ml/min/mmHg)		
TRANSPULMONARY PRESSURE (cm H_2O) (PTP) @ FRC	4-7					TOTAL LUNG CAP. (NEON DILUTION METHOD) (L)		
@ TLC	> 20							

THE CHILDREN'S HOSPITAL MEDICAL CENTER, BOSTON, MASS.

* WHEN THIS VALUE IS REPORTED, IT IS USED TO CALCULATE TOTAL LUNG CAPACITY AND RESIDUAL VOLUME.
** VALUES ARE LOWER IN CHILDREN AND THE ELDERLY.
+ ON BASIS OF ACTUAL LUNG VOLUME

COMMENTS:

F 820-25C.1/66

Fig. 144.—Example of pulmonary function report sheet A. (*Continued.*)

Ⓑ

PULMONARY FUNCTION REPORT B

DATE
CLINIC OR
DIVISION ←
RECORD NO.
PT'S NAME
PARENT
ADDRESS ←

DATE OF TEST	SERIAL NUMBER

STUDIED BY_____ REFERRED BY_____

REFERRAL DIAGNOSIS_____
PULMONARY
FUNCTION DIAGNOSIS_____

AGE (YR.)_____ WT (KG.)_____ CODE #

HT., (CM.)_____ S. A. (M²)_____

ARTERIAL BLOOD	PREDICTED	Air	O2	ARTERIAL BLOOD	PREDICTED	Air	O2
TOTAL O2 CONTENT (vol. %)	AIR - 20.6 O2 - 22.9			HEMOGLOBIN (gm. %)	15.6		
				HEMATOCRIT (%)	45		
DISSOLVED O2 (vol. %)	AIR - 0.3 O2 - 1.9			CO2 CONTENT - BLOOD (mM/L)	20.5 - 23.1		
				CO2 CONTENT - PLASMA (mM/L)	25 - 28.5		
O2 CAPACITY (vol. %)	20.9			CO2 TENSION (measured) (mmHg)	38 - 42		
O2 SATURATION (%)	96 - 99						
O2 TENSION (mmHg)	AIR>80 O2>550						
				pH (units)*	7.38 - 7.42		

EXERCISE AND RECOVERY

CONDITION

BICYCLE		Load	KgM/min		Load	KgM/min		Load	KgM/min		Recovery			Stop'd exercise due to:
ARTERIAL BLOOD	REST	2'	4'	6'	2'	4'	6'	2'	4'	6'	2'	4'	6'	
O2 TENSION (mmHg)														
O2 SATURATION (%)														
O2 TENSION (mmHg)														
pH (units)														
O2 CONSUMPTION (L/min)														
R (CO2/O2)														
MIN. VOL. RESPIR. (L/min)														
RESP. RATE (breaths/min)														
HEART RATE (beats/min)														
WASTED VENTILATION (L)														
WAST. VENT/TID. VOL. (%)														

* With Asterisk - Blood determination done with patient breathing through mouthpiece.
COMMENTS:

THE CHILDREN'S HOSPITAL MEDICAL CENTER, BOSTON, MASS.

Fig. 144 (cont.).—Example of pulmonary function report sheet B.

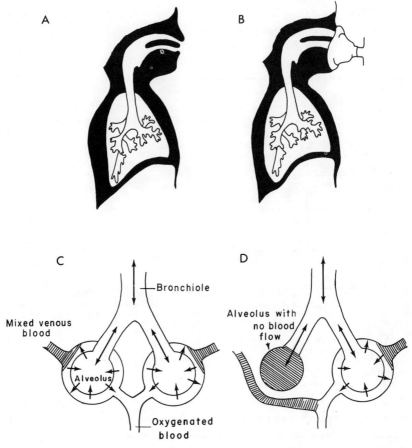

Fig. 145.—Areas in which gas exchange does not occur—"dead space." **A**, gross anatomic dead space; **B**, anatomic and equipment dead space; **C**, microanatomic dead space; **D**, physiologic dead space.

Nitrogen Wash-out Method

After normal expiration, the patient breathes 100% oxygen for 7 minutes. Since nitrogen is an inert gas, it simply diffuses across the alveolar capillary membrane. With each expiration, nitrogen is washed out of the lung. A spirometer or Douglas bag is used to collect the volume of expired gas. At the end of 7 minutes, breathing 100% oxygen, no more than 2.5% nitrogen should remain in the lung if the distribution is equal.

From the total volume of gases collected in the spirometer, the percentage of nitrogen can be readily measured with a nitrogen meter; the total amount of nitrogen existing in the lung at the end of a quiet expiration may be easily calculated. With the knowledge of this volume occupied by nitrogen and with the realization that room air is approximately 80% nitrogen, the functional residual capacity for room air may be easily calculated.

The normal values vary with age, sex and size of the patient. The actual value obtained from the patient should be considered normal if it is within 20% of the predicted, calculated normal.

In performing the routine vital capacity, the timed element is not added; thus the patient with severe ventilatory defects may show a normal vital capacity.

RESPIRATORY DEAD SPACE.—Respiratory dead space is important.

Minute volume:

The volume of air breathed per breath times the rate of breathing per minute

EXAMPLE:

$$R = 15$$
$$TV = 500$$
$$MV = 7,500 \text{ cc}$$

$$\begin{array}{cc} R & TV \\ 15 \times 500 & = 7,500 \text{ cc} \end{array}$$

Since we are interested in the volume of gas that participates in gaseous exchange in the alveoli, one must also keep in mind the anatomic dead space.

EXAMPLE: Patient "A," male, is comfortable with a respiratory rate of 10/m and tidal volume of 800 cc. The minute volume equals 8,000 cc (10 × 800 = 8,000 cc).

Patient "B," male, is dyspneic and cyanotic and has a respiratory rate of 40/m and a tidal volume of 200 cc, so that his minute volume is 8,000 cc (40 × 200 = 8,000 cc).

The minute volume for patients "A" and "B" is the same, but patient "A" is comfortable and patient "B" is in respiratory distress. The importance of calculating ventilation in terms of anatomic dead space is shown below:

Patient "A"   150 cc × 10 = 1,500 cc
              8,000 cc − 1,500 = 6,500 cc
                 6,500 cc alveolar ventilation is adequate
Patient "B"   150 cc × 40 = 6,000 cc
              8,000 cc − 6,000 cc = 2,000 cc

Alveolar ventilation is only 2,000 cc per minute and, of course, is inadequate for this patient, which accounts for the marked respiratory distress.

MECHANICS OF BREATHING

Timed vital capacity

1. The patient is instructed to exhale forcibly as rapidly as he can after a maximal inspiration.
2. The spinning drum will record the results.
3. The volume as well as the time can be calculated accurately.
4. Normally, the patient should complete 85% of his vital capacity in 2 seconds and 95% in 3 seconds.
5. Patients with bronchitis, asthma or emphysema, for example, may be able to perform the ordinary vital capacity normally; but, when the timed element is added, he will trap air in the lung so that the timed vital capacity is almost invariably abnormal.

Maximal voluntary ventilation (MVV)

1. The patient is instructed to breathe into a mouthpiece that is connected to a spirometer as deep and as fast as he can for a period of 10–15 seconds—normally 100 L per minute. Then multiply by 6 or 4 to calculate volume for 1 minute.
2. The spinning drum will record the results.
3. From the spirogram, the volume of air maximally ventilated for 1 minute may be calculated.
4. Airway obstruction will be abnormal if asthma, bronchitis or other ventilatory defects are present.
5. This test is considered normal if within 20% of the predicted calculated normal.

OXYGEN SATURATION, CONTENT AND CAPACITY OF ARTERIAL BLOOD

The blood transports oxygen in two ways:

1. In physiologic solution in the plasma
2. Chemical combination of oxygen with hemoglobin

The latter is the most important transport mechanism and in normal patients is responsible for transporting almost 20 cc of oxygen per 100 cc of blood compared with 0.3 cc of oxygen per 100 cc of plasma carried in physiologic solution.

OXYGEN IN PHYSIOLOGIC SOLUTION IN PLASMA.—The amount of oxygen carried in this manner is directly proportional to the partial pressure of

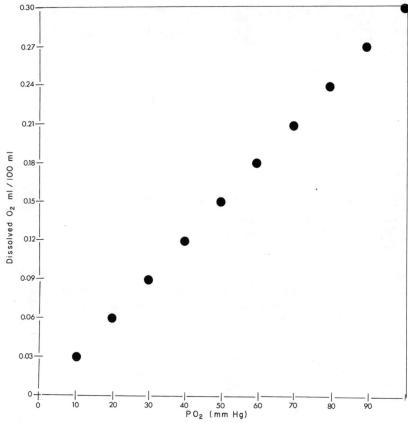

Fig. 146.—The amount of plasma dissolved with oxygen at different partial pressures.

oxygen in the alveoli. To illustrate this direct pressure-volume relationship, see Figure 146.

Plotting the curve with increasing partial pressure of oxygen in the alveoli (flasks), there is a straight line relationship between pressure and volume.

OXYGEN COMBINATION WITH HEMOGLOBIN.—If we substitute whole blood for plasma, repeat the above procedure and plot graphically, we find an S-shaped curve rather than a straight line (Fig. 148).

This S-shaped oxygen dissociation curve permits a wide range of adaptability. If an individual goes from sea level, where P_{O_2} in the alveolar is 100 mm Hg, to 8,000 feet, where P_{O_2} may fall to 80 or 85 mm Hg, very little decrease in volume of oxygen in arterial blood occurs. But, if

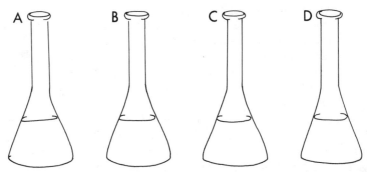

Fig. 147.—Oxygen in physiologic solution in plasma. Each flask (A, B, C and D) contains 100 ml of plasma at partial pressures of 10, 10, 90 and 100 mm Hg. **A,** the amount of oxygen carried in 100 ml of plasma at 10 mm Hg is 0.03 cc; **B,** the amount of oxygen carried in 100 ml of plasma at 20 mm Hg is 0.06 cc; **C,** the amount of oxygen carried in 100 ml of plasma at 90 mm Hg is 0.27 cc; **D,** the amount of oxygen carried in 100 ml of plasma at 100 mm Hg is 0.3 cc.

he climbs to 14,000 feet, the decrease in partial pressure of oxygen at the alveolar level may be to 70 or 65 mm Hg, and a marked drop in volume of oxygen per 100 cc of arterial blood will be evidenced.

One gram of hemoglobin when fully saturated with oxygen is capable of carrying 1.34 cc of oxygen, the normal hemoglobin being about 15.6 Gm per 100 cc of blood. Thus, we can predict:

$$15.6 \times 1.34 = 20.9 \text{ cc } O_2/100 \text{ of whole blood}$$

Diffusion.—This is the exchange of gases across the alveolar capillary membrane. Diffusion insufficiency means impairment of alveolar capillary gaseous exchange. The evaluation of diffusion insufficiency most widely used in clinical laboratories is the carbon monoxide method. This evaluation may be performed in two ways—namely, the single-breath method (Forester modification) and the steady-state method. Because of the simplicity of carbon dioxide measurement with an infrared analyzer, the single-breath method is probably the most commonly used.

In both the single-breath and the steady-state methods, the principle is the same; that is, carbon monoxide reaching the blood is combined with hemoglobin with none remaining in plasma, as does oxygen. The implication is that the mean alveolar-capillary gradient is equal to the alveolar carbon monoxide tension. (The affinity of hemoglobin for carbon monoxide is approximately 200 times as great as the affinity for oxygen.)

In the single-breath method (Forester modification), the patient is asked to exhale maximally then inspire a gas mixture containing 10% helium, 0.3%

carbon monoxide and 21% oxygen, the balance being nitrogen. After an apneic period of about 30 seconds, the patient exhales into an infrared analyzer where carbon monoxide and helium concentration are recorded. The alveolar carbon monoxide concentration at the beginning of apnea may be calculated, and the alveolar volume during the test may be calculated likewise from the helium dilution which occurs during the period of apnea. The diffusion capacity for carbon monoxide may be found easily, using simple algebraic formulas. Defects will show a widened oxygen tension gradient between alveolar and pulmonary capillary. Knowing the diffusion capacity for carbon monoxide across the alveolar capillary membrane by calculation or nomogram, one may obtain the diffusion capacity for oxygen.

Diffusion insufficiency may occur due to an abnormal membrane or when a shortened contact time occurs between alveolar gas and the blood. The latter may happen with a normal alveolar capillary membrane, but impaired pulmonary capillary blood flow is always present when the pulmonary capillary bed is decreased to less than about one-third its normal capacity with normal cardiac output. In such instances, the velocity of

Fig. 148.—Oxygen dissociation curves for human blood.

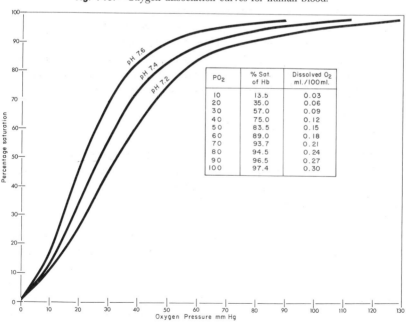

blood flow is increased so that contact time between alveolar air and capillary blood is so shortened that equilibration of alveolar and pulmonary capillary oxygen is not possible, thus showing a "diffusion defect."

PULMONARY CIRCULATION

It is often just as important to know the volume and distribution of pulmonary capillary blood flow as it is to know the volume and distribution of alveolar ventilation. Similarly, the mechanical factors involved in pumping an adequate volume of blood through the pulmonary capillaries are important to respiration.

The systolic and diastolic pressure in major vessels, cardiac chambers and pulmonary capillary pressure are listed below:

Aorta pressure: 120 mm Hg systolic, 80 mm Hg diastolic
Atrium (left): (mean) 5 mm Hg
Pulmonary artery: 24 mm Hg systolic, 10 mm Hg diastolic
Pulmonary capillary (wedge) pressure: 10 mm Hg
Left ventricle: 120 mm Hg systolic, 5 mm Hg diastolic
Right ventricle: 25 mm Hg systolic, 0 mm Hg diastolic
Venous: 70–140 mm H_2O

It is noteworthy that the right ventricular and pulmonary arterial pressures do not rise in a normal individual, even when pulmonary blood flow is increased twofold by exercise. Thus, the pulmonary vascular resistance must decrease due to dilatation of existing pulmonary capillaries or to opening of new vessels or both. The pulmonary vascular channels normally may be reduced markedly without increase in right ventricular pressure.

BLOOD GAS DETERMINATION

Problems in respiratory physiology and in clinical research concerned with human subjects and mammalian laboratory animals involve analysis of gas mixtures. Most of this work has been done with chemical methods of gas analysis by Peters, Van Slyke, Sorensen, Astrup, Severinghaus, Riley and Hasselbalch.

Certain physical properties have unique values for the gases present during respiration. Such properties are mass numbers (molecular weight), ionic mass-charge ratio, atomic and molecular emission spectra and atomic nuclear properties.

Other physical properties that have less typical values for each gas can be used for analysis with caution. Such properties are heat conductivity, magnetic susceptibility, refractive index, using visible light, viscosity, density, absorption of sound energy and velocity of sound. In general, use of these properties requires molecular separation of the species of the unanalyzed mixture by chemical absorption, then physical absorption or condensation before the method of analysis can be applied. To properly evaluate patients with respiratory impairments, it is important to have and use blood gas and acid-base balance measurement. Recent advancement in polarographic technique has made it possible to measure oxygen tension in whole blood and other fluids quite rapidly and accurately. In 1956, Clark introduced the membrane-covered electrode (Fig. 149), separating the blood or other unknown from the electrolytic cell by a membrane permeable to oxygen (polyethylene) but impermeable to ions, proteins and solutes. When whole blood is in direct contact with a platinum electrode, it coats the electrode with a precipitated protein, resulting in rapid deterioration of electrode performance. Clark overcame this problem by

Fig. 149.—Clark oxygen electrode. *A,* polyethylene membrane over tip; *B,* AgCl-Ag reference anode; *C,* braid of wire soldered to anode; *D,* anode; *E,* cathode; *F,* saturated KCl; *G,* rubber of "O" ring; *H,* platinum tip of cathode.

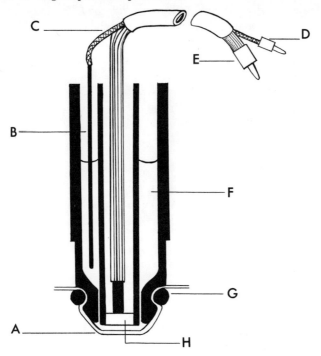

introducing the use of a plastic gas-permeable membrane to separate the blood from the platinum electrode and surrounding electrolyte. The Clark electrode measures the oxygen dissolved in the electrolyte after diffusion from the sample through the plastic membrane.

Partial pressure is the fraction of the total gas pressure exerted by a gas. For example, if the total pressure is 713 mm Hg (total atmospheric pressure minus water-vapor pressure) and the gas fraction is 0.05 (5%), then the partial pressure equals 713 × 0.05 equals 36 mm Hg at equilibration across surfaces which allow for diffusion when partial pressures are equal, thus the pK in a closed gas space above a liquid is the same as the pK in the liquid. The total gas dissolved in the liquid is related to, but not the same as, the partial pressure. The quantity is determined by the pressure and the solubility of the gas. In addition, the quantity of gas which can be carried in, and released from, a solution may represent that which is in the chemical combination in solution. Carbon dioxide in blood exists mostly as bicarbonate and oxygen mostly as oxyhemoglobin. The relationship between partial pressure and total content is given by the dissociation curves. The total oxygen combined with hemoglobin compared with the maximal oxygen in the blood when exposed to air is the oxygen saturation.

Carbon dioxide dissolved in blood undergoes the following reaction: The tension and the content of carbon dioxide and the concentration of hydrogen ions in the blood are related through the Henderson-Hasselbalch equation, which is derived by application of carbonic acid (H_2CO_3) of the law of mass

$$CO_2 \times H_2O \quad H_2CO_3 \quad H^+ + HCO_3^-$$

at equilibration $[H_2CO_3] = K[H^+][HCO_3^-]$

$$[H^+] = \frac{[H_2CO_3]}{[HCO_3^-]} = K$$

$$\log [H^+] = \log \frac{[H_2CO_3]}{[HCO_3^-]} + \log K$$

$$pH = pK + \log \frac{[HCO_3^-]}{[H_2CO_3]}$$

pH

When a solution of known $[H^+]$ is on one side of a special glass membrane and unknown $[H^-]$ on the other, an electromotor force is established. Two half cells connect this source of voltage to the voltmeter to read the pH. Since the voltage developed by these half cells, plus the junction voltage, are added and must remain constant at all times, they must remain clean and properly filled with fluid.

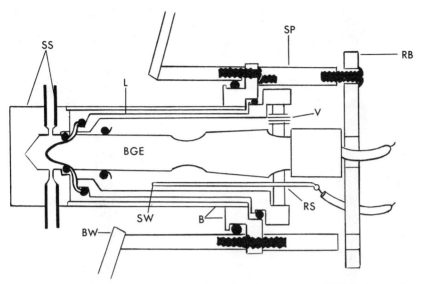

Fig. 150.—Design of a carbon dioxide electrode and its curvette. *BGE*, Beckman glass electrode; *B*, brass; *BW*, bath wall; *L*, lucite solution; *RB*, retaining bracket; *RS*, ring seal; *SP*, spacer posts; *SS*, stainless steel; *SW*, silver wire; *V*, vent.

The pH control balance shifts the entire scale recording to standardize the direct readout against a known buffer. Temperature changes the slope response to conform to the temperature characteristics of the glass electrode.

P_{CO_2}

The measurement of P_{CO_2} is actually made by a pH meter which is separated from the blood by a thin membrane which is permeable to gas, but not to liquid. Surrounding this pH electrode is the buffer solution, and, as the CO_2 equilibrates across the membrane, the pH of this buffer changes in proportion to the P_{CO_2}.

We shall try to cover briefly the problem of the interpretation of blood gases in relation to patient care on respirators. We would like to emphasize, of course, that blood gases have been analyzed for a long time by various methods: Riley bubble, the dissociation curve, Henderson-Hasselbalch relationship, the Astrup technique (Fig. 151), CO_2 electrode gas chromatography (Fig. 152) and various indirect techniques. But as we begin to use these more frequently and begin to study the physiology of the organism, we realize that the answers are probably not straightforward and that sometimes we are faced with paradoxes that are difficult to understand

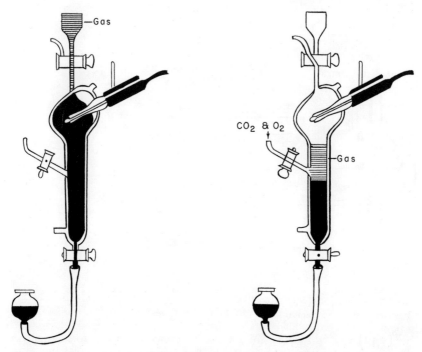

Fig. 151.—Illustration of an Astrup apparatus. This technique utilizes the plasma carbon dioxide dissociation curve to determine the Pco_2. The pH of the blood is measured, plasma is then separated from the whole blood sample and is equilibrated with a known Pco_2 and the pH measured. Reference is then made to the standard dissociation curve and a linear plot of log Pco_2 is made against pH. The blood Pco_2 is read at the intersection of this curve with the blood pH.

on the surface but have very definite physiologic meaning. Graphic representation of multiple variables is possible within certain limits (Fig. 153).

Let us look at the areas in which relevant information may be found in many postoperative surgical patients: First, at the physiologic dead space which is the V_d/V_t ratio, then, at the venous admixture, certainly at the cardiac output, which is not very frequently mentioned here but which very definitely influences the gas exchange in the lungs, and, lastly, at the problems of acid-base balance.

A common way by which to approach the patient who is to receive respiratory support in the postoperative period is through sedation and, from our experiences, we prefer intravenous morphine and, eventually, d-Tubocurare. The reason for the curare is not, as some people think, just to enable the patient to tolerate the respirator, but quite often to produce essential basal conditions. The syndrome to be counteracted is one in which the patient thrashes, becomes quite agitated and then shows a markedly elevated oxygen consumption.

How do we wean a patient from respiratory support? (See Chapter 10, p. 149.) A practical method for weaning the patient who, in the post-operative period, has been on the respirator for 12, 24 or 48 hours is as follows: First of all, check the arterial P_{O_2} on a 100% oxygen, as this will give some idea as to what the alveolar oxygen gradient is. Then check the arterial P_{O_2} with the patient breathing oxygen spontaneously. In common usage now for this purpose is the Briggs adaptor, which is a local fabrication and is essentially a "T" tube with no valves, so that the patient may inspire approximately 60–70% oxygen from a wall or tank source. The "T" tube is connected to the tracheal tube. Then, the tidal volume and the vital capacity are checked. Now if the P_{O_2} on the 60–70% mixture of oxygen and air with the patient breathing spontaneously is above 150 mm Hg and if the vital capacity is greater than 10 ml per kilo, then the patient is extubated.

Now this does not mean that all is well. The preceding is a procedure generally used in deciding whether the endotracheal tube can be removed at all. Usually in about 5% of the cases, in an hour or so the tube will have to be put back down again, which means that the patient has to be checked and rechecked quite carefully, even though the patient has been extubated.

Fig. 152.—Schematic circuit of katharometer (gas chromatography). *A*, air; *IM*, indicating meter; *MA*, milliammeter; *PC*, power and current control; *T*, test.

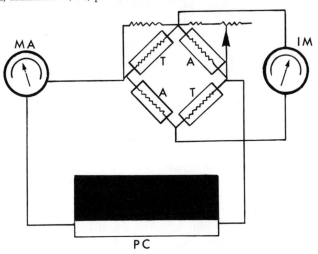

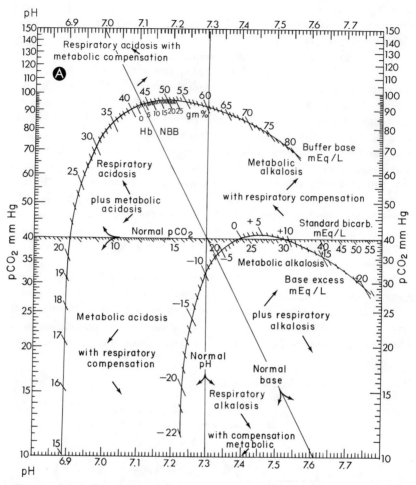

Fig. 153.—A, acid-base balance interpretation chart. Acid-base balance as described by Siggaard-Andersen measures the pH of the blood in the body of man and compares it with the pH of an equilibrated sample at known pressures of carbon dioxide. These two known Pco_2 values make up a log Pco_2-pH titration line for each sample. Normal bicarbonate value is the actual bicarbonate concentration. (*Continued.*)

A reasonable follow-up to this approach is to administer oxygen by mask 8–10 L per minute for 3–4 days.

We are all familiar with the patient who, the night before he is ready to be discharged, sits up, gasps, turns blue and later is found dead. The autopsy shows nothing which can identify the cause. The reason for this

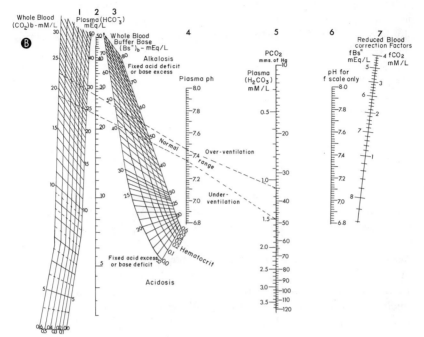

Fig. 153 (cont.).—B, represents different graphic means of determining a variable when given two known values. Nomogram for the acid-base balance of human blood at 37° C. For oxygenated blood (scales 1–5), a straight line through points given on two of the scales intersects the remaining scales at simultaneously occurring values of the other variables. The position of the line indicates the kind and magnitude of any disturbance of the acid-base balance. The normal range is for arterial, not venous, blood. Use scales 6 and 7 with P_{CO_2} only to obtain factors for correction of $(Bs'')_b$ from scale 3 and (CO_2) from scale 1 when blood is not fully oxygenated. V_6 = hematocrit = RBSs/100; U = O_2 unsaturation = $1 - (\%$ sat./ 100) corr. $(CO_2)_b = (CO_2)_b + (fCO_2 \cdot U \cdot V_6)$ corr. $(Bs'')_b = (Bs'')_b - (fBs + \cdot U \cdot V_6)$.

type of arrest is that these patients after a predischarge excursion in the corridors often go to their rooms breathing ambient air and become hypoxemic, in which case as soon as they start to move or walk about again their hypoxemia may get the better of them.

Now what do all these facts tell us? Basically what we must be interested in achieving is to determine individual needs as precisely as possible. A maximal flow or maximal oxygenation is obtained at a normal tidal volume. Generally, the rate of breathing should be slow, especially if one is using 15 ml per kg of body weight as a means of achieving a normal P_{CO_2}. It has been generally agreed clinically that one can maintain maximal oxygenation in mammals who breath 100% oxygen at tidal volumes somewhere in the range of 12–15 ml per kilo. Also, it has been documented that as one enlarges the tidal volume, all one is doing is essentially increasing the physiologic dead space so that the larger tidal volume is of little consequence.

It is of little informative value to know the particular P_{O_2}, regardless of the tidal volume, because it tells absolutely nothing about functional residual capacity. One of the important factors we have begun to recognize is that when we increase the tidal volume we may redistribute it so that the functional residual capacity may rise and the lung may be fully expanded but certainly may still be a very inefficient lung in terms of gas exchange. The V_d/V_t gives an idea of the efficiency of the lung in terms of excretion of carbon dioxide, but, since the respiratory therapist or physician has little influence on the cardiac output generally and on the distribution of blood flow but only on ventilation, the V_d/V_t may stay constant regardless of what is done and improve simply as the patient's over-all condition improves.

One fact that perhaps clinicians fail to realize is that the arterial P_{O_2} is primarily determined by the level of the hemoglobin that is available during circulation. That has been demonstrated in dogs with anatomic shunts in which the inferior vena cava was surgically anastomosed to the pulmonary veins, producing a 50% shunt. When these dogs were allowed to breathe 100% oxygen 2 weeks later, it was found that even with a hematocrit of 40, these dogs had an arterial P_{O_2} of 60 mm Hg. It is not unusual to see in patients who are suffering from severe pulmonary dysfunction that as the hemoglobin is decreased to a considerable degree, an increase in P_{O_2} results. This obviously must happen since the dissociation curve has been taken away and what is left is an oxygen solution alone. There is still a 50% shunt, but the P_{O_2} and the alveolar arterial gradient are considerably smaller on 100% oxygen when there is decreased hemoglobin present.

When the dogs were allowed to breathe room air with no hemoglobin, their P_{O_2} was the same as it was at the onset on 100% oxygen with hemoglobin present.

Of course, the first objection here is that the subject cannot carry any oxygen since hemoglobin is present. This is true, but a practical situation in which this occurs should be pointed out, the complete repair of tetralogy of Fallot. It has been debated as to whether these patients should maintain their preoperative hematocrit in order to maintain their oxygen-carrying capacity or whether keeping the hematocrit at a lower level while maintaining P_{O_2} at higher levels is perhaps beneficial.

We believe there is no value in having a hemoglobin of 15 that is 60% saturated when a hemoglobin of 10 that is 95% saturated will give the same oxygen content. This situation will always apply when the patient has an anatomic shunt or when there is a pulmonary circulation situation in which a patient has a large gradient on 100% oxygen.

THE TECHNIQUE OF DETERMINING ARTERIAL CARBON DIOXIDE TENSION BY THE REBREATHING METHOD

This method is designed to provide simple, but accurate, clinical measurements of carbon dioxide tension (P_{CO_2}) of the mixed venous blood in the absence of arterial blood gas determinations to distinguish or assess the clinical progress of patients who are in mild respiratory failure.

The actual mixed venous carbon dioxide tension (Pv_{CO_2}), normally 46 mm Hg in healthy individuals, can be directly determined by this method. The arterial carbon dioxide tension (Pa_{CO_2}), normally 40 mm Hg, is calculated from the prior knowledge of the Pv_{CO_2}.

The apparatus that is most often used for this procedure is the Goddard "capnograph," an infrared carbon dioxide analyzer system. The infrared analyzer operates on a principle of electromagnetic radiation. This instrument has a wavelength from 0.4 to 0.8 cc. As the infrared beam passes through a gas mixture containing CO_2, certain wavelengths will be absorbed by carbon dioxide. The degree of intensity loss is proportional to the concentration of gas in the mixture.

Carbon dioxide is drawn through an analyzer cell by the action of a suction pump incorporated in the system. A breathing valve and bag is connected to a continuous graphic record which gives a direct readout in percentage of carbon dioxide. Precise calibration of this instrument requires at least two known concentrations of carbon dioxide. The cylinders containing the calibrating gases can be analyzed by the Haldane technique.

PROCEDURE.—The procedure is as follows:

1. Calibrate the capnograph with the known mixtures of carbon dioxide gases. Record or obtain the barometric pressure in mm Hg. The barometric pressure in inches of mercury is converted to millimeters of mercury by multiplying it by the conversion factor 25.4. For instance, if the barometric pressure in inches of mercury was 30.1, it would be 764.54 millimeters of mercury after the conversion ($30.1 \times 25.4 = 764.54$).

2. Record and calculate the water vapor pressure in relation to the patient's body temperature. The water vapor tension of a patient's exhaled gas is normally about 47 mm Hg at 37° C. For every degree rise or fall in body temperature, there is a proportional increase or decrease in water vapor pressure (see Glossary).

3. Instruct the patient to breathe in and out of the closed system for

20–40 seconds, using either a mouthpiece and nose clip, a tight-fitting rubber anesthesia mask or by connection to an endotracheal or a tracheostomy tube. It is important to insure a good seal in order to prevent any leaks from occurring in the system. If leakage should occur in the system, equilibration will not occur, and this will be easily recognized by watching the graph pen excursions. They will often be erratic while indicating a rather high percentage of carbon dioxide. Coughing will give incorrect readings during this procedure.

4. Since the patient is breathing in a closed system with a carbon dioxide gas that approximates the per cent of carbon dioxide within his lung, eventually the carbon dioxide in the bag will equilibrate with that within the subject's lung, provided there are no leaks in the system.

5. After equilibration has occurred, the per cent of carbon dioxide in the patient's lung can be determined by noting at which point on the graph a plateau is reached.

6. Since the highest concentration of carbon dioxide present in the alveoli is the same as that of the mixed venous blood before pulmonary gas exchange has occurred, the per cent of carbon dioxide recorded at the plateau is assumed to be equal to that of the mixed venous blood.

7. The per cent of mixed venous carbon dioxide is then converted to a partial pressure of carbon dioxide in millimeters of mercury and corrected for the barometric pressure (PB) in millimeters of mercury and exhaled water vapor tension (pH_2OT) at the subject's body temperature in millimeters of mercury by the following formula:

$$Pv_{CO_2} = \%CO_2 \times \frac{PB - pH_2OT}{100}$$

In the equation, per cent carbon dioxide is the per cent of carbon dioxide recorded on the graph at the plateau, PB is the barometric pressure in millimeters of mercury and pH_2OT is the tension of the subject's exhaled water vapor in millimeters of mercury at his body temperature at the time of the test. After determining the Pv_{CO_2}, the PA_{CO_2} is calculated by subtracting 6 mm Hg from the Pv_{CO_2}.

EXAMPLE: A patient whose temperature is normal 37° C. is instructed to rebreathe from a bag and valve, the bag containing around 7% of carbon dioxide. The barometric pressure is normal at 760 mm Hg. As the patient rebreathes, a continuous record is inscribed on the graph of the per cent carbon dioxide in the system. After about 10 seconds, the graph pen no longer moves and a plateau is reached.

The plateau is recorded as 6.50% carbon dioxide. Since the patient's temperature is normal, his exhaled water tension is 47 mm Hg. With these figures, the formula is constructed:

$$Pv_{CO_2} = \%CO_2 \times \frac{PB - pH_2OT}{100}$$

$$Pv_{CO_2} = 6.50 \times \frac{760 - 47}{100}$$

$$Pv_{CO_2} = 6.50 \times \frac{713}{100}$$

$$Pv_{CO_2} = 6.50 \times 7.13$$

$$Pv_{CO_2} = 46.3 \text{ mm Hg}$$

General comments.—Some patients may have a mixed venous Pv_{CO_2} higher than that capable of being recorded on the graph. In this case, the analyzer should be recalibrated electrically to read off in higher percentages. However, accuracy is sacrificed in the higher ranges and more reliable information will be found by arterial blood gas determination.

The rebreathing technique is a practical method that has sufficient accuracy for clinical purposes even when the physiologic dead space is increased to approximately 60–70% of the tidal volume.

COLLINS 9-LITER RESPIROMETER (FIG. 154)

OBJECTIVE.—This is a means of measuring respiratory excursions and lung volumes (Fig. 155). The recordings and interpretation of pulmonary function studies are a valuable aid to the physician in determining the patient's pulmonary status.

Pulmonary function terms:

Vital capacity (VC): The greatest volume of gas that can be expelled by voluntary efforts after maximal inspiration.

Inspiratory capacity (IC): The maximal volume that can be inspired from the resting end-expiratory position.

Expiratory reserve volume (ERV): The maximal volume that can be exhaled from the resting end-expiratory position.

Functional residual capacity (FRC): The volume of gas remaining in the lungs at the end of a quiet exhalation.

Residual volume (RV): The volume of gas remaining in the lungs after forced expiration.

Total lung capacity (TLC): The volume of gas in the lungs at the time of maximal inspiration.

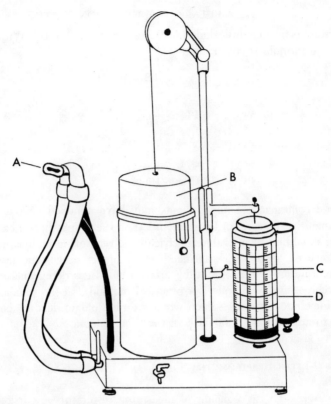

Fig. 154.—Collins respirometer. *A*, breathing tubes and bite block; *B*, water-air displacement drum; *C*, pen writer; *D*, recording drum.

Fig. 155.—Volumes of the lung.

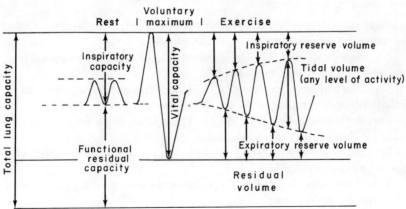

Maximal voluntary ventilation (MVV): The volume of gas exchanged per minute at a stated exercise activity.

EQUIPMENT NEEDED.—Collins 9-Liter Respirometer, graphing paper, ink, distilled water, mouthpiece and oxygen.

RESPIROMETER PREPARATION.—This procedure is carried out as follows:

1. Place respirometer on level surface.

2. Fill with distilled water by raising bell 3–4 inches and pouring water against side of the bell until level registers one half way up on the water level gauge. The water-drain petcock must be closed and the handle turned at a right angle to the body of the petcock.

3. Both pens must be in working order and filled with ink. One color ink for the ventilator pen.

4. There must be an adequate supply of paper on the kymograph.

5. The respirometer is then filled with oxygen until the recording pen is near the baseline. Pull the knob on the pulley, and the ventilograph pen is lowered to a position 4–5 cm above the respirometer pen and the knob is allowed to snap back.

6. The motor should be turned on and the speed selector adjusted to "slow." This is to make sure the drum is rotating properly.

PATIENT PREPARATION.—This is carried out as follows:

1. Procedure must be carefully explained to the patient.

2. The patient should be taught how to keep lips tightly around mouthpiece.

3. The patient should be allowed to acquaint himself with breathing through the mouthpiece for a few minutes.

4. The patient should be sitting in a hard-back chair if possible.

OPERATION.—The purpose of the operation is to measure tidal volume, maximal breathing capacity, vital capacity and timed vital capacity.

1. The rubber mouthpiece is attached to the valve and is placed between lips and teeth and a nose clip is applied. The valve is turned to "free breathing" until the patient adjusts to the mouthpiece.

2. The spirometer is turned on and the speed selector is adjusted to "slow."

3. The free-breathing valve at the mouth is turned to the respirometer and a tracing is obtained.

4. For recording timed vital capacity, the speed selector is changed from "slow" to "fast" and several vital capacity maneuvers are repeated with instructions to inspire as deeply as possible and then to exhale as completely and as rapidly as possible.

5. When measuring the maximal breathing capacity, the spirometer bell is filled three quarters full of oxygen or air. The ventilograph pen is lowered

as much as possible, with the kymograph on fast speed. The patient is asked to breathe as deeply and as rapidly as possible 12–15 seconds. The patient should be constantly and emphatically urged to do his utmost. The patient will usually choose a rate between 40 and 70 respirations per minute, with a tidal volume of about half of the vital capacity.

COMMENTS.—It has been noted that the patient's familiarity with the testing procedures can have a definite effect on the test results. The technician should consider trial testing to fully orientate the patient to what is expected of him.

PARKINSON-GOWEN DRY GAS METER

OBJECTIVE.—The objective is to monitor periodically the expired tidal volume on patients who are being ventilated continuously with mechanical ventilators.

EQUIPMENT.—The Parkinson-Gowen Meter measures the flow rate of gas in terms of liters. The dial is calibrated in liters and tenths of liters (0.1 L = 100 cc.)

TECHNIQUE.—This is carried out as follows:
1. Turn off secondary gas flow to the nebulizer, if in use.
2. Attach tubing from the meter to the exhalation port of the respirator.
3. Set the red needle on the zero point.
4. Allow 10 breaths to be exhaled into the meter. This will give the tidal volume for 10 breaths in terms of liters. Divide this figure by 10 to obtain the average tidal volume per breath in terms of cc.

EXAMPLE: 6.5 liters for 10 breaths is the same as 6,500 cc for 10 breaths. Dividing this figure by 10 will give an average of 650 cc tidal volume for each breath.

5. Disconnect the meter tubing from the ventilator exhalation port, and drain the tubing to remove excess moisture.
6. Turn on the secondary gas flow to the nebulizer, if in use.

COMMENT.—Expired tidal volume should be measured on all patients who are receiving continuous ventilation.

BENNETT MONITORING SPIROMETER

OBJECTIVES.—The objectives are to monitor and control the tidal volume during assisted or controlled ventilation. The spirometer needs no secondary power source and does not add to source gas consumption. It fills by very small force from the patient, and empties by gravitational force.

It is valved closed to receive expiration and valved open to dump its contents by the pressures in the ventilator main tube.

The spirometer is clinically accurate. Its capacity is 2,200 ml corrected at room temperature (72° F.) saturated to body temperature (98.6° F.). Under these conditions, its accuracy is affected only by ventilator flow during expiration and by tube system expansion and gas compression.

OPERATING TECHNIQUE.—A collecting tube and adaptor is placed on the expirator which then leads to the condensor tube. In its passage from the exhalation manifold to the spirometer, the expired gas condenses and is deposited in the flex tube and is drawn into a removable vial. This condensing system minimizes water collection in the bellows assembly.

The bellows, made of a thin and flexible silicone, is seated on a base which contains the valving mechanism and is encased by a transparent dome. The excursion of the bellows is guided and aided by a post which is attached to the top of the bellows.

At the beginning of expiration, the bellows and valve are positioned on the housing of the dome. Then, as expired gas flows past the one-way leaflet, it raises the bellows. The total movement of the bellows is read against a scale calibrated in milliliters, indicating the tidal volume of air from the lungs of the patient. Static resistance to expiration and thus positive pressure remaining during the expiratory pause derive from the weight and cross-sectional area of the bellows assembly. It, too, is low—less than 0.75 cm water over the entire range of the bellows.

If the tidal volume is greater than the capacity of the bellows or if misassembly or malfunction restrains the bellows, a poppet in the valve and bellows circuit serves as a relief. The poppet unseats at less than 3 cm water.

When the bellows rises, the weight of the disc and post are removed from a floating pushrod in the base. This relief allows a padded lever, aided by a spring, to seal a small bleed hole in the valve.

The bellows maintains its filled position during the expiratory pause. When inspiration begins, system pressure is conducted to the spirometer valve; there it fills a chamber to lift a diaphragm and unseat the poppet. When the poppet rises, the bellows falls, and its contents are dumped into the room.

Meanwhile, system pressure more slowly fills a second chamber in the spirometer valve to lift a second diaphragm. Lifting of this diaphragm seals the first chamber from system pressure, but the poppet has been already unseated, and the first chamber remains pressurized until the bellows completes its descent. At this moment, the weight of the bellows assembly presses against the floating pushrod in the base. This causes the rod to push down the lever and unseat the bleed hole in the valve. Pressure in the first chamber is dumped into the room and the poppet reseats. The spirometer is now prepared to receive another volume of expired gas.

COMMENTS AND PRECAUTIONS.—The following precautions should be noted:

1. Any leak in the expiratory system will cause the spirometer to under-read.

2. The ventilator tubes expand slightly during inspiration, and the gas contained in the tubes is compressed. This gas does not enter the patient's lungs, but when the tubes contract and the gas expands during expiration that volume appears as part of the expired gas volume, thus causing the spirometer to overread.

3. Any flow during expiration will be recorded by the spirometer as expired gas with consequent overreading. This addition may result from the expiratory portion of continuous nebulizer flow from an additional gas flow in the circuit during expiration.

4. Gas in the lungs is at body temperature; gas in the spirometer is at nearly room temperature and saturated with water vapor. In its passage from the patient to the spirometer, the gas volume and the cooling of the gas itself causes a further reduction in the volume because the increase lies in the volume that was in the patient's lungs, not that volume now in the spirometer. A spirometer volume is usually corrected to body temperature, saturated.

5. When expiration is retarded by a device which restricts flow from the exhalation valve, the decay of expiratory system pressure will be slowed. Extreme restriction of expiratory flow may cause the spirometer valve mechanism momentarily to underread.

6. Negative expiratory pressure cannot be used with the spirometer.

7. Every 8 hours, unscrew the vial and empty the condensate. Do not allow the condensate to fill the vial and rise into the tube, as this would impede expiration.

WRIGHT RESPIROMETER

The indications for this respirometer are the monitoring of tidal volume during controlled or assisted ventilation and the measuring of lung volume during spontaneous breathing.

OBJECTIVES.—The objectives of the Wright Respirometer are to measure the ventilation in anesthesia, inhalation therapy and also to provide a research tool of general application in respiratory physiology.

EQUIPMENT.—The chromium-plated brass housing has over-all dimensions of $2\frac{1}{2}'' \times 2\frac{1}{4}''$ and the meter has a $1\frac{1}{2}''$ diameter watch face dial protected by a clear cover plate. The periphery of the dial is marked by 100 divisions with numerals 10, 20, etc., at the appropriate intervals. One complete revolution of the hand sweeping this dial indicates a volume 100 L. In addition to the main dial, there is a smaller scale which resembles the seconds dial fitted to many watches. This dial is marked in 100 divisions with the numerals 1, 2, etc., at the appropriate intervals. One complete revolution of this hand of the small dial indicates a volume of 1 L. A button is fitted to the instrument for resetting the hands to zero and an "on-off" button in the form of a sliding stud is mounted on the outside of the housing.

TECHNIQUE.—The technique is carried out as follows:

1. Turn off secondary gas flow to the nebulizer of the respirator, if in use.

2. Attach $\frac{7}{8}''$ (inside diameter) chimney opening to the exhalation port of the respirator or a $\frac{9}{16}$ adaptor to a tracheotomy tube.

3. With the button on the left side of the meter, press in to zero point.

4. Allow 10 breaths to be exhaled into the meter. This will give the tidal volume for 10 breaths in terms of liters. Divide this figure by 10 to obtain the average tidal volume per breath in terms of cc.

EXAMPLE: 6.5 liters for 10 breaths is the same as 6,500 cc for ten breaths. Division of this figure by 10 will give an average of 650 cc tidal volume per each breath.

5. Disconnect the meter from the ventilator exhalation port and drain it to remove an excess of moisture which could damage the delicate inner rotors and gears.

GENERAL COMMENTS.—Expired tidal volumes should be measured on all patients who are on continuous ventilation. The frequency of these measurements should be determined by the physician.

With reasonable care and handling, the instrument will give many years of service. It is advisable to blow a gentle current of dry air or oxygen from a cylinder through the instrument's inlet or exit opening for a few minutes after each use in order to remove any trace of water vapor. The instrument can also be dried in a warm oven up to 140° C.

REFERENCES

Cherniack, R. M., and Cherniack, L.: *Respiration in Health and Disease* (Philadelphia: W. B. Saunders Company, 1961).

Davenport, H. W.: *The ABC of Acid-Base Chemistry* (4th ed.) (Chicago: University of Chicago Press, 1958).

Gaensler, E. A.: Evaluation of pulmonary function: Methods, Ann. Rev. Med. 12:385, 1961.

Anderson, W. H.: A comparison of various segments of the forced expirogram with the maximum breathing capacity, Dis. Chest 38:370, 1960.

Kory, R. C.; Callahan, R.; Boren, H. G., and Snyder, J. C.: The Veterans Administration Army cooperative study of pulmonary function, clinical spirometry in normal men, Am. J. Med. 30:243, 1961.

Comroe, J. H., Jr., and Fowler, W. S.: Lung function studies, VI. Detection of uneven alveolar ventilation during a single breath of oxygen: A new test of pulmonary disease, Am. J. Med. 10:408, 1951.

Severinghaus, J. W.; Mitchell, R. A.; Richardson, B. W., and Singer, M. M.: Respiratory control at high altitude suggesting active transport regulation of CSF pH, J. Appl. Physiol. 18:1155, 1963.

Bjure, J.: Spirometric studies in normal subjects IV. Ventilatory capacities in healthy children 7–17 years of age, Acta pediat. 52:232, 1963.

Campbell, E. J. N.: Disordered pulmonary function in emphysema, Postgrad. M. J. 34:30, 1958.

Cotes, J. E.: *Lung Function Assessment and Application in Medicine* (Philadelphia: F. A. Davis Company, 1965).

CHAPTER 16

Environmental Control Systems

THE FACTORS involved in environment are as follows:

1. Gas content and percentage
2. Pressure
3. Temperature
4. Humidification
5. Radiation

In this chapter we shall discuss the first four of these as they relate to inhalation therapy. At present, radiation, aside from x-ray, usually is not a factor requiring control in relation to patients within hospital environments.

An ever-increasing number and variety of toxic substances in the general atmospheric environment threaten man's health, even though he may be in the hospital. To bring these conditions under control requires a refined knowledge of the relationship of man to his environment.

The approximate necessary constancy of the internal temperature of the body, even under wide variations of atmospheric conditions, is the result of the balance between the heat of oxidation and the loss of heat from the body, a balance itself the product of a sophisticated control system.

Lavoisier in his 18th century studies of man and environment found that man absorbed the least amount of oxygen in the fasting state at comfortable temperatures. He proved that when the temperature was low, consumption of oxygen was increased slightly. Ingestion of food caused a definite increase in the oxygen absorbed, and physical labor resulted in tripling the amount of oxygen used.

Numerous recent investigations emphasize the fundamental importance of the problems of the thermal exchanges between man and his environment.

TEMPERATURE REGULATION

As the state of the art of "inhalation therapy" progresses, many more factors become involved in patient care which depend on mechanical devices. Due to the therapist's association with extremely ill patients and his special knowledge of mechanical devices, an area which is becoming increasingly associated with inhalation therapy is that of temperature-regulating devices.

When an elevation in temperature occurs, the basal metabolic rate is elevated about 7% for each degree Fahrenheit rise in temperature. At a temperature of 105° F, metabolism is elevated about 50% above normal. The biochemical disturbances associated with this include negative nitrogen balance, dehydration, loss of potassium and cellular water, and acidosis. In order to compensate for the acidosis, respiration is increased, and the work of breathing is increased.

The source of body heat must be carefully balanced against the loss of body heat in order to maintain a relatively constant body temperature.

The principal source of body heat is from combustion of foodstuffs within the body. Although the contribution of each organic system varies widely, the following are approximately correct in the resting state:

	% of Total
Liver	50
Brain	20
Muscle	20
Respiration and circulation	10

Loss of body heat occurs in three principal ways—radiation, vaporization and convection. Radiation is the transfer of heat by means of electromagnetic waves. Vaporization causes heat transfer due to the amount of heat required for the conversion of a liquid to a vapor. Convection is the principle whereby heat is lost to gas circulating over the body or within the respiratory passages. In addition, a small amount of heat is lost by conduction directly to cooler objects and by warming ingested food.

In the resting state, the normal heat loss as a percentage of the total is as follows:

	% of Total
Radiation	60
Vaporization	20–27
Convection	12–15

In the case of increased body temperature, mechanisms are actuated for heat loss. More blood is supplied to the skin and the subcutaneous tissues, permitting greater heat loss by radiation, vaporization and convection. In addition to the greater blood flow to the surface, increased heat loss by vaporization may be facilitated by sweating.

In 1938, Temple Fay investigated the use of cold in the therapy of terminal cancer. With advances in medicine, especially beginning in 1952, surface temperature-regulating devices have come into widespread use in thoracic, cardiac, cardiovascular and neurologic surgery. In the more recent past, electrically activated surface coolant units have been used with great benefit in intensive care areas, pediatrics and general medicine (Fig. 156).

There are several commercial units available at present, but their principal operation may be described in general terms. They consist of a tank which contains the coolant, a refrigeration coil and an electric immersion heater. They have either single or dual thermostat controls which can regulate both the refrigerating and heating units.

The coolant may be water, propylene glycol or ethyl alcohol. After the reservoir tank is charged with coolant, it is circulated via connecting tubes

Fig. 156.—Seriously ill infant on a temperature-regulating mattress. A, mattress; B, gastrostomy tube to drainage; C, infusion of whole blood; D, continuous intravenous feeding; E, temperature-regulating machine; F, polyethylene tubing into saphenous vein; G, nasal sump suction.

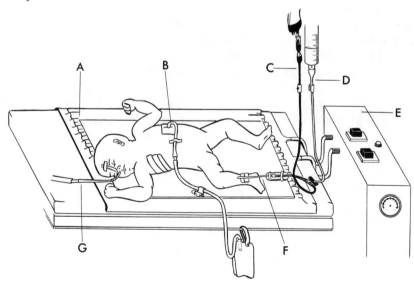

(usually plastic or rubber) to a coil contained within the surface applicators or blankets.

CAUTION: The orders for duration of use, temperature range desired and precautions to be observed must be written by the physician.

The control and regulation of body temperature as a portion of environmental control system will undergo much development and greater application as further advances are made. It is an area that anyone interested in inhalation therapy should keep closely abreast of.

HYPERBARIC OXYGEN CHAMBER

The second factor involved in environmental control affecting patients is ambient pressure. A method of increasing available oxygen in a controlled environment which has become more widely used recently is that of hyperbaric oxygen chambers (Fig. 157). The basic principle involved here is quite simple and easily understood. By raising the atmospheric pressure above normal ambient pressure (average 760), the amount of dissolved gases in the blood, more specifically in the plasma, is increased.

For example, if the patient is breathing 100% oxygen at 760 mm atmospheric pressure, the possible oxygen which could be in his arterial blood stream after subtracting the partial pressure of carbon dioxide and water vapor would be approximately 700 mm Hg P_{O_2}. If the environmental pressure was raised to three atmospheres pressure absolute, the resultant ambient pressure would be 3×760 or 2,280. If then the patient is allowed to breathe oxygen, the resultant oxygen in the arterial blood could theoretically be as great as 2,100 mm Hg P_{O_2}.

There are many possible dangers associated with hyperbaric oxygen chambers, such as rapid decompression, sickness of personnel, oxygen toxicity, fire hazards and adverse drug responses. The total problem of hyperbaric chambers is too complex to discuss in great detail here, and the reader is referred to the excellent texts by Paul Bert, and by Haldane.

EQUIPMENT AND METHODS USED TO CONTROL GAS CONTENT, HUMIDIFICATION AND TEMPERATURE

Environmental control systems are indicated when moderate-to-high concentrations of oxygen and mist are desired. Tents or hoodlike devices are extremely beneficial to infants, children and some adults. It is important to be able to monitor this environment. In order to accomplish this, we must understand the effects of air movement, temperature changes and the oxygen demand.

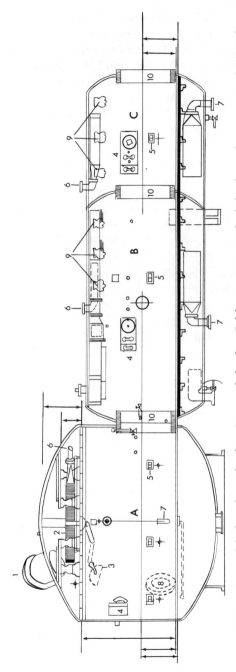

Fig. 157.—Schema of the hyperbaric chamber. *A,* surgical chamber; *B,* laboratory area, medical chamber and recompression lock; *C,* decompression chamber for change of personnel. *1,* air conditioning; *2,* filter; *3,* surgical light; *4,* telephone and intercom system; *5,* conductive electrical outlets; *6,* air inlet; *7,* air exhaust system; *8,* exchange port; *9,* lights; *10,* pressure-tight doors.

OXYGEN TENTS.—The adult oxygen tent was used considerably in the past for oxygen administration. The advantages of using the oxygen tent for adults at present seem to be those of comfort, isolation and air conditioning. Perhaps a change in mechanical design could make this an extremely useful and needed tool in inhalation therapy. A possible attempt at such modification is the face tent (Fig. 158). With the older models, because of the tent's low temperature range, it is difficult to administer the desired humidity when the inspired gas attains body temperature.

In order to fully saturate the contents of an oxygen tent at 70° F, it would take 111 gr of moisture per pound of dry air. When the inspired gas is raised to body temperature (98.6° F), this gas would be only 40% saturated with water vapor as it requires 290 gr of moisture per pound of dry gas to produce saturation at body temperature. It is quite evident that temperature is the major limiting factor in the amount of water vapor that is available for delivery to the patient. Water must be given up by the body to bring the partially saturated gas mixture up to full saturation. The water is given up from the mucous membranes in the respiratory tract. The secretions tend to thicken as they lose water and become difficult to raise. The inspissated crusted mucus and cellular debris create a situation in which bacteria may multiply rapidly.

The temperature on the control panel of the tent may not accurately show the temperature in the tent: A thermometer should be placed in the tent and checked periodically.

Because of the tent's weight and size, it not only constitutes a storage and moving problem but also takes up valuable bedside space.

Hazards are present due to the nature of the tent's canopy and electrical

Fig. 158.—Translucent polypropylene face tent with large bore adaptor and tubing for aerosol therapy.

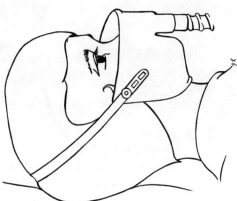

circuits. Of all the methods of delivering oxygen, the tent poses the greatest risk due to the high oxygen flow required for it and impregnation of the bed clothes with condensed water droplets.

Even with the most expert care, the oxygen tent is difficult to clean and may serve as a source of bacterial contamination and growth.

Use of oxygen tent.—The equipment needed for the correct setup of an oxygen tent are a flowmeter, canopy, thermometer, oxygen analyzer and an aerosol unit.

Preparation of patient.—After taking the tent to the patient's room do the following:

1. Check the canopy for leaks.
2. Attach the canopy to the oxygen tent and check the regulator or flowmeter at the bedside.

Technique.—The following points should be carried out:

1. Place "No Smoking" signs in the patient's room and the immediate area.
2. Place the canopy over the upper part of the bed, tucking it well under the mattress at the sides and back. Bring the front of the canopy down toward the foot of the bed—avoid dragging the canopy over the patient's face. Warn the patient about rushing noises as the tent is flooded with oxygen. Fold the cotton sheet in fourths; place the canopy within the folds of the sheet and tuck under the mattress on both sides.
3. Direct the inflow of oxygen away from the patient's head and neck. Reduce the flow rate to 10–12 L after 10–15 minutes.

General comments.—Every time the tent is opened, oxygen is lost; therefore, one should try to consolidate care and treatments. The tent sleeves should be used rather than opening the entire canopy. The temperature of the tent should be maintained at 68° F to 70° F, unless the physician has instructed otherwise. An oxygen analyzer should be used for the periodic check of the oxygen concentration in the tent. The tent should be drained periodically and cleaned according to the individual specifications.

Pediatric tents (Fig. 159) differ slightly from adult oxygen tents. Speed is often a vital factor in administering oxygen with adequate humidity to the respiratory tract. Most pediatric oxygen tents can be assembled quickly. Because of the small size of the enclosed area, moderate saturation, recirculation of gases and cool vapor can be provided usually in 60 seconds.

Pediatric oxygen tents can be powered by either a gas source or with the use of an oil-free air compressor. When oxygen is indicated, the air compressor or piped compressed gas is used as a power source.

The method used to cool pediatric tents is to circulate the atmosphere in the canopy over a cooling element such as ice. Circulation is usually produced by a gas source such as oxygen or compressed air. In some gas-

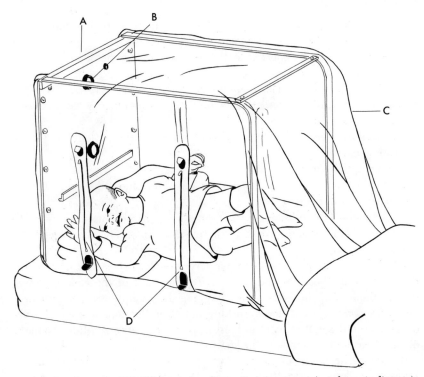

Fig. 159.—Croupette-type oxygen and cooling unit. A, ice storage (not shown in diagram); B, humidity and cooling ports; C, plastic canopy; D, entry ports.

powered tents, opening of a damper, which bypasses the atmosphere around the ice, allows maintenance of the circulation but reduces the cooling effects.

INCUBATORS (FIGS. 160 AND 161).—The objectives are as follows:

1. To provide a constant atmosphere with a controlled amount of humidity.

2. To provide protection from the constant attack of airborne microorganisms.

3. To provide enriched oxygen tensions when indicated.

4. To maintain the infant's body temperature.

5. To monitor various physiologic parameters of the infant.

6. To provide, in certain instances, environmental light radiation of the correct frequency.

Modern-day incubators are equipped to provide varying concentrations of oxygen. One or two inlets are incorporated for controlled administration of oxygen.

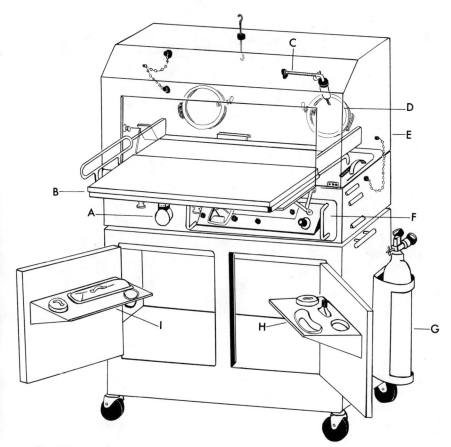

Fig. 160.—Incubator used for newborn intensive care. *A*, water level; *B*, slide-out support tray; *C*, mercury thermometer; *D*, entry ports; *E*, flip-forward top; *F*, power pack and temperature control unit; *G*, oxygen cylinder rack; *H* and *I*, accessory trays.

Oxygen is administered in all incubators by using a "back pressure compensated" flowmeter. Tubing from the flowmeter is attached to the oxygen inlet valve. Incubators such as the Armstrong 190A have two oxygen inlet valves for 40 and 100% oxygen concentrations. In other units such as the Air-Shields Isolette, the concentration of oxygen varies with the liter flow. High liter flows will yield increased oxygen tensions. When using oxygen in any concentration, one should monitor the tension with an accurate oxygen analyzer.

When oxygen is used with nebulizers incorporated into the system for the purpose of increasing humidity, an adequate flow rate in liters per minute should be used. Some incubators will have oxygen-limiting devices

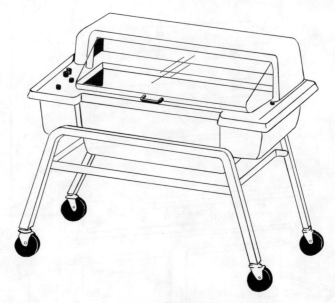

Fig. 161.—Transport incubator.

on the nebulizer. One should be aware that this type of system could introduce airborne bacteria into the water and hence into the entire system. An alternate method would be to use compressed air and oxygen mixtures.

The servo-controlled incubator is used as a primary unit to control the temperature of the environment at the normal physiologic level, utilizing a modulating heat principle whereby the amount of heat varies according to the need of the infant. This principle allows improved stabilization of the infant temperature and reduces variations in air temperature within the incubator (Fig. 162).

A highly sensitive and accurate temperature-sensing thermistor (patient probe) is attached directly to the skin of the infant's abdomen with paper tape. The patient probe detects temperature changes as small as $\pm 0.1°$ F. These minute variations in skin temperatures are amplified and relayed through the power unit, causing the heater temperature to modulate for the amount of heat necessary to stabilize the infant's body temperature at the desired set control point.

Use of incubators.—The use of incubators is outlined as follows:

1. The incubator must be preheated. Turn the heater control knob to the start position to monitor the inside temperature. When the desired level is reached inside, turn the control knob until the heater light goes off.

2. Fill the humidity reservoir with sterile distilled water and select the desired humidity on the humidity control panel.

3. For aerosol therapy, attach the nebulizer to the hood of the incubator. Use only sterile distilled water in the nebulizer.

4. Most incubators have cooling features to be used when the temperature in the room or incubator is at a critical level or is higher than the desired level. In the Isolette, an ice chamber is filled with 15–20 lb of ice with about 1 quart of water for maximal cooling effect. The heater control knob is turned clockwise when minimal desired temperature has been reached. Turn the control knob counterclockwise enough to turn on the indicating light. This maneuver sets the thermostat to maintain the temperature shown on the thermometer and prevents overcooling. Turn the humidity control knob to "full open."

5. If the built-in alarm should sound, the hood temperature has exceeded 100° F. The hood door should be opened and the unit checked for malfunction.

Cleaning and maintenance.—These procedures should be carried out as outlined below:

1. All sleeves should be removed and washed with a detergent after each use.

2. The hood should be cleaned with a mild detergent or chemical germicide that is not harmful to the plexiglass.

3. Between patient use, remove and clean the mattress, the mattress support frame, hood seal gasket, main deck assembly and the humidity reservoir.

Fig. 162.—Incubator temperature monitoring and regulation pack. *A*, control and red line adjustment; *B*, thermometer; *C*, high-temperature alarm; *D*, thermostat-control light; *E*, heater light; *F*, thermostat control; *G*, thermocouple.

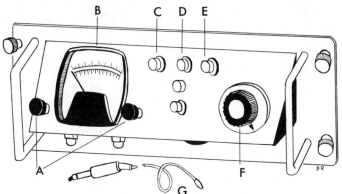

4. Drain water from the humidity reservoir chamber.

5. Fill the reservoir with chemical germicide.

6. Remove power pack unit and use compressed air to blow out any dust or foreign particles. Clean with germicide.

7. Change filters as necessary. Always keep in mind that a dirty filter will result in an increased oxygen concentration or a reduced circulation of air.

8. Replace parts as necessary.

9. Lubricate motor as necessary. Use only the oil designated by the manufacturer.

10. Aerate for 12–24 or more hours if ethylene oxide gas is used for sterilization of parts or the entire unit.

REFERENCES

DiGiovanni, C., Jr., and Birkhead, N. C.: Effect of minimal dehydration or orthostatic tolerance following short-term bed rest, Aerospace Med. 35:225, 1964.

Hale, H. B.: Human cardioaccelerative responses to hypoxia in combination with heat, Aerospace Med. 31:276, 1960.

Bullard, R. W.: Effects of hypoxia on shivering in man, Aerospace Med. 32:1143, 1961.

Stiehm, E. R.: Different effects of hypothermia on two syndromes of positive acceleration, J. Appl. Physiol. 18:387, 1963.

Welch, B. E.; Cutler, R. G.; Herlucher, J. E.; Hargreaves, J. J.; Ulvedal, F.; Shaw, E. G.; Smith, G. B.; McMann, H. J., and Bell, L.: Effect of ventilating air flow on human water requirements, Aerospace Med. 34:383, 1963.

Macpherson, R. K.: Physiological Responses to Hot Environments, Medical Research Council Special Report Series, No. 298. Her Majesty's Stationery Office, London, 1960.

Welch, B. E.; Morgan, T. E., and Clamann, H. G.: Time concentration effects in relation to oxygen toxicity in man, Fed. Proc. 22: 1053, 1963.

King, B. G.: High concentration—Short time exposures and toxicity, J. Indust. Hyg. & Toxicol. 31:365, 1949.

CHAPTER 17

Writing Orders for Inhalation Therapy

ONE OF THE MANY PROBLEMS associated with the administration of inhalation therapy to patients is the communication of exact information of what the physician wants the patient to receive. When the patient is in the hospital, specific orders in the doctor's order book should be written so that there can be no doubt in mind as to the therapy prescribed. In the past, on many occasions we have seen "IPPB for patient p.r.n.," or "O₂ and suction p.r.n.," or worst of all "Inhalation Therapy to see patient."

ORDERING OXYGEN

One of the most commonly administered drugs used in inhalation therapy is oxygen. In ordering oxygen, five factors must be considered:

1. *Source.* In most hospitals today, piping systems provide a wall outlet for oxygen. Some, however, still require that cylinders be used to administer oxygen. When this is so, care should be taken to use the proper size of cylinder for each treatment, as cost of oxygen bears definite relationship to cylinder size.

2. *Flow rate in liters per minute and/or percentage oxygen desired.* This is dependent on the disease state or degree of hypoxia which the individual patient is experiencing. If a physician prescribes in liter flow per minute, he should always bear in mind the percentage of oxygen he desires the patient to receive.

3. *How the oxygen is to be administered.* The possibilities here are many and varied, and depend, too, on the size of the patient, his disease state and the capabilities of the inhalation therapy department. Some possibilities would include nasal catheter, nasal cannula, face mask, tent, incubator, tracheostomy mask, and funnel.

4. *Type of aerosol mist equipment or humidifier desired.* It should be constantly re-emphasized that oxygen is very drying to mucous membranes. This produces toxic results in itself and probably susceptibility to infection. If relative humidity is desired, then heated nebulizers will be required. Spinning discs, Venturi-type or ultrasonic nebulizers have advantages and disadvantages which the physician should evaluate before he prescribes what he thinks is most indicated.

5. *How long the oxygen is to be administered.* This depends on the physician's judgment as to the improvement or deterioration of the patient's condition.

ORDERING SUCTION

An area where specific orders are needed and not always written is that in which suctioning of the patient is requested. Due to manifold respiratory problems, debility and sometimes neural loss, inhalation therapy implies suctioning in a great percentage of patients. Suctioning is a complex procedure; it should be approached with thorough knowledge and great caution as it may induce cardiac arrest. Many factors must be considered:

1. *How often the patient should be suctioned.* Often "p.r.n." is enough. In relation to intermittent positive-pressure breathing therapy, suctioning after administration of aerosol treatments by time intervals such as t.i.d. or when the patient is awake in cases of tracheostomies will require specific ordering by the physician.

2. *Whether preoxygenation or atropinization is required.* Many patients suffer from chronic hypoxia and require suctioning; however, line suctioning removes oxygen as well as mucus. Oxygen administration prior to suctioning will be beneficial; the patient's arterial saturation will not be lowered as much. In some patients, particularly children or patients with increased vagal nerve tone, suctioning may produce a marked decrease in heart rate and, in some instances, cardiac arrest. The use of atropine to block the action of the vagus nerve may be very beneficial in these patients.

3. *Whether sterile technique is required.* In most cases, it is advisable to perform suctioning by means of sterile technique, and certainly in all instances of suctioning endotracheal and tracheostomy tubes. This would include the use of sterile gloves and sterile suction catheter, and the avoidance of first suctioning the mouth and then the trachea.

4. *The proper size of suction catheter, dependent on the size of the patient, should be stated in the physician's order.* It is important to remember that too large a catheter may remove oxygen too rapidly, causing hypoxia or promoting atelectasis.

5. *The position of the patient's head while suctioning.* This is extremely important when performing endotracheal suctioning in an attempt to remove material from either the left or right main stem bronchus. Rotation of the head to the right will allow easier access to the left bronchus, and vice versa.

6. In patients who have a tracheostomy tube with an inner cannula, how often the inner cannula should be removed and what solution should be used for cleaning of the inner cannula are of extreme importance.

7. If drugs are to be instilled via a tracheostomy or an endotracheal tube, how often they should be used, dosage of the drug and how long they should remain before suction can be carried out are necessary considerations.

Ordering IPPB

Perhaps among the most frequently incomplete orders are those written to request the use of positive-pressure breathing devices; whether they are to be used for intermittent treatments or if they are to be used for continuous ventilation, either assisted or controlled. Let us first examine the possibilities for orders for intermittent treatments, commonly abbreviated IPPB.

1. *The type of apparatus to be used.* This has been discussed earlier in the text. See Chapter 13 (p. 211). There are various advantages and disadvantages to all types of apparatus; the proper piece of equipment should be chosen to produce the desired result.

2. *The type of gas to be administered to the patient.* Oxygen, compressed air, helium-oxygen mixtures are but a few examples of the types of gases which may be used. The exact percentage concentration of the gas desired should also be written.

3. *How often the therapy is to be administered.* Included here should be the duration of each treatment and the total days of therapy prescribed. For example, t.i.d. for 15 minutes each for 3 days. It is also important when postoperative IPPB is used that the patient be allowed sufficient time for rest. Often therapy is prescribed "when awake."

4. *The peak inspiratory pressure desired, usually written in centimeters of water pressure.* Included here as well should be the type of respiration desired, such as "prolong inspiration," or "prolong expiration."

5. *Whether the treatment is to be associated with physiotherapy and/or suctioning.* Usually chest physiotherapy is given before the IPPB treatment and suctioning follows.

6. *If drugs are to be nebulized, the specific drug and amount must be written.* See Chapter 14 (p. 234).

ORDERING OF VENTILATORS

For continuous ventilatory support, either assisted or controlled, there are a number of factors which the therapist must consider before the maximal benefit can be derived from therapy.

1. Whether ventilation is to be assisted or controlled. (This depends on yet other factors, most important of which is the patient's disease state.)

2. The type of ventilator best suited to the patient's needs. See Chapter 10 (p. 149).

3. Inspired gas mixture, preferably given in percentage concentration of each gas, e.g., oxygen, air, helium, nitrous oxide and carbon dioxide.

4. The respiratory rate best suited to the patient's requirements.

5. The tidal volume and minute volume, which depend on the pneumographic analysis of the patient's requirements.

6. Peak inspiratory pressure, which should not be exceeded. This again will depend on disease state and lung compliance.

7. If a tracheostomy or an endotracheal tube is used which is equipped with one or two balloon cuffs, how often the cuffs should be deflated, the amount of cubic centimeters of air which should be used to inflate the cuffs and how long the cuffs should remain deflated are also considerations.

8. Medications, if any, also have to be considered: the type, the percentage concentration, how often the medication is to be used, the total volume to be administered and whether the medication is to be instilled or nebulized.

9. How often the tidal volume, minute volume and percentage oxygen should be measured are further considerations.

ORDERING CHEST PHYSIOTHERAPY

Another area of special interest to inhalation therapists and physiotherapists which is intimately involved in over-all patient care is the writing of orders concerning chest physiotherapy.

1. *How often the physiotherapy should be administered.* It should be carefully kept in mind what the patient will tolerate depending on the degree of illness.

2. *The positions that the patient should be placed in.* Very often one lobe or one lung will require more drainage and therapy than another.

3. *The type of physiotherapy to be performed.* These might include percussion, vibration, cupping or expiratory assistance.

Orders for outpatients or home care are written in the same general manner but usually in the form of a prescription.

EXAMPLE:

Jones, John

IPPB 15 min. t.i.d. with AP 5 air 100% for 3 days. 0.5 ml Isuprel 1:1000 and 1.5 ml normal saline in nebulizer each time. Peak insp. pressure 25 cm H_2O—prolong expiration, encourage cough and deep breath.

It is important to remember that therapy should be prescribed for a period of time and either discontinued or reinstated. In the writing of orders or prescriptions, it is common practice to use latin abbreviations, of which a brief list is presented, with their meanings.

ABBREVIATIONS

Abbreviation	*English Definition*
a or āā	of each
a.c.	before meals
ad.	to; up to
ad lib.	as desired
alt. diem	every other day
alt. hor.	every other hour
alt. noc.	every other night
aq.	water
aq. com.	common water
aq. dest.	distilled water
aq. tep.	tepid water
arg.	silver
av.	avoirdupois
bib.	drink
b.i.d.	twice a day
b.i.n.	twice a night
č	with
C	centigrade
cap.	capsule
cc	cubic centimeter
cg	centigram
cm	centimeter
dil.	dilute
dr	dram or drams

Abbreviation	*English Definition*
et	and
F	Fahrenheit
Gm	gram
gtt.	drops
H	hour
h.n.	tonight
hor. interm.	at intermediate hours
h.s.	at bedtime
kg	kilogram
L	liter
lb	pound
M	meter
mEq	milliequivalent
mg	milligram
mist.	mixture
μ	micron
ml	milliliter
mm	millimeter
N_2	nitrogen
n.b.	note well
no.	number
non rep.	don't repeat
O_2	oxygen
omn. hor.	every hour
omn. noct.	every night
os	mouth
p.c.	after meals
per	through or by
p.o.	by mouth
p.r.n.	as needed
Q.h.	every hour
$Q._2h.$	every two hours
$Q._3h.$	every three hours
q.i.d.	four times a day
Q.s.	a sufficient quantity
quotid.	every day
Q.v.	as much as you will
Rx	take
š.	without
s.o.b.	shortness of breath
sol.	solution
solv.	dissolve

Abbreviation	English Definition
s.o.s.	if necessary
stat.	immediately
T.	temperature
t.i.d.	three times a day
t.i.n.	three times a night
vol.%	volume percent
Wt.	weight
w/v	weight by volume

CHAPTER 18

Organizational Structure of Inhalation Therapy in U.S.A.

CONSTITUTION OF THE AMERICAN ASSOCIATION
FOR INHALATION THERAPY

1966 Revision

ARTICLE I

NAME

This organization shall be known as the American Association for Inhalation Therapy, incorporated under the General Not for Profit Corporation Act of the State of Illinois.

ARTICLE II

OBJECT

Section A. Purpose

1. To encourage and develop educational programs for those persons interested in the field of inhalation therapy.

2. To advance the science, technology and art of inhalation therapy through institutes, meetings, lectures, and the preparation and distribution of a newsletter, a journal, and other materials.

3. To facilitate cooperation between inhalation therapy personnel and the medical profession, hospitals, service companies, industry, and other agencies interested in inhalation therapy; except that this corporation shall not commit any act which shall constitute unauthorized practice of medicine under the laws of the state of Illinois, or any other state.

Section B. Intent

1. No part of the net earnings of the corporation shall inure to the benefit of any private member or individual, nor shall the corporation perform particular services for individual members thereof.

2. Distribution of the funds, income, and property of the corporation may be made to charitable, educational, scientific or religious corporations, organizations, community chests, foundations, or other kindred institutions maintained and created for one or more of the foregoing purposes if at the time of distribution the payees or distributees are exempt from income taxation, and if gifts or transfers to the payees or distributees are then exempt from taxation under the provisions of Sections 501, 2055, and 2522 of the Internal Revenue Code, or any later or other sections of the Internal Revenue Code which amend or supersede the said sections.

ARTICLE III

MEMBERSHIP

Section A. Classes

The membership of this Association shall include two (2) classes; active member and associate member.

Section B. Provisions

The procedure with respect to admission to membership, categories of membership, qualifications, and the exercises of privileges thereof, shall be specified in the Bylaws.

ARTICLE IV

GOVERNMENT

Section A. Board of Directors

The Government of this Association shall be vested in a Board of eighteen (18) active members consisting of the immediate Past President, President, President Elect, Vice President, Secretary, Treasurer, and twelve (12) others.

Section B. House of Delegates

1. There shall be a House of Delegates consisting of elected representatives from each chapter as specified in the Bylaws. The Vice President of the AAIT shall be the Speaker of the House of Delegates.

2. The function of the House of Delegates shall be to aid in the direction and operation of the Association.

Section C. Board of Medical Advisors

1. The Board of Medical Advisors of the American Association for Inhalation Therapy shall consist of sixteen (16) member physicians as follows: four (4) from the American College of Chest Physicians; four (4) from the American Society of Anesthesiologists; two (2) from the American Academy of Pediatrics; two (2) from the American Association of Thoracic Surgeons; two (2) from the American Thoracic Society, and two (2) from the American College of Allergists.

2. Each member shall be appointed by his parent society to serve a four (4) year term, nonrecurring except after a two (2) year absence from the Board. The

appointment of members to the Board shall be so staggered that the ACCP and ASA shall appoint a new member every year, and the other parent societies shall appoint a new member every two (2) years. Terms shall begin January 1.

3. Appointees to the Board of Medical Advisors shall not be members of the Board of Schools of Inhalation Therapy of the AMA or of the Board of the American Registry of Inhalation Therapists.

4. The Board of Medical Advisors shall have only such powers as are granted to them by the Bylaws of this Constitution.

5. They shall elect their own officers and be responsible for such organizational policies as they may otherwise require.

6. The Board of Directors of the AAIT and all of its standing committees will consult with the Board of Medical Advisors in regard to all matters of medical policy and ethics.

7. The Chairman of the Board of Medical Advisors or his designate shall attend all the meetings of the Board of Directors as a nonvoting advisor.

8. An annual meeting of the Board of Medical Advisors shall be held at the time and place of the annual meeting of the AAIT and also at such other times as may be determined by the Chairman and Vice Chairman of the Board of Medical Advisors.

Section D. Executive Secretary

The Board of Directors shall employ a business counsel to be identified as the Executive Secretary who will establish a Headquarters Office from which he will assist in the conduct of the business of the Association.

Section E. Emeritus Board

There shall be an Emeritus Board consisting of all past members of the Board of Directors. Its function shall be purely advisory except as otherwise specified in the Bylaws.

Section F. Elections

The procedure with respect to nominating and electing officers and board members shall be provided in the Bylaws.

ARTICLE V

MEETINGS

The American Association for Inhalation Therapy shall hold an annual meeting as specified in the Bylaws, and such other meetings during the year as provided in the Bylaws, in order to fulfill the objectives of the organization.

ARTICLE VI

CHAPTERS

A local or regional group of ten (10) or more active members of the AAIT meeting the requirements for affiliation as outlined in the Bylaws, may become a Chapter of the Association upon approval of the Chapter Affairs Committee subject to ratification by the Board of Directors of the AAIT.

ARTICLE VII

AMENDMENTS

This Constitution may be amended at any annual meeting or by mail vote of the American Association for Inhalation Therapy by a two-thirds (²⁄₃) majority of those voting, provided that at least 50% of the qualified membership votes, and provided that the amendment has been presented in writing to the membership at least sixty (60) days prior to the vote. The number of members representing 50% of those qualified to vote shall be certified by the Executive Secretary and the Chairman of the Membership Committee and that number indicated at the time of the vote.

PROPOSED REVISIONS OF THE BYLAWS OF THE AMERICAN ASSOCIATION FOR INHALATION THERAPY

ARTICLE I

MEMBERSHIP

Section A. Active Member

An individual is eligible to be an active member if he has had one and one-half (1½) years of experience in inhalation therapy in a recognized institution or organization, provided his primary function is directly related to patient care under medical supervision and provided he is not directly involved with the manufacture of, nor profits from, the sale of gases, equipment or drugs, and is not a physician.

Section B. Associate Member

An individual is eligible to be an associate member if he holds a position related to inhalation therapy and does not have the requirements to become an active member. Associate members shall have all of the rights and privileges of the Association except that they shall not be entitled to hold office, committee chairmanships, or vote.

Section C. Special Membership Status

1. Life Status—Life membership may be conferred by a two-thirds (²⁄₃) majority vote of the Board of Directors as recommended by the House of Delegates. To be eligible for life membership, a person must have been an active member or associate member. Life members shall have all the rights and privileges of the Association except that they shall not be entitled to hold office, committee chairmanships, or vote; and they shall be exempt from the payment of dues.

2. Honorary Status—Honorary membership may be conferred by a two-thirds ($^2/_3$) majority vote of the Board of Directors as recommended by the House of Delegates upon persons who have rendered distinguished service to inhalation therapy. Honorary members shall have all the rights and privileges of the Association except that they shall not be entitled to hold office, committee chairmanships, or vote; and they shall be exempt from the payment of dues.

3. Foreign Associate Status—An individual is also eligible for associate membership if he is a member in good standing of an inhalation therapy association of any foreign country.

4. Student Status—An individual is eligible for associate membership as a student if he is enrolled in a formal training program in inhalation therapy. Student status is for a period of one and one-half ($1^1/_2$) years from the date of acceptance. Members in a student status shall have all the rights and privileges of the Association except that they shall not be entitled to hold office, committee chairmanships, vote, or wear official AAIT shoulder patches or insignia.

Section D. Prerequisites

Each applicant for membership must either be a high school graduate or have evidence of equivalent education and must meet other qualifications of ethical practice and suitable moral standards as determined by the Membership Committee.

Section E. Application for Membership

(see also, Article X, Section A, Bylaws)

1. An applicant for membership shall complete an approved application form in duplicate, sending one (1) copy directly to the Headquarters Office for the Membership Committee and send the second copy to the appropriate local Chapter for its investigation and recommendation to the Membership Committee. The duplicate copy shall also serve as application for membership in the Chapter.

2. The names and addresses of all applicants shall be submitted by the Executive Secretary to be published in the next Newsletter after receipt of the application in the Headquarters Office.

3. Any member or members may object to approval of an applicant for membership by filing written objection with the Chairman of the Membership Committee through the Headquarters Office within thirty (30) days after publication of the applicant's name.

Section F. Annual Registration

Each active member and associate member must complete annually a questionnaire reasserting his qualifications for membership. This questionnaire shall be returned with the dues payment and membership will not be renewed unless this is done.

ARTICLE II

NOMINATIONS AND ELECTIONS

Section A. Nominating Committee

The President, with the approval of the Board of Directors, shall appoint a Nominating Committee each year at the annual meeting to present a slate of nominees for the following year. The Chairman of this Committee shall report the slate of nominees to the Board of Directors at the board meeting the following spring, and not later than June 1.

Section B. Nominations

The Nominating Committee may place in nomination the names of more than one (1) person for the Offices of President Elect, Vice President, Secretary, and Treasurer, and shall place in nomination for each of the four (4) Board Members to be elected, the names of two (2) or more persons who have been recommended by the House of Delegates. (See Article X, Section G and Article VIII, Section E, 5.) Only active members in good standing shall be eligible for nomination. The Nominating Committee shall provide a pertinent biographical sketch of each nominee's professional activities and services to the organization, all of which shall be a part of the ballot.

Section C. Ballot

The Nominating Committee's slate shall be mailed to every active member in good standing and eligible to vote at least sixty (60) days prior to the annual meeting. The list of nominees shall be so designed as to be a secret mail ballot with provisions for write-in votes for each office. Ballots, to be acceptable, must be postmarked at least ten (10) days before the annual meeting. The deadline date and time shall be clearly indicated on the ballot.

Section D. Election Committee

The President shall appoint an impartial election committee which shall check the eligibility of each ballot and tally the votes forty-eight (48) hours prior to the annual business meeting. The results of the election shall be announced at the annual business meeting.

ARTICLE III

OFFICERS

Section A. Officers

The officers of this Association shall be: President, President Elect (who shall automatically succeed to the presidency), Vice President, Secretary, and Treasurer.

Section B. Term of Office

The term of office shall begin immediately following the annual meeting at which the respective officers are elected. The incumbent officers shall remain in office until such date and until their respective successors assume office.

Section C. Succession

No officer may serve more than three (3) consecutive terms in the same office, except the Treasurer.

ARTICLE IV

DUTIES OF OFFICERS

Section A. The President shall:

1. Preside at the annual business meeting and all meetings of the Board of Directors.

2. Prepare an agenda for the annual business meeting and submit it to the membership not less than thirty (30) days prior to such a meeting in accordance with Article 12, Section B of the Bylaws.

3. Prepare an agenda for each meeting of the Board of Directors and submit it to the members of the Board not less than fifteen (15) days prior to such a meeting.

4. Appoint Standing Committees subject to the approval of the Board of Directors; appoint Special Committees.

5. Be an ex-officio member of all committees.

6. Present to the Board of Directors an annual report of the Association.

Section B. The President Elect shall:

Become acting President and shall assume the duties of the President in the event of the President's absence, resignation, or disability.

Section C. The Vice President shall:

1. Be speaker of the House of Delegates.

2. Report the activities of the House of Delegates and present their recommendations to the Board of Directors.

3. Assume the duties but not the office of the President Elect in the event of the President Elect's absence, resignation, or disability but will also continue to carry out the duties of the office of the Vice President.

Section D. The Treasurer shall:

1. Account for the moneys of this Association, approve payment of bills and disburse funds under the direction of the Board of Directors in accordance with the approved budget.

2. Be responsible for the continuing record of all income and disbursements

and provide for the President and the Chairman of the Board of Medical Advisors a quarterly financial report.

3. Prepare and submit in writing at the spring meeting of the Board of Directors a complete report of the finances of the Association for the preceding year and such other audits as may be directed by the Board of Directors. A copy of these reports is to be directed to the Chairman of the Board of Medical Advisors.

Section E. The Secretary shall:

Keep the minutes of the Board of Directors and annual business meetings; attest the signature of the officers of this Association; affix the corporate seal on documents so requiring, and, in general, perform all duties as from time to time may be assigned by the President or the Board of Directors.

Section F. Additional Duties

In addition to the foregoing specific duties, the duties of the officers shall be such as stated in Robert's Rules of Order, Revised, except when in conflict with the Constitution or Bylaws of this Association.

ARTICLE V

BOARD OF DIRECTORS

Section A. Composition

1. Members of the Board of Directors (with the exception of the Past President, President, President Elect, Vice President, Secretary, and Treasurer, who are members of the Board of Directors pursuant to Article IV of the Constitution) shall be elected for a three (3) year nonrecurring term of office. Members of the Board of Schools of Inhalation Therapy of the AMA and Trustees of the ARIT shall not be directors of the AAIT.

2. Four (4) Directors shall be elected each year except that at the time of adoption of this Constitution, the entire Board shall be reconstituted in accordance with these Bylaws.

3. The President shall be Chairman and presiding officer of the Board of Directors and Executive Committee. He shall invite in writing such individuals to the meetings of the Board as he shall deem necessary. The invitations shall be presented to the Sergeant at Arms at the time of the meeting.

4. The President shall appoint a member of the Association to serve as Parliamentarian and Sergeant at Arms who shall attend all Board meetings without a vote.

Section B. Meetings

1. The Board of Directors shall meet preceding and immediately following the annual meeting of this Association and shall hold not less than two (2) additional and separate meetings during the course of the year.

2. Additional meetings of the Board of Directors may be called by the President

at such times as the business of this Association may require, or upon written request of ten (10) members of the Board of Directors filed with the President and the Executive Secretary of this Association.

3. Members of the Board of Directors shall be reimbursed for reasonable expenses incurred at the discretion of the Budget and Audit Committee and with the majority approval of the entire Board.

Section C. Duties of the Board of Directors

1. Supervise all the business and activities of the Association within the limitations of the Constitution and Bylaws.

2. Direct the activities of the Executive Secretary.

3. Notify the Board of Medical Advisors of all such meetings and actions as are deemed pertinent or otherwise indicated by Article IV, Section C, of the Constitution.

Section D. Executive Committee

The Executive Committee of the Board of Directors shall consist of the Past President, President, President Elect, Vice President, Secretary, and Treasurer. They shall have the power to act for the Board of Directors in the absence of the Board and such action shall be subject to ratification by the full Board at its next meeting. They will also function as the Budget and Audit Committee. (See Article X, Section B, Bylaws.)

ARTICLE VI

VACANCIES

Section A. Board of Directors

Any vacancy that occurs on the Board of Directors and any vacancy occurring in any office, with the exception of the President and President Elect, shall be filled from the list of available candidates provided by the House of Delegates, by the Board of Directors to serve until the next annual election.

Section B. President

In the event of a vacancy in the office of the President, the President Elect shall become acting President to serve the unexpired term followed by his own term as President.

Section C. President Elect

In the event of a vacancy in the office of the President Elect, the Vice President shall assume the duties of the President Elect as well as his own until the next election.

Section D. Committees

In the event of vacancies occurring in any committee, the President shall appoint members to fill such vacancies subject to the approval of the Board of Directors.

ARTICLE VII

QUORUMS

Section A. Business Meeting

A majority of the active members registered and present at a duly called business meeting shall constitute a quorum.

Section B. Board Meeting

A majority of the Board of Directors shall constitute a quorum at any meeting of the Board.

ARTICLE VIII

HOUSE OF DELEGATES

Section A. Election of Delegates

1. The House of Delegates shall be composed of one (1) representative of each chartered Chapter of this Association.

2. The delegates shall be elected by a majority of the active members of their respective Chapters each year at least ninety (90) days before the annual meeting and shall serve as their Chapter's respresentative to the House of Delegates from the time of their election until they are replaced or re-elected the following year.

3. An Alternate Delegate is also to be elected to serve in the absence of the Delegate. The alternate delegate may attend the House of Delegates meeting but is not eligible to cast the votes for his Chapter unless the Delegate is absent.

4. Only active members in good standing who are not on the Board of Directors of AAIT shall be eligible to represent their Chapter.

Section B. Voting

1. Each Delegate shall have one (1) vote for each active member of his Chapter as certified by the Executive Secretary and the Chairman of the Membership Committee to the House of Delegates' Credentials Committee.

2. The number of votes claimed by each Chapter shall be submitted to the Speaker of the House of Delegates at the time of reporting the newly elected delegate ninety (90) days before the annual House of Delegates meeting.

3. The Speaker shall appoint a Credentials Committee to certify the Delegates, Alternate Delegates, and the number of votes each Delegate may cast.

Section C. Meeting

The House of Delegates shall meet on the day preceding the official beginning of the annual meeting and at other times as called by their Speaker.

Section D. Speaker

The Vice President of this Association shall be the Speaker of the House of Delegates and the Chairman of their Credentials Committee. The House of Delegates shall elect such other officers as they require.

Section E. Purpose

The purpose of the House of Delegates is to provide a working liaison between the Board of Directors and the members through the Chapter representatives. The Delegate shall:

1. Attend all meetings of the House of Delegates and report the activities to their Chapters.

2. Attend the annual meeting.

3. Submit a written summary report not to exceed three hundred (300) words, of the activities of their Chapters for the preceding year. A financial report is also to be submitted by the Delegate for each Chapter's Board of Directors.

4. Furnish the Nominating Committee with the names, biographical sketches, and pictures of at least two (2) deserving and qualified members for each vacancy on the Board of Directors and such other names as they deem advisable for consideration for nomination for other offices.

5. Attend all meetings of their Chapter's Board of Directors.

6. Through their Speaker, present recommendations of their Chapter to the Board of Directors of this Association.

ARTICLE IX

COMMITTEES

Section A. Standing Committees

The members of the following standing committees shall be appointed by the President, subject to the approval of the Board of Directors, to serve for a term of one (1) year, except as otherwise specified in these Bylaws.

1. Membership
2. Budget and Audit
3. Chapter Affairs
4. Research and Education Fund
5. Elections
6. Judicial
7. Nominating
8. Program
9. Safety and Technical Information
10. Constitution and Bylaws
11. Public Relations and Liaison

Section B. Special Committees and Other Appointments

1. Special Committees may be appointed by the President.

2. Representatives of the AAIT to the Board of Schools of Inhalation Therapy of the AMA, the ARIT, and to such other organizations as request representation, shall be appointed by the President with the approval of the Board of Directors.

The term of appointment shall be for the same number of years as there are representatives of the AAIT. One (1) new appointment shall be made each year to each organization except as necessary to establish and maintain this rotation.

Section C. Committee Chairmen's Duties

1. The President shall appoint the Chairman of each Committee.

2. The Chairman of each committee shall confer promptly with the members of his committee on work assignments.

3. The Chairman of each committee may recommend prospective committee members to the President. When possible the Chairman of the previous year shall serve as a member of the new committee.

4. Pertinent committee correspondence shall be submitted by the committee chairmen to the Secretary of this Association. He shall forward copies to the Executive Committee. The President may direct the Secretary to send additional copies to other persons as deemed necessary.

5. All committee reports will be made in writing and submitted to the Secretary of the Association through the Headquarters Office at least thirty-five (35) days prior to the meeting at which the report is to be read. Copies will be made at Headquarters Office for each member of the Board.

6. Nonmembers or physician members may be appointed as consultants to committees. The President shall request recommendations for such appointments from the Board of Medical Advisors.

7. Each committee Chairman requiring operating expenses shall submit a budget for the next fiscal year to the Budget and Audit Committee at the time of the Spring meeting of the Board of Directors.

ARTICLE X

DUTIES OF THE COMMITTEES

Section A. Membership Committees

1. This Committee shall consist of three (3) members of the Board of Directors, one (1) new member being appointed each year for a term of three (3) years except as necessary to establish and maintain this rotation.

2. This Committee shall evaluate the background and experience of applicants for qualification and classification for membership guided by local Chapter evaluation and verification.

3. The Chapter will be given a maximum of sixty (60) days in which to report its recommendation. At this time, separate reminders will be sent by the Executive Secretary to the Chapter President and Chapter Secretary. Failure on the part of the Chapter to report within an additional thirty (30) days will leave the sole decision in regard to admission to the national Membership Committee.

Section B. Budget and Audit Committee

1. This Committee shall be composed of the Executive Committee and the Chairman of the Board of Medical Advisors or his designate.

2. They shall propose an annual budget for approval by the Board at the fall

meeting of the Board of Directors. The proposed budget shall then be submitted to the membership at least sixty (60) days prior to the annual business meeting. The budget shall then be ratified by the House of Delegates at the annual meeting.

3. They shall review and audit the quarterly financial reports and recommend approval or necessary action to the Board.

4. They shall require that the Treasurer and Executive Secretary not exceed the budget in any category without the consent of the Budget and Audit Committee and the approval of the full Board.

Section C. Chapter Affairs Committee

1. This Committee shall consist of the Vice President as Chairman and four (4) other members. Two (2) shall be appointed each year to serve for a two (2) year term of office except as necessary to establish and maintain this rotation.

2. This Committee shall receive applications for Chapter charters and shall review the Constitution and Bylaws of the proposed Chapter for compliance with the national objectives of this Association and report its findings to the Board of Directors.

3. This Committee shall review proposed amendments to existing Chapter Constitutions and Bylaws.

4. This Committee shall review the minutes of all the meetings of the Chapters and advise the Chapter President and Secretary in writing of any irregularities or other recommendations.

5. This Committee shall maintain the official list of approved Chapters, their current officers and Delegates and their Medical Advisors.

Section D. Research and Education Fund Committee

1. This Committee shall consist of four (4) members of the Emeritus Board. One (1) member may be reappointed annually, the other three (3) will rotate. One (1) new member will be appointed each year. The Chairman of the Board of Medical Advisors or his designate will serve as an ex-officio member of this Committee.

2. It will be the function of this Committee to accept, acknowledge, and administer any funds given to the Association for the purpose of research or education, in accordance with a set of rules to be drafted and kept current by the Committee and approved by the Board of Directors.

Section E. Elections Committee

1. This Committee shall prepare, receive, verify, and count all ballots.

2. The Committee shall consist of three (3) members who will serve for a one (1) year term of office.

Section F. Judicial Committee

1. This Committee shall consist of six (6) members from the Emeritus Board or the Board of Directors. Two (2) members shall be appointed each year for a three (3) year term of office, except as is necessary to establish and maintain this rotation.

2. This Committee shall review formal, written complaints against any individual AAIT member charged with any violation of the AAIT Constitution, Bylaws, or Code of Ethics or otherwise with any conduct deemed detrimental to the Association.

3. If the Committee determines that the complaint justifies an investigation, a written copy of the charges shall be prepared for the Chairman of the Board of Medical Advisors or his designate with benefit of legal counsel if deemed advisable.

4. A statement of charges shall then be served upon the member and an opportunity given that member to be heard before the Committee.

5. After careful review of the results of the hearing conducted with benefit of legal counsel when the Chairman of the Committee deems counsel to be necessary or desirable, the Committee shall make recommendations for action to the Board of Directors.

Section G. Nominating Committee

1. This Committee shall prepare for approval by the Board of Directors, a slate of officers and directors for the annual election. The recommendations for directors shall come to this Committee from the House of Delegates.

2. The Committee shall serve for a one (1) year term of office, and shall be appointed from members of the Board of Directors or Emeritus Board.

3. It shall be the duty of this Committee to make the final critical appraisal of candidates to see that the nominations are in the best interests of the Association, through a consideration of personal qualifications and geographic representation.

Section H. Program Committee

1. This Committee shall consist of six (6) members and be so constructed as to provide experienced members for program planning.

2. The Chairman shall be the member who was Chairman of the Local Arrangements Committee the previous year, unless deemed otherwise by the Board of Directors.

3. The other members shall include the Chairman of the Local Arrangements Committee of the immediate year and of the upcoming year, unless deemed otherwise by the Board of Directors.

4. The Chairman of the Board of Medical Advisors or his designate, the Chairman of the local Board of Medical Advisors, and the Executive Secretary will be consultant members to this Committee.

5. This Committee shall, with the assistance of a Local Arrangements Committee, prepare the program for the annual meeting.

Section I. Safety and Technical Information Committee

1. This Committee shall consist of four (4) members, two (2) to be appointed each year for a two (2) year term except as is necessary to establish and maintain this rotation.

2. This Committee shall make recommendations on safe inhalation therapy practices to be followed by members of the Association.

Section J. Constitution and Bylaws Committee

1. This Committee shall consist of five (5) members, one (1) of whom shall be a past President, with one (1) member being appointed annually for a five (5) year term except as is necessary to establish and maintain this rotation.

2. The Committee shall receive and prepare all amendments to the Constitution and Bylaws for submission to the Board of Directors. The Committee may also initiate such amendments for submission to the Board of Directors.

Section K. Public Relations and Liaison Committee

1. This Committee shall consist of the Editor-at-Large as chairman and four (4) other members who will serve for one (1) year terms subject to reappointment.

2. This Committee shall concern itself with the relations of this Association with public, hospitals, and other organizations through the dissemination of information concerning inhalation therapy.

3. The Committee shall maintain such liaison as has been established by the Board of Directors with other organizations whose activities may be of interest to the members of this Association.

4. This Committee shall prepare exhibits and pamphlets to bring the message of AAIT to medical, nursing, and hospital groups as well as educational facilities where use of such material can be expected to recruit new people to the field of inhalation therapy. Such material shall be subject to the approval of the Board of Medical Advisors.

ARTICLE XI

EDITORIAL BOARD

Section A. Members

The Editorial Board shall consist of four (4) members appointed by the Board of Directors for one (1) year terms and subject to reappointment. The chairman of the Board of Medical Advisors or his designate shall be a member of the Editorial Board as the Medical Consulting Editor.

Section B. Titles

One (1) member shall be designated Editor-in-Chief of all AAIT publications and the Chairman of the Editorial Board. One (1) member shall be appointed Editor of the "Newsletter." One (1) shall be appointed Editor of "Inhalation Therapy." One (1) member shall be appointed Editor-at-Large in charge of other publications of the AAIT and be Chairman of the Public Relations and Liaison Committee.

Section C. Remuneration

The remuneration for editorial services shall be determined by the Board of Directors.

Section D. Other Members

The Editorial Board may select such associate and consulting editors as they deem necessary, subject to the approval of the Board of Directors of the AAIT.

Section E. Editorial Policy

The Editorial Board shall establish and maintain a written set of rules defining their operating policies, subject to the approval of the Board of Directors. This policy statement shall be published at least once each year in the Journal.

Section F. Newsletter

The "Newsletter" shall be published at least bimonthly. Communications from the President, the Chairman of the Board of Medical Advisors, and Executive Secretary shall take priority over other available material.

Section G. Budget

The Editorial Board shall prepare and submit to the Budget and Audit Committee at the time of the spring meeting of the Board of Directors a proposed budget for the next fiscal year.

Section H. Report

The Editor-in-Chief shall submit an annual written report to the President thirty-five (35) days prior to the annual meeting of the Board of Directors.

Section I. Publisher

The Editorial Board shall, with the approval of the Board of Directors, select a publisher and a managing editor.

Section J. Editor-at-Large

1. He shall be in charge of the tapes of lectures.
2. He shall with the help of the entire Editorial Board review the tapes annually to keep them current.
3. He shall with the Editorial Board review proposed educational programs to determine which lectures should be taped. After review of these tapes, he will determine which are worthy of duplication.
4. He shall be in charge of all other unspecified educational material.
5. He shall maintain a current catalog of all the above items.
6. He shall be Chairman of the Public Relations and Liaison Committee.

ARTICLE XII

ANNUAL MEETING

Section A. Site

At each annual meeting, the Board shall decide the location and time of the annual meeting to be held five (5) years hence.

Section B. Notification

Not less than ninety (90) days prior to the annual meeting, written notice of the time and place of the annual meeting shall be sent to all members of the Association. Not less than thirty (30) days prior to the annual meeting, an agenda for the annual business meeting will be sent to all members.

ARTICLE XIII

MAIL VOTE

Whenever, in the judgment of the Board of Directors, it is necessary to present to the membership, prior to the next annual meeting any question that may arise, the Board of Directors may, unless otherwise required by these Bylaws, instruct the Elections Committee to prepare a ballot for submission to the membership by mail. The question thus presented shall be determined according to a majority of the valid votes received by mail within thirty (30) days after date of such submission to the membership, except in the case of a constitutional amendment or a change in the Bylaws when a two-thirds ($\frac{2}{3}$) majority of the valid votes received is required, provided that in each case at least one-half ($\frac{1}{2}$) of the active members have submitted a ballot. Any and all action approved by the members in accordance with the requirements of this Article shall be binding upon the Association and upon each member thereof. Any amendment to the Constitution or Bylaws of this Association shall be presented to the membership at least ninety (90) days prior to a mail vote.

ARTICLE XIV

CHAPTERS

Section A. Composition

All members of Chapters must be members of the American Association for Inhalation Therapy.

Section B. Chapter Admission Procedure

1. The formal application for a charter shall be directed to the Headquarters Office of the Association and shall consist of six (6) copies of a list of officers, membership, minutes of the organizational meeting, and the proposed Constitution and Bylaws, as well as the application for approval of the proposed Medical Advisor or Advisors. (See Article XIV, Section E, Bylaws.)

2. Applications will be considered by the Chapter Affairs Committee and, if approved, submitted to the Board of Directors for ratification.

Section C. Minutes

A copy of the minutes of every Chapter meeting shall be sent to the Headquarters Office of the Association within ten (10) days following the meeting at which they are approved. This copy will in turn be sent to the Chairman of the Chapter Affairs Committee.

Section D. Withdrawal of a Chapter's Charter

1. The Board of Directors of the American Association for Inhalation Therapy may withdraw the charter of any Chapter with due and sufficient cause.

2. Action for the withdrawal of the charter of any Chapter may be initiated for cause upon written complaint filed by any two (2) or more members of this Association with the Chairman of the Chapter Affairs Committee. Before any charter can be withdrawn, the officers, if known, of the Chapter shall be given written notice of the charges filed against such Chapter and shall be given opportunity to appear at a hearing before the Chapter Affairs Committee of this Association at a time and place designated in the notice. The hearing will not be held sooner than thirty (30) days after the mailing of such notice. If the officers of the Chapter are not known to the Chapter Affairs Committee, then such notice shall be given to all the known members of the Association in that Chapter. Representatives of the Chapter in question shall be permitted to give testimony and introduce evidence in support of the continuance of the Chapter Charter at the hearing before the Chapter Affairs Committee.

Section E. Chapter Medical Advisor

1. Each Chapter shall have at least one (1) Medical Advisor, who shall be approved by the Board of Medical Advisors. Any subsequent change in advisors must be approved by the Board of Medical Advisors.

2. To receive approval of a Chapter Medical Advisor, a letter shall be sent to the Chairman of the Board of Medical Advisors to include the reasons for selecting the advisor, his curriculum vitae, and publications.

3. No member of the Board of Schools of Inhalation Therapy of the AMA, Board of the American Registry of Inhalation Therapists, or Board of Medical Advisors shall serve as a Chapter Medical Advisor.

4. Chapter Medical Advisors shall be elected by the Chapter membership at their annual election. Tenure of office shall not exceed three (3) years followed by a minimal absence of one (1) year from the advisory group.

5. The term of office of the Chapter Medical Advisor may be terminated at any time by a two-thirds (⅔) majority vote of the Chapter's membership. Notification of this action shall also be submitted to the Board of Medical Advisors.

ARTICLE XV
Fiscal Year

The fiscal year of this Association shall be from January 1 through December 31.

ARTICLE XVI
Dues

Section A. Amount

Annual dues for each category of membership other than Honorary and Life shall be determined for the following year by the Board of Directors after consideration of the budget.

Section B. Payment

Dues shall be payable on or before January 10 and become delinquent on April 10. Any member whose dues are not paid by April 10 shall be dropped from membership after suitable notification. Any member who has been dropped may be reinstated during the calendar year by the payment of his current dues plus a reinstatement fee determined by the Board of Directors on an annual basis.

ARTICLE XVII

ETHICS

If the conduct of any member shall appear, by report of the Judicial Committee, to be in willful violation of the Constitution, Bylaws, or standing rules of this Association or prejudicial to the Association's interests as defined in the Association's Code of Ethics, the Board of Directors may, by two-thirds ($\frac{2}{3}$) vote of its entire membership, suspend or expel such a member. A motion to reconsider the suspension or expulsion of a member may be made at the next regular meeting of the Board of Directors. Thereafter, readmission shall proceed as prescribed for new members.

ARTICLE XVIII

AMENDMENTS

These Bylaws may be amended at any annual meeting or by mail vote of the American Association for Inhalation Therapy by a two-thirds ($\frac{2}{3}$) majority of those voting provided that at least 50% of the qualified membership votes.

ARTICLE XIX

PARLIAMENTARY PROCEDURE

Questions of parliamentary procedure shall be settled according to Robert's Rules of Order, Revised, whenever they are not in conflict with the Constitution and Bylaws of this Association.

CHAPTER 19

Requirements of an Approved School of Inhalation Therapy

IN THE ORGANIZATION of a formal school of inhalation therapy which is either hospital based or college affiliated, it is mandatory that the already existing department of inhalation therapy be under medical administration. By "medical administration," we mean having a full-time medical director who may be either an anesthesiologist, chest physician or a physician of internal medicine. The medical director is usually chosen from one of these three fields because of their common foundation in pulmonary physiology, and also because physicians in these specialties focus their practice within the hospital. The medical director must be well versed in chest diseases, with considerable clinical experience in treating respiratory disease.

Equally important in the establishment of a formal school of inhalation therapy is the quality of the services being rendered to the patients by the existing department. To have an effective school, the department should be adequately staffed at all times so as to provide the necessary care to the patient. The students enrolled in the school should not be used as "slave help": They are there to learn, not to fulfill the duties of the departmental staff in providing patient care.

For teaching purposes, the ratio between students and instructor should be close. This is important because of the nature of instruction. It is impossible to provide the necessary quality when this ratio of students to instructor is exceeded. *We cannot emphasize this too much.* It is important to the student, and it should be a matter of concern to the medical director, the technical director and the clinical instructors. The students who are receiving this formal training, upon graduation, will be providing respiratory care to patients who are critically ill, and the lives of these patients are at the mercy of each individual providing this care. It is the case that each formal school in the past has been evaluated according to the number of students passing the registry examination. Whether this should be the ultimate standard by which to evaluate schools remains a question.

Provision should be made for each student enrolled to receive clinical experience, adequate in kind and amount, under the direction of the teaching staff.

321

Equipment of all types and models in current accepted use should be available for demonstration and clinical use. When affiliation with other hospitals is necessary, it should be emphasized that these hospitals must provide adequate supervision and meet all the requirements of the Board of Schools.

A library containing references, texts and scientific periodicals pertaining to inhalation therapy should be maintained. This area has been vastly neglected in the past. Students must be required to write research papers; they must read and keep up with the current literature within the field of inhalation therapy as well as within other allied health professions. The goal is to provide these individuals with an integrated approach to the problem of caring for the ill.

A school of inhalation therapy approved by the Council on Medical Education and the Board of Schools for Inhalation Therapy has adopted the following plan:

CURRICULUM

FIRST YEAR
Quarter 1

COURSE NO.	COURSE TITLE	LECTURE (LAB) HOURS	CREDIT
18.107	Integrated Science	4(3)	5
20.100	Social Anthropology	4	4
30.101	English	3	3
86.101	Medical Terminology	2	2
89.191	Intro. to Inhalation Therapy	4	3

Quarter 2

18.108	Integrated Science	4(3)	5
19.102	Intro. Psychology	4	4
20.102	English	3	3
86.102	Hospital Law, Ethics	2	2
86.192	Intro. to Inhalation Therapy	4	3

FIRST YEAR
Quarter 3

18.109	Integrated Science	4(3)	5
21.100	Princ. of Sociology	4	4
30.103	English	3	3
86.511	Personal, Community Health	2	2
86.193	Intro. to Inhalation Therapy	2(2)	3

Summer Session (Part I)

86.589	Basic Nursing Procedures	(150 clock hours)	nc

(Continued)

CURRICULUM (*cont.*)

SECOND YEAR
Quarter 4 or 5 (alternating with the "Internship" quarter)

COURSE NO.	COURSE TITLE	LECTURE (LAB) HOURS	CREDIT
29.100	Public Speaking	3	3
60.101	Physical Education	(2)	nc
86.194	Procedures in Inhalation Therapy	3(6)	5
86.104	Foundations of Medical Science	3	3

SECOND YEAR
Quarter 6 or 7 (alternating with one quarter of co-op work assignment)

19.201	Abnormal Psychology	4	4
60.102	Physical Education	(2)	nc
86.195	Procedures in Inhalation Therapy	3(6)	5
86.105	Foundations of Medical Science	3	3

THIRD YEAR
Quarter 8 or 9 (alternating with one quarter of co-op work assignment)

23.201	U.S. History to 1865	4	4
86.196	Procedures in Inhalation Therapy	2(6)	4
86.103	Emergency Procedures	1(2)	2
	Elective	3	3

Quarter 10

23.211	U.S. History from 1865	4	4
86.197	Procedures in Inhalation Therapy	2(6)	4
86.124	Health Education	2	2
	Elective	3	3

Total quarter hours of credit in the program 100

This program was carefully planned to coordinate and integrate technical training and experience with liberal arts courses to lead to an Associate in Science degree and to provide additional clinical experience under the cooperative plan of education. All students are required to spend the first academic year in the classroom, receiving instructions in applied and social sciences as well as taking theory courses in inhalation therapy.

During the summer of the first academic year, all students receive 150 hours of classroom instruction, demonstration and clinical practice in nursing arts.

During the second and third years, 12-week academic quarters alternate with 12-week quarters of clinical practice under supervision. One of these quarters (500 hours) is counted as a required internship. During the other two clinical quarters, the students are designated as "co-operatives" and each receive a stipend.

Classroom and clinical practice hours in all areas meet or exceed the recommended minimal criteria for an approved school of inhalation therapy.

ROTATION OF STUDENTS FOR CLINICAL HOSPITAL EXPERIENCE

YEAR	GROUP	FALL	WINTER	SPRING	SUMMER
I	All	Academic #1	Academic #2	Academic #3	Nursing/arts Vacation
II	Group A	Academic #4	Co-op work	Academic #5	Co-op work/ Vacation
	Group B	Co-op work	Academic #4	Co-op work Vacation	Academic #5
III	Group A	Academic #6	Internship	Academic #7	(graduation in June of third year)
	Group B	Internship	Academic #6	Academic #7	

Because of the co-operative plan, not more than one third of the total student body is in the clinical practice setting at any given time. (First year students are not assigned to clinical duty, except as observers or for demonstration with their own instructors.)

"The Essentials and Guidelines for an Approved School of Inhalation Therapy"

FOREWORD

The Board of Schools of Inhalation Therapy is organized under the auspices of the Council on Medical Education of the American Medical Association and sponsored by the following organizations:

1. American Society of Anesthesiologists
2. American College of Chest Physicians
3. American Association of Inhalation Therapists

Its primary purpose is to maintain a high standard of education among schools of inhalation therapy and to encourage further development of these schools.

HISTORY

In June, 1956, the House of Delegates of the AMA considered a resolution introduced by the New York State Medical Society regarding the field of inhalation therapy and recommending the establishment of "Essentials" to stimulate the development of Schools. This was adopted in principle and referred to the Council on Medical Education for study. After preliminary study, an exploratory conference was held in Chicago in September, 1957, of all organizations interested in inhalation therapy. It was unanimously agreed that minimal standards for training should be developed. The "Essentials" proposed by the New York State Society of Anesthesiologists in May, 1956, were approved as a basic document for study and exploration. The American Society of Anesthesiologists and the American College of Chest Physicians were delegated to evaluate the proposed curriculum and to obtain experience in inhalation therapy training.

From September, 1957, to January, 1962, several pilot schools adopted the proposed curriculum to varying degrees and found that the minimal standards represented a realistic approach in training. Thereupon, a report was made to the Council on Medical Education in February, 1962, recommending the earlier "Essentials" with minor modification, and the establishment of a mechanism for approving schools. In March, 1962, the Council approved the "Essentials" as submitted. These were subsequently approved by the AMA House of Delegates in December, 1962, in Los Angeles.

COMPOSITION OF THE BOARD

The Board consists of 7 members appointed by the organizations sponsoring it. Two physicians each are appointed by the American Society of Anesthesiologists and American College of Chest Physicians, and three technicians are designated by the American Association of Inhalation Therapists. This Board, responsible for the evaluation of schools of inhalation therapy, held its first meeting in January, 1963, at AMA headquarters.

BASIC CONCEPTS

An approved school for training inhalation therapy technicians must have the following:

1. *A medical director,* active in the field of inhalation therapy and concerned with the proper education of therapy technicians. Ordinarily, this physician will be a board-certified anesthesiologist or a board-certified chest physician.

2. *A technician supervisor,* experienced in the field of inhalation therapy and interested in training technicians. This supervisor should be certified as a registered therapy technician. He should have an adequate number of assistants.

3. *A hospital facility* with an active, well-organized inhalation therapy service and an administration sympathetic to the needs of inhalation therapy.

4. *A program* to provide or to integrate the knowledge essential to practice in the field of inhalation therapy and to provide the practical skills needed by competent technicians.

I. *Administration*

1. Acceptable schools for training inhalation therapy technicians may be established only in medical schools approved by the Council on Medical Education of the American Medical Association or in accredited hospitals. An acceptable hospital may affiliate with a college or university accredited by their respective regional association of colleges and secondary schools.

2. All training of technicans shall be under competent medical control. Though the basic sciences may be taught in a college setting, it should be recognized that this is preliminary or preclinical in nature and that inhalation therapy itself is a clinical discipline.

3. Resources for continued operation of the school should be insured through regular budgets, gifts or endowments but not entirely through students' tuition fees.

4. Records of high school or college work or other credentials of students must be on file. Attendance and grades of students together with a detailed analysis of their clinical experience shall be recorded systematically.

a) Attendance record: An attendance record should be kept for each student showing daily hours, sick time, holiday time and vacation, leave of absence and absence without leave.

b) Records of classes and grades earned should be kept for each student and compiled in transcript form on completion of the course.

c) Each student should keep a notebook and record daily his or her clinical experiences and the time utilized in performing each experience.

d) The director or instructor should keep a record patterned after the suggested curriculum which shows a weekly and monthly composite of the student's experience. This will facilitate preparation of a transcript of his work.

5. At least four students should be enrolled in each class. Approval may be withdrawn if a school does not have any students for a period of 2 years.

a) The student capacity for which a school is approved shall not be exceeded without obtaining approval from the Council on Medical Education.

b) A request to increase student capacity should include the following supporting data in duplicate:

1. The last annual statistical report of clinical procedures performed by the department of inhalation therapy.

2. A complete list of all faculty and technical personnel working in inhalation therapy with qualifications and years of experience of each.

II. *Faculty*

6. The school should have a competent teaching staff. The director must be a licensed physician who has had specific training or experience in inhalation therapy acceptable to the Council. He shall take regular part in and be responsible for the actual conduct of the training program. Basic science instructors must be competent in their respective fields and be properly qualified or certified.

a) Physicians who have been certified by American College of Chest Physicians or who have been certified by the American Board of Anesthesiology may be considered to have acceptable experience in inhalation therapy.

b) If the director is not so certified or eligible for such certification, he must submit to the Council, as a part of the school's application for approval, his curriculum vitae emphasizing his training and experience in clinical physiology.

7. In clinical practice, the enrollment shall not exceed five students to each instructor. In order to be considered an instructor, a technician should be a registered inhalation therapist and have not less than 3 years' experience.

a) The teaching supervisor and the instructors must be well qualified to instruct students and must have a keen interest in teaching and producing well-trained technicians.

b) Besides listing the instructors, a complete list of the inhalation therapy personnel employed by the department providing the clinical training should accompany the application form for an approved school. This should include their education, training and duties in inhalation therapy.

c) There should be a sufficient staff of therapists to insure that the work of the department is carried out without help from the students.

III. *Facilities*

8. Provision should be made for each student enrolled to receive a foundation in the basic sciences and adequate clinical experience in kind and amount under the supervision of the teaching staff.

a) Experience should be gained with a sufficient number of patients in all of the major hospital departments, namely, medicine, surgery, obstetrics and pediatrics. In these patients, a wide variety of clinical problems should be represented requiring different forms of inhalation therapy.

b) If the variety of clinical material is such that experience in some procedures is limited, then arrangement should be made to provide these experiences in other institutions. For example, a hospital without pediatrics or obstetrics may not be able to furnish training in inhalation therapy utilizing incubators and pediatric resuscitation devices.

9. Affiliation of the Clinical Program with a community college or educational program beyond the high school level for the purpose of providing the basic science courses is encouraged. The number of students in the collegiate basic science program should not exceed the number of students that can be clinically

supervised and trained. The hospital primarily responsible for the training program shall make the affiliation. The affiliated school or college must be accredited by the regional association of secondary schools or colleges.

10. Adequate equipment should be available for demonstration and clinical use. This should include all types of modalities in current accepted use.

11. Where affiliation with other hospitals is deemed necessary or important, it should be permitted only if adequate supervision is possible. Such affiliation must be approved by the Council.

12. A library of adequate space and availability and containing references, texts and scientific periodicals pertaining to inhalation therapy should be maintained.

   a) Reference and text materials should be in the departmental quarters readily available to the student.

   b) Reference materials should include standard textbooks in anatomy, physiology, physics, chemistry, pharmacology, psychology, microbiology and basic nursing arts.

   c) In addition to library facilities, adequate classroom space with regular classroom appointments and facilities for storing and using visual aids should be available to the school.

IV. *Requirements for Admission*

13. Candidates for admission must have completed 4 years of high school or have passed a standard equivalency test. Courses in biology, physics, chemistry, algebra and geometry are recommended. Education beyond high school, at the vocational, nursing or collegiate level, is desirable. A pre-entrance examination of candidates is also recommended.

GENERAL COMMENTS ON ADMISSION REQUIREMENTS

Data from which to determine that a prospective student has satisfied at least one of the requirements for admission to an approved school should be available from the school's application form filled in and submitted by the prospect.

An application form for prospective students should contain the following minimum information:

1. *Personal History*

   a) Name, permanent address, present address, telephone number, parent or guardian or next of kin with the address and phone number of the named person.

   b) Birth date, birth place, citizenship status, marital status, number and kind of dependents (children or parents or others).

   c) A general statement as to how the applicant rates his own health.

2. *Scholastic Record*

   a) Name and address of secondary school, high school, academy, or other attended; number of years attended, diploma or certificate granted, and the last year school was attended or date of diploma or certificate.

b) Query about college entrance exams.

c) Name and address of university, college, nursing school, junior college, trade school, other attended; dates of attendance, degree, diploma, certificate or credits earned.

d) The prospective student should be instructed to forward a copy of a transcript of his prior academic record to the director of the school of inhalation therapy.

3. *Employment*

A list of positions held since high school including type of work, length of time employed, name of the employer, reason for leaving.

4. Statement of military service status or record.

5. The names and addresses of two adults, not related, knowing applicant well enough to give an appraisal of candidate in connection with application to school. One of these should be a former teacher.

6. A brief statement describing the applicant's interest in inhalation therapy in the applicant's own handwriting.

7. Space should be clearly indicated on the application form for a recent photograph, not a snapshot.

V. *Health*

14. Applicants shall be required to submit evidence of good health and successful vaccination. All students shall be given a medical examination, as soon as practicable after admission, by a physician designated by the school. This examination shall include a roentgen examination of the chest. There shall be periodic medical examination of the student.

a) Every precaution should be taken to prevent any health hazard in the department or during clinical practice.

b) The personnel health service of the hospital should be available to the student.

c) Any injuries on duty should be taken care of at once as an emergency.

d) Hospitalization for a limited time should be made available by the hospital either directly or through hospitalization insurance.

VI. *Curriculum*

15. Length of course should include not less than 18 months of theoretical instruction and practical hospital experience.

a) Interruptions in attendance for valid health reasons shall be evaluated on an individual basis.

b) Credit for courses completed should not be lost by interruption of the program.

c) Time cannot be made up or the course shortened by evening or weekend attendance.

16. The basic curriculum should include no less than the subjects and clock hours presented in the accompanying table. The applied sciences may be taught in an affiliated university, medical center or accredited college. The sciences should be oriented to make clinical application smooth. All subjects under practice must be taught in the hospital environment as should the subjects under clinical application.

a) The suggested basic curriculum is intended as a guide to a suitable teaching program. Each school should prepare a formal course outline and schedule following the recommendations set forth in the basic curriculum. The course outline for each subject should list in each category suggested:

1. Topics to be presented
2. The outlines, syllabi, texts, visual aids, and equipment needed to supplement lectures or demonstrations
3. Instructor scheduled to conduct the class
4. The amount of time allotted for the class

b) Each student should have a check list of procedures he is expected to perform with spaces provided to show each day's work in each listed category and the amount of time spent on each. The student's check list should make provision for entering the area of work, character of ward assignment, i.e., Pediatrics, Obstetrics, etc.

c) An evaluation record should be maintained on each student.

d) Registered nurses who have graduated from accredited schools of nursing may be granted credit for basic science subjects which are common to the curriculum of the School of Nursing and the School of Inhalation Therapy. Graduate nurses (R.N.) may be expected to have had a broad education in anatomy, microbiology, chemistry, pathology, physiology, physics, psychology, nursing arts, and ethics. This education amounts to about 600 hours.

BASIC CURRICULUM FOR INHALATION THERAPY TECHNICIANS

SUBJECT	CLOCK–HOURS
A. *Applied Sciences*	
Anatomy	50
Microbiology	25
Chemistry	50
Pathology	25
Pharmacology	35
Physiology	50
Psychology	15
Physics	50
	300

Subject	Clock Hours Theory	Practice
B. Procedures		
Analysis, Gas	5	5
Airway Management	10	20
Administration, Oxygen	30	50
Administration, Other Gases	10	10
Humidification	30	25
Humidification, Aerosols		
Ventilation, Assisted	50	100
Ventilation, Controlled		
Resuscitation	20	20
Lung Physiotherapy	10	10
Spirometry	5	10
Equipment, Maintenance	30	50
	200	300
C. Clinical Application		
Emergency	10	50
Medicine	30	80
Obstetrics	5	10
Pediatrics	20	50
Surgery, General	10	60
Surgery, Thoracic		
Neurosurgery		
Pulmonary Function	5	30
	80	280
D. Ethics and Administration	20	20
E. Nursing Arts	— 100°	—
F. Clinical Practice	— 500°	—
TOTALS	600 600	600
GRAND TOTAL	1,800 Clock hours of instruction	

° Theory and Practice

VII. Ethics

17. Excessive tuition or other student fees and commercial advertising shall be considered unethical.

18. Schools substituting students for paid technicians to meet the work load of a department will not be considered for approval.

a) Students should not take the responsibility or the place of qualified inhalation therapy technicians.

b) The staff of inhalation therapy should be adequate to perform the work of the department without the students being present.

c) Any indication of exploitation of students will result in disapproval of a school.

VIII. *Admission to the Approved List*

19. Admission for approval of a school for inhalation therapy technicians should be made to the Council on Medical Education, Department of Allied Medical Professions, American Medical Association, 535 North Dearborn Street, Chicago, Illinois 60610. Forms will be supplied for this purpose on request. They should be completed by the administrator of the institution requesting approval and signed by the physician-director of the program.

20. Approval may be withdrawn whenever in the opinion of the Council a school does not maintain an educational program in accordance with the above standards.

21. Approved schools should notify the Council whenever a change occurs in the directorship or teaching supervisor of the school.

a) When there is a change in the director, information concerning the qualifications of the new medical director must be submitted in duplicate to the Council as soon as possible. If the new director's credentials are in order, the school's approval will be continued.

b) If there is an extended interval during which there is no director, the students already enrolled will be permitted to complete the course but no new students may be enrolled until a medical director is appointed and approved.

22. Inquiries regarding registration of qualified inhalation therapists should be addressed to the American Registry of Inhalation Therapists, 122 South Michigan Avenue, Chicago, Illinois 60603.

CERTIFICATE

Each school should present to a successful student, on completion of the educational program, a suitable certificate. This should show the name of the school, the location, the name of the student and the date of graduation. It should be suitably endorsed by the director of the school, the administrator of the institution and the supervisor technician.

REFERENCES

Essentials of an Acceptable School for Inhalation Therapy Technicians, Council on Medical Education of the American Association, 535 North Dearborn Street, Chicago, Illinois 60610.

Egan, D. F.: Inhalation therapy department: Staffing and services, J. Am. Hosp. A., Sept. 1, 1968.

Starkweather, D. B.: Inhalation therapy department: Administrative organization hospital, J. Am. Hosp. A., Sept. 1, 1968.

Appendix

A. Glossary

Absolute Pressure: The total pressure above a vacuum or true zero pressure. Absolute pressure is atmospheric pressure plus the gauge pressure.

Acapnia: Reduced carbon dioxide content of the blood.

Acid-Base Balance: A condition in which the reaction of acids and bases are maintained in equilibrium by physiologic processes.

Acidosis: (1) An excess of acid in the blood. (2) Reduced alkaline (bicarbonate) reserve of the blood.

Aerosol: A fine suspension of liquid or solid particles in an atmosphere of gas.

Air Content, Alveolar, Dry: 14% (100 mm Hg) O_2; 80.4% (565 mm Hg) N_2; 5.6% (40 mm Hg) CO_2; = 100% (713 mm Hg water pressure of 47 mm Hg removed from these data).

Air Content, Atmospheric, Dry: 20.94% (159.2 mm Hg) O_2; 79.02% (600.5 mm Hg) N_2; 0.04% (0.3 mm Hg) CO_2; = 100% (760 mm Hg).

Air Content, Expired, Dry: 16.3% (116 mm Hg) O_2; 79.2% (565 mm Hg) N_2; 4.5% (32 mm Hg) CO_2; = 100% (713 mm Hg water vapor pressure of 47 mm Hg removed from these data).

Airway: (1) The path which air travels from the atmosphere to the alveoli. (2) Any of the several devices used in securing a clear respiratory passage.

Alkalosis: An elevated alkaline (bicarbonate) reserve of the blood or reduction in acids in the blood.

Alveolar Membrane: Thin layer of tissue which partitions the air in the alveoli and the capillary blood.

Alveolar Ventilation: Tidal volume minus the physiologic dead space.

Alveoli: Singular *alveolus*; air sacs at the end of the respiratory channels.

Ammeter: A device for measuring the flow of electrical current.

Amplitude Modulation: A technique of amplifying and/or broadcasting of electrical signals. The electrical signal is made to alter or modulate the amplitude of a carrier current. The carrier current thus modulated is amplified or broadcast and the original signal then retrieved by demodulation.

Aneroid Manometer: A pressure-measuring device which compares the pressure in the system to that of a vacuum. Such a device measures true total pressure.

Anoxemia: Oxygen deficiency in the blood. Literally, without oxygen. See Hypoxia.

Anthracosilicosis: Chronic lung disease found in coal miners. Diffused fibrosis of the lungs accompanied by black pigmentation; caused by prolonged inhalation of dust containing silicon dioxide and carbon. A form of pneumonoconiosis.

Anthracosis: Black pigmentation of the lungs associated with a mild degree of chronic inflammation from inhalation of carbon dust. A form of pneumonoconiosis.

Apnea: Cessation of breathing.

Apneusis: Abnormal respiration characterized by a prolonged inspiration, unrelieved by expiration.

Arrhythmia: Irregularity of heart beats.

Asphyxia: Suffocation, coma, from lack of oxygen and accumulation of carbon dioxide.

Asphyxia Neonatorum: Suffocation of the newborn. Inability to breathe immediately following birth.

Aspiration: Removal of accumulated mucus and foreign bodies by suction.

Asthma: Recurrent attacks of difficult breathing, with dyspnea, cough, wheezing and a sense of constriction of the chest.

Atelectasis: Partial or complete collapse or imperfect expansion of the air sacs of the lungs.

Atmosphere (atm): The pressure exerted by 76 cm mercury with a density of 13.5951 Gm/cm³ at 1 g (the standard barometric pressure at sea level).

$$1 \text{ atm} = 1.01325 \times 10^6 \text{ dynes/cm}^2$$
$$= 1033.2 \text{ Gm/cm}^2$$
$$= 760 \text{ mm Hg}$$
$$= 14.696 \text{ psi}$$

Atmospheric Pressure: At sea level, 760 mm Hg (millimeters of mercury) or 14.7.

Atomizer: Device to reduce a liquid or solid to small droplets in the form of a spray.

Barometer: A pressure-measuring device which senses atmospheric pressure.

Bradycardia: Decreased heart rate.

Bradypnea: Decreased respiratory rate.

Bridge Circuit: The Wheatstone bridge circuit is an electrical circuit designed to indicate the resistance in a given circuit by comparing it to known resistance.

Bronchi: Singular *bronchus*. The two primary divisions of the trachea or windpipe.

Bronchia: Subdivision of bronchi.

Bronchiectasis: Abnormal and chronic dilation of bronchial tubes.

Bronchiole: Very small bronchial tubes.

Bronchiolitis: Inflammation of the bronchioles; capillary bronchitis.

Bronchitis: Inflammation of the mucous membrane of the bronchial tubes.

Bronchoconstrictor: An agent which narrows the air passages of the lungs.

Bronchodilator: An agent which dilates the air passages of the lungs.

Bronchospasm: Spasmotic narrowing of the lumen of a bronchus.

Capacitance: The ability to retain an electrical charge.

Capillary: A minute thin-walled blood vessel, smallest of the blood-transport system. Capillaries constitute the exchange point between the red blood (arterial blood) and returned blood (venous blood).

Carbon Button Transducer: A transducer composed of carbon granules contained within an enclosure covered with a diaphragm. Pressure on the diaphragm compresses the granules decreasing the electrical resistance across the granules.

Cardiac Catheterization: The insertion of a tube into the chambers of the heart as a method for studying the flow, pressure and oxygen content of blood in the heart.

Carrier Current: An alternating current of moderately fast frequency employed in amplitude and frequency modulation. This current is modulated by, and by this method carries, the electrical signal to be broadcast or amplified.

Cheyne-Stokes Respiration: Abnormal breathing, intermittently deep and shallow and ceasing temporarily.

Chromatography: A technique for the separation of mixtures of substances for quantitative analysis.

Colorimetry: Quantitative analysis of the color present in a sample.

Compliance: A measure of the elastic properties of the lung or thorax alone, or together, in volume change per unit pressure change, usually liter per centimeter of water (L/cm H_2O). See Elastance.

Conductance: A measure of the nonelastic properties of the airway, lungs and thorax expressed in unit of volume in time change per pressure change, usually liters per second per centimeter of water ($L/sec/cm$ H_2O). See Resistance.

Constantan: A metallic alloy employed in thermocouples and in the resistance wire of strain gauge manometers.

Coronary Occlusion: Shutting or closing off of one of the arteries of the heart.

Coronary Thrombosis: A blood clot forming in the arteries supplying the heart muscle and blocking the proper blood supply to an area of the heart muscle.

Cor Pulmonale: Dilation of the right side of the heart, secondary to an obstructing pulmonary disease or to obstruction of the pulmonary artery.

Costal Breathing: Respiration produced solely by the intercostal muscles.

Cyanosis: Bluish gray pallor associated with blood oxygen deficiency. It is caused by color of the reduced hemoglobin in the capillaries.

Cystic Fibrosis of the Pancreas: See Fibrocystic Disease of the Pancreas.

Damping: A mechanical (or electrical) interference with the oscillations of a mechanical (or electrical) system.

Dead Space, Anatomic: The internal volume of the airway, from the nose and mouth to the alveoli.

Dead Space, Mechanical: Space in breathing apparatus, outside the patient where the expired air is trapped and then reinhaled.

Dead Space, Physiologic: The anatomic dead space plus the volume of inspired gas ventilating the alveoli, which have no capillary blood flow; *plus* the volume of inspired gas ventilating alveoli in excess of that required to arterialize the pulmonary capillary blood flowing around them.

d'Arsonval Movement: A moving coil galvanometer. Electrical current applied to the galvanometer is conducted to a coil suspended between the poles of the permanent magnet. The entire coil moves with passage of current through it.

Density: The relationship between the volume of a gas and its weight.

Diaphragm: The muscular sheath which separates the thorax from the abdomen.

Diaphragmatic Breathing: Respiration produced solely by use of the diaphragm.

Diffusion: Transfer of gases across the alveolar capillary membrane.

Displacement Plethysmograph: An instrument for measuring the volume of a portion of the body directly by enclosing it in an inelastic container and measuring displacement of the medium immediately surrounding the part of the body.

Dynamic Pressure: Pressure which changes rapidly.

Dyspnea: Consciousness of air want; shortness of breath; labored breathing, subjective difficulty in breathing.

Edema, Pulmonary: An excess accumulation of fluid in the lungs.

Elastance: A measure of the elastic properties of the lung or thorax alone, or together, expressed in unit pressure change per volume change, usually centimeters of water per liter (cm H_2O/L). See Compliance.

Emphysema: A term used to describe many different pulmonary conditions. Chronic pulmonary emphysema is marked by diffused bronchial obstruction, by changes in and destruction of alveolar walls producing enlarged air sacs of varying size, by diffused interstitial involvement, by changes in pulmonary vessels and a decrease of the capillary bed. It often follows some other chronic bronchopulmonary disease.

Esophagus: The portion of the digestive canal between the pharynx and the stomach.

Fibrillation, Ventricular: Heart condition in which the beat is rapid, irregular and ineffective. The spontaneous contraction of individual muscle fibers (fibrils) leads to irregular and ineffective beats. Fibrillary twitching without propulsion of blood.

Fibrocystic Disease of the Pancreas: A disease of children, probably congenital, involving many glands throughout the body, including the mucus-secreting glands in the lungs. It can produce many types of lung disease.

Fibrosis: Pathologic formation of fibrous tissue.

Frequency Modulation: A method of amplifying and/or broadcasting (telemetry) electrical signals. The signals are made to modulate or alter the frequency of a carrier current. The modulated carrier current then is amplified or transmitted and the original signal is retrieved by demodulation.

Galvanometer: A device that converts changes in electrical current into movement of a portion of the unit.

Hematocrit: The height of the column of red blood cells in a tube of whole blood which has settled or has been centrifuged to separate cells from plasma, usually expressed in per cent.

Hemoglobin: The chemical compound in red blood cells which carries oxygen.

Hemoptysis: Expectorating blood or blood-stained sputum from the lungs.

Hemothorax: An effusion of blood into the pleural cavity.

Hering-Breuer Reflex: Pulmonary nerve impulses which help to regulate the depth and rate of respiration.

Hydraulic: Pertaining to fluid.

Hypercapnia: Excess carbon dioxide in the blood, usually causing increased ventilation.

Hyperpnea: Increased ventilation, regardless of cause.

Hypertension: High arterial blood pressure.

Hyperventilation: Excessive air exchange.

Hypocapnia: Deficiency of carbon dioxide in the blood, usually causing decreased ventilation.

Hypopnea: Decreased ventilation, regardless of cause.

Hypotension: Low arterial blood pressure.

Hypoventilation: Insufficient air exchange.

Hypovolemia: Deficiency in the volume of blood in the body.

Hypoxemia: Oxygen deficiency in the oxygen content of the blood.

Hypoxia: The capacity of the blood to carry oxygen is normal, but deficient oxygenation of the arterial blood is present.

Impedance: Interference with the passage of some form of physical energy through a medium. Electrical impedance refers to the interference with the passage of electrical current through a conducting medium. If a signal is a truly direct current signal, impedance would be synonymous with resistance. Since many physiologic signals, although of direct current nature, occur repetitively with fairly rapid frequency, the impedance of the tissues through which they pass would be a factor of the resistance, capacitance and inductance of those tissues. When utilizing alternating current to produce physiologic effects such as electrical anesthesia, capacitance and conductance would assume major factors in the impedance of the tissues through which such a current is made to pass.

Impedance Plethysmograph: A device for measuring the volume of a portion of the body by checking the electrical impedance of that portion.

Infrared Analyzer: An instrument which measures the concentration of a specific gas present in a sample by analyzing the amount of absorption of infrared energy by that sample.

Internal Respiration: The exchange of gases between the blood and the tissues.

Interstitial: Between cells.

Intrapleural Pressure: Pressure of the air between the layers of the pleura, normally below atmospheric.

Intrapulmonary Pressure: Pressure of air within the lungs, normally below atmospheric on inspiration, above atmospheric on expiration.

Laminar Flow: Smooth flow of a gas, in which all the particles making up the gas move along lines parallel to the walls of the tubes.

Larynx: Upper part of the trachea containing the vocal cords.

Lobectomy: Removal of a lobe of the lung.

Lumen: The space in the interior of a tubular structure.

Lung Capacities and Volumes:

TLC = Total Lung Capacity. Volume of air in the lungs after a maximum inspiration.

VC = Vital Capacity. Volume of air which can be expelled from the lungs with maximal effort after a maximal inspiration.

IC = Inspiratory Capacity. Maximal volume of air which can be inspired after a normal expiration.

FRC = Functional Residual Capacity. Volume of air present in the lungs after abnormal expiration.

TV = Tidal Volume. Volume of air moving in or out of the lungs during each cycle.

IRV = Inspiratory Reserve Volume. Maximal volume of air which can be inspired following a normal inspiration.

ERV = Expiratory Reserve Volume. Maximal volume of air which can be expired following a normal expiration.

RV = Residual Volume. Volume of air remaining in the lungs after a maximal expiration.

MV = Minute Volume. Volume of air passing in or out of the lungs in one minute (Rate × TV).

Manometer: A pressure-measuring device

Mediastinum: The median dividing wall of the thoracic cavity, covered by the mediastinal pleura and containing all the thoracic viscera and structures except the lungs.

Metric Measurements: 2.54 cm = 1 inch
$$1 \text{ cm} = 0.39 \text{ inch}$$
$$1.37 \text{ cm } H_2O = 1 \text{ mm Hg}$$
$$1 \text{ liter} = 1000.028 \text{ cc}$$
$$1 \text{ liter} = 1000 \text{ ml}$$
$$1 \text{ gal.} = 3.79 \text{ liters}$$

Micron: 1/1000 millimeter; approximately 1/25000 inch.

Microphone: A transducer which converts sound or related vibratory phenomenon into electrical signals.

Modulate: To alter the characteristics of.

Modulation: The process or result of the process whereby some characteristic of a wave form is varied in accordance with another signal. See Frequency Modulation and also Amplitude Modulation.

Mucoviscidosis: See Fibrocystic Disease of the Pancreas.

Myocardium: Heart muscle.

Natural Frequency: The frequency at which a mechanical device or an electrical current tends to oscillate or vibrate.

Nebulizer: Type of atomizer which removes the large droplets, usually by baffling.

Noise: Interference superimposed upon the signal being monitored.

Oscillator: When applied to electronics, an electrical circuit which produces an oscillating, rhythmically changing electrical impulse.

Oximeter: A means of measuring the ratio between oxygenated and reduced hemoglobin in a peripheral vascular bed or in the blood contained in a cuvette.

Oxygen Dissociation Curve: A graph which indicates the amount of oxygen which will be taken up by the hemoglobin at different oxygen tensions. This varies with pH, CO_2 tension and body temperature.

Oxygen Saturation: The ratio of the volume of oxygen (at STP) in a given unit volume of blood, to the maximal value of O_2 that can be absorbed by that unit volume of blood at high partial pressures of O_2 (e.g., 760 mm Hg), usually expressed in per cent.

Oxyhemoglobin: The combination of oxygen and hemoglobin. pH: Symbol denoting hydrogen ion concentration. A solution with pH 7.00 is neutral, one with a pH of more than 7.00 is alkaline, and one with a pH lower than 7.00 is acid.

Partial Pressure: The pressure exerted by one gas in a mixture of gases.

Pericardium: The membranous sac covering the heart.

Permeability: The capacity of a membrane to allow another substance to pass through it.

Pharynx: The area between the cavity of the mouth and the larynx and esophagus.

Photoelectric Cell: An electronic device which converts visible light or electromagnetic radiations in the frequency range of light into electrical current or changes in an electrical circuit.

Physiology: The science which treats of the functions of the living organisms and its parts.

Plethysmograph: An instrument for measuring the volume of a portion of the body.

Pleura: A membrane enveloping the lungs and covering the inside of the thorax. There is a pleura for each lung.

Pleural Cavity: Potential space between the pleura of the thorax.

Pneumatic: Pertaining to gas.

Pneumonectomy: Operative removal of a portion of the lung tissue.

Pneumonia: Inflammation of the lung.

Pneumonoconiosis (also Pneumoconiosis): Chronic inflammation of the lungs caused by inhalation of dust.

Pneumonomycosis: Any disease of the lung due to an infection by a fungus.

Pneumonosis: Any noninfective degenerative disease of the lungs.

Pneumonotomy: Surgical incision of the lung.

Pneumotachograph: A device which senses the velocity of a gas stream.

Pneumothorax: Pressure of air or other gases in the pleural cavity.

Potentiometer: An instrument which indicates voltage in a circuit.

Relative Humidity: The ratio between the amount of water vapor actually present in the atmosphere at a given temperature to that which it is capable of holding if saturated with water vapor at the same temperature, usually expressed as percentage.

Resistance: A measure of the nonelastic properties of the airway, lung and thorax expressed in pressure change per unit of volume in time change, usually centimeters of water per liter per second (cm H_2O/L/sec). Resistance is not constant but varies with the flow rate, gas, airway changes and point in the ventilation cycle; it frequently is expressed as a standard flow rate, such as 0.5 L per second in the midvolume range. Resistance includes frictional resistance to air flow, and the smaller elements of frictional resistance to tissue flow and inertial reaction to acceleration. See Conductance.

Respiratory Exchange Ratio or Respiratory Quotient: The ratio between the volume of carbon dioxide eliminated over the volume of oxygen consumed.

Respiratory Quotient (R.Q.): The ratio of the rate of production of carbon dioxide (volume at STP per unit time) to the rate of uptake of oxygen (volume at STP per unit time).

Semiconductor: A material that will pass more current than an insulator but not as much as a conductor. Germanium and silicon are the two materials now being utilized for the manufacture of semiconductors. By imposing the proper electrical charge on a certain phase of the semiconductor, the conductance through the semiconductor is altered.

Shunt: Passage of blood through other than the usual channels.

Signal-Noise Ratio: The ratio between the magnitude of the electrical signal being monitored and the magnitude of the interference from other sources which is superimposed upon the signal being monitored. The higher the ratio, the greater will be the fidelity of the signal; the lower the ratio, the more likely will the interference affect the fidelity of the signal. One major problem in regard to noise is to be able to distinguish it from the signal itself.

Signal Strength: The strength of an electrical signal or any other type of signal when measured at a given point. When applied to radio, it refers to the strength of the radio signal as measured a given distance from the antenna.

Solid State Device: A component of electronic equipment consisting of a solid block of special material designed to handle electrical signals in a special way. The transistor is an example of a solid state device. See also Semiconductor.

Standard Deviation (S.D.): The square root of the average of the squares of deviation from the mean. Also called root mean square deviation. Same as *standard error.*

Static Pressure: Slowly changing or constant pressure.

Stenosis: Narrowing of a tube.

String Galvanometer: A galvanometer, the moving part of which consists of a string or fiber.

Tachycardia: Increased heart rate.

Tachypnea: Increased respiratory rate.

Temperature Coefficient: The change in a physical property of a substance produced by the change in temperature of that substance.

Tension: The partial pressure of a gas in a liquid.

Thermistor: A semiconductor that changes in resistance with reference to its change in temperature.

Thermocouple: A junction of dissimilar metallic conductors which, when placed at a temperature different than the reference junction, will generate an electrical potential and can be used to measure temperature.

Thorax: The chest; the upper part of the trunk between the neck and the abdomen.

Trachea: The windpipe leading from the larynx to the bronchi.

Transducer: A device which transduces or translates energy from one physical form into another.

Transistor: A semiconductor which possesses the same function as the vacuum tube.

Turbulent Flow: Irregular and disorderly flow of a gas, in which the particles making up the gas do not move along lines parallel to the walls of the tube.

Vasoconstrictor: An agent which causes narrowing of the blood vessels.

Vasodilator: An agent which causes dilation of the blood vessels.

Ventilation: Movement of air into and out of the lung.

Viscosity: Property of gas, resulting from molecular friction, which causes it to offer more or less resistance to change its shape; internal friction.

Voltmeter: A device designed to measure voltage.

Water Vapor Pressure: The partial pressure exerted by the water vapor present in a gas.

B. Water Content of Saturated Air at Varying Temperatures

Temperature, Degrees Centigrade	Temperature, Degrees Fahrenheit	Grams per Cubic Meter
0	32	4.85
1	33.8	5.19
2	35.6	5.56
3	37.4	5.95
4	39.2	6.36
5	41	6.80
6	42.8	7.26
7	44.6	7.75
8	46.4	8.27
9	48.2	8.82
10	50	9.41
11	51.8	10.02
12	53.6	10.67
13	55.4	11.35
14	57.2	12.06
15	59.0	12.83
16	60.8	13.64
17	62.6	14.47
18	64.4	15.36
19	66.2	16.31
20	68	17.30
21	69.8	18.35
22	71.6	19.42
23	73.4	20.58
24	75.2	21.78
25	77	23.04
26	78.8	24.36
27	80.6	25.75
28	82.4	27.22
29	84.2	28.75
30	86	30.35
35	95	39.60
37	98.6	43.90

C. Conversion Factors

British Thermal Unit (Btu):

$$1 \text{ Btu} = 1.0559 \times 10^{10} \text{ ergs}$$
$$= 251.995 \text{ Gm-cal}$$
$$= 778.77 \text{ ft-lb}$$
$$= 0.25199 \text{ kcal}$$
$$1 \text{ Btu/hr} = 0.1667 \text{ Btu/min}$$
$$= 0.04199 \text{ kcal/min}$$
$$= 0.2932 \text{ watt}$$
$$1 \text{ Btu/min} = 0.25199 \text{ kcal/min}$$
$$= 0.023599 \text{ hp}$$
$$= 17.595 \text{ watts}$$
$$1 \text{ Btu/ft}^2, \text{ hr} = 2.7125 \text{ kcal/m}^2, \text{ hr}$$

BPTS: Body Temperature ($= 37$ degrees C), ambient pressure and saturated (water vapor pressure $= 47$ mm Hg)

Caloric Equivalent of Oxygen: One liter of oxygen (STPD) consumed is equivalent to 4.825 kcal of metabolic heat produced, when the R.Q. is 0.82.

Centimeter (cm): $1 \text{ cm} = 0.03280 \text{ ft}$
$$= 0.3937 \text{ inch}$$
$$= 0.01 \text{ m}$$
$$= 10 \text{ mm}$$
$$= 1 \times 10^4 \ \mu$$

Centimeters per Second per Second: $1 \text{ cm/sec}^2 = 0.0328 \text{ ft/sec}^2$

Centipoise: Unit of absolute viscosity; 1 centipoise $= 0.01$ poise

CLO (clo): The unit of insulation resistance for clothing.

$$1 \text{ clo} = 0.18 \text{ degrees C m}^2\text{hr/kcal}$$
$$= 0.88 \text{ degrees F ft}^2\text{hr/Btu}$$

Cubic Centimeter (cc or cm^3): $\quad 1 \text{ cc} = 3.531 \times 10^{-5} \text{ ft}^3$
$$= 0.061023 \text{ inch}^3$$
$$= 1 \times 10^{-6} \text{ m}^3$$
$$= 1,000 \text{ mm}^3$$
$$= 2.6417 \times 10^{-4} \text{ gal. (U.S. fluid)}$$
$$= 0.0338 \text{ oz (U.S. fluid)}$$
$$= 2.113 \times 10^{-3} \text{ pint (U.S. fluid)}$$
$$1 \text{ cc/sec} = 0.0021186 \text{ ft}^3/\text{min}$$

Cubic Foot: $\quad 1 \text{ ft}^3 = 1728 \text{ inch}^3$
$$= 28.32 \text{ liters}$$
$$= 0.02832 \text{ m}^3$$
$$1 \text{ ft}^3/\text{min} = 472.0 \text{ cc/sec}$$
$$= 0.4720 \text{ liter/sec}$$
$$= 62.43 \text{ lb H}_2\text{O/min}$$
$$1 \text{ ft}^3/\text{sec} = 1699.3 \text{ liters/min}$$

Cubic Inch: 1 inch^3 = 5.787 × 10^{-4} ft^3
$\qquad$ = 1.639 × 10^{-2} liter
$\qquad$ = 1.639 × 10^{-5} m^3

Cubic Meter: 1 m^3 = 35.3144 ft^3
$\qquad$ = 6.1023 × 10^4 inch^3
$\qquad$ = 999.973 liters

Degree (angular): 1 deg = 60 min
$\qquad$ = 0.01745 radian
$\qquad$ = 3600 sec
$\qquad$ 1 deg^2 = 3.0462 × 10^{-2} steradian

Degrees Centigrade (° C): ° C = 5/9(° F − 32)
$\qquad$ 1° C = 1.8° F

Degrees Fahrenheit (° F): ° F = (9/5 × ° C) + 32
$\qquad$ 1° F = 0.556° C

Degrees per Second: 1 deg/sec = 0.017453 radian/sec
$\qquad$ = 0.1667 rpm

Dyne: $\quad$ 1 dyne = 1.0197 × 10^{-6} kg
$\qquad$ = 2.2481 × 10^{-6} lb
$\quad$ 1 dyne-cm = 1 erg

Dyne per Square Centimeter: 1 dyne/cm^2 = 9.8692 × 10^{-7} atm
$\qquad$ = 0.0010197 Gm/cm^2
$\qquad$ = 4.0148 × 10^{-4} inch H$_2$O
$\qquad$ = 7.5006 × 10^{-4} mm Hg
$\qquad$ = 1.4504 × 10^{-5} psi

Electron Charge (e): e = 1.602 × 10^{-19} coulomb

Erg: 1 erg = 9.4805 × 10^{-11} Btu
$\qquad$ = 7.3756 × 10^{-8} ft-lb
$\qquad$ = 2.3889 × 10^{-11} kcal
$\qquad$ = 8.8510 × 10^{-7} lb-inch

Foot (ft): 1 ft = 30.48 cm
$\qquad$ = 12 inches
$\qquad$ = 0.3048 m

Foot per Minute: 1 ft/min = 0.3048 m/min
$\qquad$ = 0.005080 m/sec
$\qquad$ = 0.011364 mph

Foot per Second: 1 ft/sec = 1.0973 km/hr
$\qquad$ = 0.5921 knot (per hr)
$\qquad$ = 0.6818 mph

Foot-Pound (ft-lb): $\quad$ 1 ft-lb = 0.001285 Btu
$\qquad$ = 1.3558 × 10^7 ergs
$\qquad$ = 3.2389 × 10^{-4} kcal
$\qquad$ 1 ft-lb/min = 3.0303 × 10^{-5} hp
$\qquad$ = 0.01667 ft-lb/sec
$\qquad$ = 0.022597 watt

1 ft-lb/sec = 0.001818 hp
= 0.01943 kcal/min
= 1.3558 watts

Gram (Gm):   1 Gm = 0.001 kg
= 1,000 mg
= 0.03527 oz
= 0.0022046 lb
1 Gm/cm^3 = 62.428 lb/ft^3
1 Gm/hr = 0.540 lb/day
= 0.0003757 lb/min
1 Gm/liter = 0.062427 lb/ft^3
1 Gm/cm^2 = 9.6784 × 10^{-4} atm
= 980.665 $dynes/cm^2$
= 0.9356 mm Hg
= 0.014223 psi
1 Gm/m^2, hr = 2.78 × 10^{-5} Gm/cm^2, sec
= 0.7448 lb/ft^2, hr

Gram-Calorie (Gm-cal): 1 Gm-cal = 3.0874 ft-lb
= 0.001 kcal

Horsepower (hp): 1 hp = 3.300 × 10^4 ft-lb/min
= 550 ft-lb/sec
= 10.688 kcal/min
= 745.7 watts

Inch: 1 inch = 2.540 cm
= 0.0833 ft
= 25.40 mm

Inch of water (inch H_2O). 1 inch H_2O = 0.002458 atm
(at 4° C) = 2.490.82 $dynes/cm^2$
= 0.0361 psi
= 1.868 mm Hg

Joule: 1 joule = 1 watt-sec

Kilogram (kg): 1 kg = 1,000 Gm
= 2.205 lb
= 32.1507 oz

Kilogram-Calorie (kcal or large calorie): 1 kcal = 3.9683 Btu
= 4.186 × 10^{10} ergs
= 1,000 Gm-cal
= 3087 ft-lb
1 kcal/hr = 0.0661 Btu/min
= 0.857 ft-lb/sec
= 0.1667 kcal/min
= 1.161 watts
1 $kcal/m^2$ hr = 0.3687 Btu/ft^2 hr

$$1 \text{ kcal/min} = 3.9685 \text{ Btu/min}$$
$$= 51.457 \text{ ft-lb/sec}$$
$$= 0.093557 \text{ hp}$$
$$= 69.767 \text{ watts}$$

Kilogram-Centimeter Squared: $1 \text{ kg-cm}^2 = 0.3417 \text{ lb-inch}^2$
Kilogram-Meter per Second: $1 \text{ kg-m/sec} = 7.2330 \text{ ft-lb/sec}$
$$= 9.80665 \text{ watts}$$
Kilometers per Hour: $1 \text{ km/hr} = 0.9113 \text{ ft/sec}$
$$= 0.5396 \text{ knot}$$
$$= 6214 \text{ mph}$$
Liter (L): $1 \text{ liter} = 0.03531 \text{ ft}^3$
$$= 61.02 \text{ inch}^3$$
$$= 1,000 \text{ ml}$$
$1 \text{ liter/min} = 5.886 \times 10^{-4} \text{ ft}^3/\text{sec}$
$1 \text{ liter/sec} = 2.12 \text{ ft}^3/\text{min}$
Meter (m): $1 \text{ m} = 100 \text{ cm}$
$$= 3.281 \text{ ft}$$
$$= 39.37 \text{ inch}$$
Meter per Second: $1 \text{ m/sec} = 3.281 \text{ ft/sec}$
$$= 3.600 \text{ km/hr}$$
$$= 2.2369 \text{ mph}$$
Micron (μ or mu): $1 \mu = 10^{-6} \text{ meter}$
$$= 3.937 \times 10^{-5} \text{ inch}$$
$$= 0.001 \text{ mm}$$
Mil: $1 \text{ mil} = 0.001 \text{ inch}$
$$= 0.0254 \text{ mm}$$
$$= 25.40 \mu$$
Miles per Hour (mph): $1 \text{ mph} = 88 \text{ ft/min}$
$$= 1.4667 \text{ ft/sec}$$
$$= 1.6093 \text{ km/hr}$$
$$= 0.8684 \text{ knot}$$
Milligram (mg): $1 \text{ mg} = 0.001 \text{ Gm}$
$$= 3.5274 \text{ oz}$$
$$= 2.2046 \times 10^{-6} \text{ lb}$$
$1 \text{ mg/m}^3 = 6.243 \times 10^{-4} \text{ lb/ft}^3$
Milliliter (ml): $1 \text{ ml} = 1.000028 \text{ cc}$
$$= 0.061025 \text{ inch}^3$$
$$= 0.001 \text{ liter}$$
$$= 0.0338 \text{ oz (U.S. fluid)}$$
Milliliters per Hour: $1 \text{ ml/hr} = 0.06102 \text{ inch}^3/\text{hr}$
Millimeter (mm): $1 \text{ mm} = 0.10 \text{ cm}$
$$= 0.03937 \text{ inch}$$
$$= 1,000 \mu$$

Millimeter of Mercury (mm Hg): 1 mm Hg = 0.0013158 atm
$$\text{(at } 0° \text{ C)} = 1333.22 \text{ dyne/cm}^2$$
$$= 1.3595 \text{ Gm/cm}^2$$
$$= 0.019337 \text{ psi}$$
$$= 0.535 \text{ inch H}_2\text{O}$$

Milliseconds (msec): 1 msec = 0.001 sec

Ounce (oz): 1 oz = 28.3495 Gm
$$= 0.0625 \text{ lb}$$

Parts per Million (ppm): 1 ppm = 1.0 mg/liter of H_2O
$$= 8.345 \text{ lb/million gallons}$$

Poise: Unit of viscosity; 1 poise = 1 dyne/sec, cm^2
$$= 1 \text{ Gm/cm, sec}$$
$$= 0.067196 \text{ lb/ft, sec}$$

Pound (lb): 1 lb = 453.5924 Gm
$$= 0.45359 \text{ kg}$$
$$= 16 \text{ oz}$$
1 lb/day = 18.89 Gm/hr
1 lb/hr = 0.7559 Gm/min
$$= 10.886 \text{ kg/day}$$

Pound-Inch: 1 lb-inch = 1.1298×10^6 dyne/cm

Pound-Inch Squared: Unit of moment of inertia
$$1 \text{ lb-inch}^2 = 2.9264 \text{ kg-cm}^2$$

Pound of Water per Minute: 1 lb H_2O/min = 0.01603 ft^3/min
$$= 2.670 \times 10^{-4}/\text{ft}^3/\text{sec}$$

Pound per Cubic Foot: 1 lb/ft^3 = 0.01602 Gm/cm^3

Pounds per Square Inch (psi): 1 psi = 0.06805 atm
$$= 6.8947 \times 10^4 \text{ dyne/cm}^2$$
$$= 70.307 \text{ Gm/cm}^2$$
$$= 51.715 \text{ mm Hg}$$
$$= 27.7 \text{ H}_2\text{O}$$

Pounds per Square Inch Absolute (psia): Absolute pressure, where 0 psia = vacuum

Pound Weight: 1 lb wt = 4.4482×10^5 dynes
$$= 453.59 \text{ Gm wt}$$

Radian (rad): 1 rad = $\frac{1}{2\pi}$ circumference or revolution (0.15915)
$$= 57.296 \text{ deg}$$
1 rad/sec = 57.296 deg/sec
$$= 9.549 \text{ rpm}$$
1 rad/sec^2 = 572.96 rpm^2

Revolutions per Minute (rpm): 1 rpm = 6 deg/sec
$$= 0.10472 \text{ radian/sec}$$
1 rpm^2 = 0.001745 radian/sec^2

Root Mean Square (rms): Square root of the mean of the squares of a set of numbers.

Square Centimeter: $1 cm^2 = 1.076 \times 10^{-3} ft^2$
$$= 0.1550\ n^2$$
$$= 100\ mm^2$$

Square Foot: $1\ ft^2 = 929.0\ cm^2$
$$= 144\ inch^2$$

Square Inch: $1\ inch^2 = 6.4516\ cm^2$
$$= 0.006944\ ft^2$$
$$= 645.1626\ mm^2$$

Square Millimeter: $1\ mm^2 = 0.01\ cm^2$
$$= 0.001550\ inch^2$$

Steradian: $\frac{1}{4\pi}$ solid angle around a point

$$1\ steradian = 3282.8063\ deg^2$$
$$= 0.07958\ sphere$$

STPD (Standard Temperature and Pressure, Dry): $0°$ C, 760 mm Hg, water vapor pressure $= 0$.

Watt: $1\ watt = 1\ joule/sec$
$$= 1 \times 10^7\ erg/sec$$
$$= 0.736\ ft\text{-}lb/sec$$
$$= 0.001341\ hp$$
$$= 0.01432\ kcal/min$$

SYMBOLS

Rx	Take	—	Minus; deficiency; alkaline reaction; negative
M	Mix		
āā, āa	Of each	±	Plus or minus; either positive or negative; indefinite
mμ	Millimicron, micromillimeter		
μg	Microgram	#	Number
mEq	Milliequivalent	÷	Divided by
mg	Milligram	×	Multiplied by
mg %	Milligrams percent	=	Equals
Qo$_2$	Oxygen consumption	>	Greater than
s̄s̄, ss	One-half	<	Less than
′	Foot; minute; primary accent; univalent	:	Ratio; "is to"
		::	Equality between ratios
″	Inch; second; secondary accent; bivalent	°	Birth
		†	Death
‴	Line ($\frac{1}{12}$ inch); trivalent	°	Degree
μ	Micron	%	Per cent
μμ	Micromicron	♂	Male
+	Plus; excess; acid reaction, positive	♀	Female
		⇌	Denotes a reversible reaction

Symbols Often Used in Respiratory Physiology

Primary Symbols for Gases	Suffixes

V = volume of gas or blood

$\dot{V}$ = gas volume per unit time

$\dot{v}$ = instantaneous flow rate of gas

Q = blood volume per unit time

P = pressure of gas

F = fractional concentration in dry gas

C = concentration in blood; also compliance

S = saturation

f = frequency of respiration

R = respiratory exchange ratio; also resistance

D = diffusive capacity

T = transfer factor

I = inspired gas

E = expired gas

A = alveolar gas

V_t = tidal volume

D = dead space gas

B = barometric pressure

a = arterial blood

v = venous blood

c = capillary blood

pl = plasma

m = alveolar capillary membrane

L = Lung

th = thorax

ti = tissue

aw = airway

Factor to Convert Vol. to 37° C Sat.	When Gas Temperature (C) Is	With Water Vapor Pressure (mm Hg) Of
1.102	20	17.5
1.096	21	18.7
1.091	22	19.8
1.085	23	21.1
1.080	24	22.4
1.075	25	23.8
1.068	26	25.2
1.063	27	26.7
1.057	28	28.3
1.051	29	30.0
1.045	30	31.8
1.039	31	33.7
1.032	32	35.7
1.026	33	37.7
1.020	34	39.9
1.014	35	42.2
1.007	36	44.6
1.000	37	47.0

Cylinder Style and Approximate Dimensions	Cylinder Pressure at 70 F (psig)		Carbon Dioxide 840	Oxygen 1800–2400
A (3″ o.d. × 7″)	Contents weight (lb)		0.8	0.23
	Gas volume at 70 F	cu ft	6.6	2.7
	and 14.7 psia	liters	184.0	76.5
B (3½″ o.d. × 13″)	Contents weight (lb)		1.6	0.5
	Gas volume at 70 F	cu ft	13.3	5.3
	and 14.7 psia	liters	377.0	150.0
D (4¼″ o.d. × 17″)	Contents weight (lb)		4.0	1.0
	Gas volume at 70 F	cu ft	33.0	12.6
	and 14.7 psia	liters	934.0	356.0
E (4¼″ o.d. × 26″)	Contents weight (lb)		6.6	2.0
	Gas volume at 70 F	cu ft	56.0	22.0
	and 14.7 psia	liters	1585.0	622.0
F (5½″ o.d. × 51″)	Contents weight (lb)		20.0	6.0
	Gas volume at 70 F	cu ft	170.0	73.0
	and 14.7 psia	liters	4800.0	2062.0
M (7⅛″ o.d. × 43″)	Contents weight (lb)		31.0	9.0
	Gas volume at 70 F	cu ft	266.0	106.0
	and 14.7 psia	liters	7400.0	3000.0
G (8½″ o.d. × 51″)	Contents weight (lb)		28.0	16.0
	Gas volume at 70 F	cu ft	372.0	186.0
	and 14.7 psia	liters	10500.0	5260.0

Index

P

Pancreatic dornase (*see* Dornavac)
Paramagnetic oxygen analyzer: schema of, 88
Parkinson-Gowen dry gas meter, 278
  equipment, 278
  objective, 278
  technique, 278
Pauling-type paramagnetic oxygen analyzer: schema of, 88
Percussion: vibrations due to, 198
Personnel, 15–16
Pharmacology (*see* Drugs)
Pharynx, 19–20
  clearing, in airway management, 119–120
  tubes, in airway management, 120
Phenols, 110
Physiology
  lung, clinical, 255–257
  respiratory, symbols used in, 351
Physiotherapy of chest, 187–195
  breathing, diaphragmatic and abdominal, 187
  clapping, 189
  cupping, 188
  orders for, 298–299
    frequency of physiotherapy, 298
    positions, 298
    type of physiotherapy, 298
  position of patient for, 191–195
  postural drainage, 188
  therapy cycle, 190–195
  vibrating, 188–190
Plasma: oxygen in physiologic solution in, 260–261, 262
Plastic tracheotomy tube, 129
Plethysmograph, 156
Pleura, 21
  parietal, 24
  rub, 203
  visceral, 24
"Pneumatic chamber," 156
Pneumotaxic center, 31
Pneumothorax, 25
  sound wave reflection in, 200
Polyethylene mask, 101
Polypropylene face tent, 288
Positive pressure
  in airway management, 119
  breathing (*see* Intermittent positive pressure breathing)
Postural drainage, 188

Pounds per square inch
  absolute, 39
  gauge, 39
Precautions: with gases, 62
Preoxygenation: and suction, 296
Pressure, 38–45
  atmospheric, 38
    standard, 39
  breathing (*see* Intermittent positive pressure breathing)
  compensated flowmeter, 77
  generator (*see* Generator)
  intrapleural, 25
  intrapulmonic, during quiet breathing, 25
  intrathoracic, 25
  measurement with fluids, 40
  positive (*see* Positive pressure)
  regulator
    single-stage, cross-section of, 75
    three-stage, 76
    two-stage, cross-section of, 76
  subatmospheric, 25
Program: for school of inhalation therapy, 326
PSIA, 39
PSIG, 39
Pulmonary (*see* Lung)
Pumps: for suctioning, 132
Puritan aerosol nebulizer assembly, 102

R

Racemic epinephrine (*see* Vaponefrin solution)
Radford nomogram, 171
Rales, 201–202
  coarse, 202
  high-pitch, 202
  medium-pitch, 202
Ratio: blood flow/ventilation, 35
Rebreathing
  (*See also* Face mask, oxygen)
  method, arterial carbon dioxide tension determination by, 273–275
Records, 18
  lung function and, 255, 256–257
  monitoring devices and, 206–210
Regulator (*see* Pressure regulator)
Regulatory authorities for compressed gases, 62–64
  federal, 62–64
  local, 64
  provincial, 64
  state, 64